Diet and Cancer

Series Editor
Adriana Albini
Head Oncology Research, IRCCS MultiMedica, Via Fantoli 15/16,
20138 Milano, Italy
and
MultiMedica Castellanza
21053 Castellanza (VA), Italy
Tel. +39-02-55406532
Fax +39-02-55406503
adriana.albini@multimedica.it

For further volumes:
http://www.springer.com/series/8049

Marja Mutanen · Anne-Maria Pajari
Editors

Vegetables, Whole Grains, and Their Derivatives in Cancer Prevention

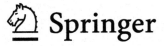 Springer

Editors
Marja Mutanen
Department of Food
 and Environmental Sciences
University of Helsinki
Helsinki 00014, Finland
marja.mutanen@helsinki.fi

Anne-Maria Pajari
Department of Food
 and Environmental Sciences
University of Helsinki
Helsinki 00014, Finland
anne-maria.pajari@helsinki.fi

ISBN 978-90-481-9799-6   e-ISBN 978-90-481-9800-9
DOI 10.1007/978-90-481-9800-9
Springer Dordrecht Heidelberg London New York

Library of Congress Control Number: 2010936635

Printed on acid-free paper

Springer is part of Springer Science+Business Media (www.springer.com)

Preface

This book aims to update our knowledge and increase our understanding on the field of vegetables and whole grains in cancer prevention. There is a long list of bioactive compounds available in vegetable kingdom such as vitamins, minerals, carotenoids, phytosterols, polyphenols etc., which have been intensely studied, often as pure compounds, by several research groups in the diet and cancer field. This book focuses not only on single compounds but aims to widen the view by including data on whole vegetables and grains, their extracts and some of their specific components.

Although epidemiological data provide a strong basis for evaluating associations between cancer and environmental factors including diet, making definitive conclusions on the role of diet in cancer prevention would require such inclusive human interventions, which are not possible to conduct. In addition, diet and cancer are two of the most difficult subjects for epidemiological studies to address due to the complex nature of eating patterns and the length of the carcinogenic process. Animal experiments and in vitro cell culture studies form the basis for our understanding in this research field today. Both of these approaches have their limitations, but three main conclusions can be drawn from the results obtained so far; foods contain several components with potential chemopreventive activity; a single component may lose its chemopreventive efficacy when isolated from the food matrix; isolated and concentrated components as supplements may actually induce tumor development.

When considering the rate and amount of accumulating new scientific knowledge, the groups of experts who have contributed to this book have managed to synthesize and summarize the current state of knowledge in their field admirably. At the moment, it seems that the mechanisms of some compounds in cancer prevention have been studied thoroughly and such data dominate over the in vivo animal data. Even though it is fundamental to understand the molecular mechanisms that underlie the effects of specific vegetable derived components, it would be of utmost importance to confirm the results from in vitro studies in animals to verify the applicably of these results in human situation.

Over the last decades, a whole range of new technologies has become available for cancer research. Knockouts, conditional knockouts, and knockins in mouse models in combination with microarray/cDNA chip technologies with pathway analyses as well as proteomic approaches will open new ways to study the effects of diet in the carcinogenic process. Exploitation of these techniques will increase our knowledge on the possibilities of diet in cancer prevention and raise our understanding to a new level.

In this book, Chapters 1 and 2 cover current knowledge of cruciferous and green leafy vegetables in cancer prevention. These vegetable classes contain several bioactive compounds, the mechanisms of which have been included. Similarly, Chapters 3 and 4 give profound reviews on tomato lycopene and carotenoids and their mechanism of action in carcinogenesis. The role of alliums and their sulphur and selenium constituents are addressed in the Chapter 5. Capsaicinoids from chilli peppers with detailed mechanisms of action are discussed in-depth in Chapter 6. The Chapter 7 represents a description of an experimental model utilized to study the genotoxicity and carcinogenicity of soy isoflavones, and Chapter 8 summarizes the current understanding on wide issue in cancer fields, i.e. dietary seeds and their phytochemicals in carcinogenesis. Whole nuts in cancer prevention are discussed in Chapter 9 and Chapter 10 summaries the current knowledge on whole grains.

We warmly thank all the authors for their outstanding contributions.

Helsinki, Finland   Marja Mutanen
                                                                      Anne-Maria Pajari

Contents

Contributors

Anane Aidoo FDA Jefferson Laboratories, National Center for Toxicological Research, Division of Genetic & Reproductive Toxicology, Jefferson, AR 72079, USA, anane.aidoo@fda.hhs.gov

Charlotte Armah Institute of Food Research, Colney Lane, Norwich NR4 7UA, UK, Charlotte.armah@bbsrc.ac.uk

Andrea Atzmon Department of Clinical Biochemistry and the Colorectal Unit, Faculty of Health Sciences, Ben-Gurion University and Soroka Medical Center of Kupat Holim, Beer-Sheva, Israel, andi_s79@hotmail.com

Arthur J.L. Cooper Department of Biochemistry and Molecular Biology, New York Medical College, Valhalla, NY, USA, arthur_cooper@nymc.edu

Michael Danilenko Department of Clinical Biochemistry and the Colorectal Unit, Faculty of Health Sciences, Ben-Gurion University and Soroka Medical Center of Kupat Holim, Beer-Sheva, Israel, misha@bgu.ac.il

Paul A. Davis Department of Nutrition, College of Agricultural and Environmental Sciences, University of California, Davis, Davis, CA 95616, USA, padavis@ucdavis.edu

Karam El-Bayoumy Department of Biochemistry and Molecular Biology, Penn State College of Medicine, Penn State Hershey Cancer Institute, Hershey, PA, USA, kee2@psu.edu

Keren Hirsch Department of Clinical Biochemistry and the Colorectal Unit, Faculty of Health Sciences, Ben-Gurion University and Soroka Medical Center of Kupat Holim, Beer-Sheva, Israel

Marina Khanin Department of Clinical Biochemistry and the Colorectal Unit, Faculty of Health Sciences, Ben-Gurion University and Soroka Medical Center of Kupat Holim, Beer-Sheva, Israel, hanin@bgu.ac.il

Joydeb Kumar Kundu National Research Laboratory of Molecular Carcinogenesis and Chemoprevention, College of Pharmacy, Seoul National University, Seoul 151 742, South Korea, kundujk@yahoo.com

Joseph Levy Department of Clinical Biochemistry and the Colorectal Unit, Faculty of Health Sciences, Ben-Gurion University and Soroka Medical Center of Kupat Holim, Beer-Sheva, Israel, lyossi@bgu.ac.il

Karin Linnewiel Department of Clinical Biochemistry and the Colorectal Unit, Faculty of Health Sciences, Ben-Gurion University and Soroka Medical Center of Kupat Holim, Beer-Sheva, Israel, khermoni@gmail.com

Mugimane G. Manjanatha FDA Jefferson Laboratories, National Center for Toxicological Research, Division of Genetic & Reproductive Toxicology, Jefferson, AR 72079, USA, mugimane.manjanatha@fda.hhs.gov

Richard Mithen Institute of Food Research, Colney Lane, Norwich NR4 7UA, UK, Richard.mithen@bbsrc.ac.uk

Yael Morag Department of Clinical Biochemistry and the Colorectal Unit, Faculty of Health Sciences, Ben-Gurion University and Soroka Medical Center of Kupat Holim, Beer-Sheva, Israel, morag.yael@gmail.com

Marja Mutanen Department of Food and Environmental Sciences, (Nutrition), University of Helsinki, Helsinki, Finland, marja.mutanen@helsinki.fi

Mikael Niku Division of Veterinary Biosciences, Faculty of Veterinary Medicine, University of Helsinki, Helsinki, Finland, mikael.niku@helsinki.fi

Seija Oikarinen Department of Food and Environmental Sciences, (Nutrition), University of Helsinki, Helsinki, Finland, seija.oikarinen@helsinki.fi

Anne-Maria Pajari Division of Nutrition, Department of Food and Environmental Sciences, University of Helsinki, Helsinki, Finland, anne-maria.pajari@helsinki.fi

John T. Pinto Department of Biochemistry and Molecular Biology, New York Medical College, Valhalla, NY, USA, John_Pinto@nymc.edu

Krista A. Power Guelph Food Research Centre, Agriculture and Agri-food Canada, Guelph, ON, Canada, krista.power@agr.gc.ca

Hagar Salman Department of Clinical Biochemistry and the Colorectal Unit, Faculty of Health Sciences, Ben-Gurion University and Soroka Medical Center of Kupat Holim, Beer-Sheva, Israel, hagarsal@gmail.com

Yoav Sharoni Department of Clinical Biochemistry and the Colorectal Unit, Faculty of Health Sciences, Ben-Gurion University and Soroka Medical Center of Kupat Holim, Beer-Sheva, Israel, yoav@bgu.ac.il

Raghu Sinha Department of Biochemistry and Molecular Biology, Penn State College of Medicine, Penn State Hershey Cancer Institute, Hershey, PA, USA, rus15@psu.edu

Young-Joon Surh National Research Laboratory of Molecular Carcinogenesis and Chemoprevention, College of Pharmacy, Seoul National University, Seoul 151 742, South Korea, surh@plaza.snu.ac.kr

Lilian U. Thompson Department of Nutritional Sciences, University of Toronto, Toronto, ON, Canada, lilian.thompson@utoronto.ca

Maria Traka Institute of Food Research, Colney Lane, Norwich NR4 7UA, UK, Maria.traka@bbsrc.ac.uk

Anna Veprik Department of Clinical Biochemistry and the Colorectal Unit, Faculty of Health Sciences, Ben-Gurion University and Soroka Medical Center of Kupat Holim, Beer-Sheva, Israel, annave@bgu.ac.il

Shlomo Walfisch Department of Clinical Biochemistry and the Colorectal Unit, Faculty of Health Sciences, Ben-Gurion University and Soroka Medical Center of Kupat Holim, Beer-Sheva, Israel, walfisch@bgu.ac.il

Xiang-Dong Wang Nutrition and Cancer Biology Laboratory, Jean Mayer United States Department of Agriculture Human Nutrition Research Center on Aging at Tufts University, Boston, MA 02111, USA, xiang-dong.wang@tufts.edu

Yan Wang Department of Pharmacology at University of Virginia, Charlottesville, VA 22908, USA, yw7u@cms.mail.virginia.edu

Diet and Cancer, How to Prevent or Cure Tumors with the Help of Food, Beverages and Their Derivatives

Adriana Albini

The World Health Organization (WHO) reports that cancer is a leading cause of death worldwide. Deaths from cancer were 7.4 million in 2004 and are projected to continue rising, with an estimated 12 million deaths in 2030 if we do not take specific actions. However our lifestyle alone could change things. Health and disease are the result of the combination of our genetic background and the effects on our DNA and molecules from the surrounding environment. Carcinogenesis is a multi-step process originating from an alteration of DNA, or regulatory RNA, that can be inherited or caused by exposition to external mutagenic agents (viral, physical and chemical), leading to corruption of self-repair systems and mutation rate increases. One single mutation is not enough for tumor insurgence (Sugimura et al. 1992), further alterations of cell cycle check points, resulting in uncontrolled proliferation and programmed cell death inhibition, are needed.

Several epidemiological studies have recorded and analyzed incidence and mortality rates per country (Parkin 2004; Coleman et al. 2008; Berrino et al. 2007), considering diverse major types of cancer: lung, breast and female genital tract cancers (uterine, cervix, ovary), colorectal cancer, and other gastrointestinal tract cancers (esophagus, stomach, liver, pancreas), prostate cancer, and other urologic tract cancers (kidney, bladder), head and neck cancers (such as oral cavity and larynx) non-Hodgkin lymphomas, leukemias, brain and nervous system cancers, malignant melanoma and other cutaneous neoplasms. These studies highlighted that different tumor types have different geographical distributions. For example, breast cancer, colon cancer and prostate cancer incidence is higher in Denmark (Ewertz and Gill 1990) and lower in China. The first intriguing question was whether this difference was due to genetic background (predisposition or protection from cancer) or to environmental factors. Very useful for the understanding of the role of genetics and environment were the 'migrant studies', in which populations migrating to a new and distant country, and their offspring, are monitored. Tumor incidence of migrants was compared with those still living in their country of origin and those in the

A. Albini (✉)
Head Oncology Research, IRCCS MultiMedica, Via Fantoli 15/16, 20138 Milano, Italy
e-mail: adriana.albini@multimedica.it

destination country. The results indicate that, for almost all types of cancer, migrated people acquired the same cancer incidence rate of the host country, even after only one or two generations (Nomura et al. 1991). These findings clearly sustain that the environment and-or life style plays a fundamental role in cancer insurgence.

But how does the environment get in touch and influence the outcome of our genetic inheritance? The term environment indicates all we experience and we are exposed to during lifetime. Consequently, everything we get in touch with and we introduce into our organism (i.e. food) can modulate our molecular behavior.

The interest in influence of diet on cancer incidence rate is testified by the numerous studies published on this topic (Riboli 1992). Investigations comparing different habits found that diet is clearly an important factor for cancer risk.

A diet characterized by high animal fat intake, such as the Scandinavian or US diet, is more likely to favor breast cancer (Doll and Peto 1981), prostate cancer and colon cancer, whereas soy and green tea consumption, a common habit in China, seems to exert a protective effect on these same tumors (Wu et al. 2008). The diet is one of the components of our lifestyle that in turn is usually a mirror of the habits 'inherited' from the family. Parents who do not habitually eat vegetables, for instance, tend to not prepare them for their children, leading to inadequate eating habits. From this point of view the family may be considered as a macroenvironment.

The relationship between nutrition and cancer should be considered from two different points of view. On the one hand, there is the quantity of food intake, on the other hand there is the quality of nutrients and non-nutrient components housed in food.

The ratio between energy intake and energy consumption is critical, when unbalanced, as frequently found in the western countries and increasing in the rest of the world, overweight and obesity are the consequence. Adipose tissue is an important repository of hormones and other molecules, and an excess of body fat and obesity are considered a risk factor not only for diabetes and cardiovascular disease, but also for cancer.

In terms of quality, on the other hand, the food we eat may provide the organism with nutrients and other substances able to create an inner microenvironment protective towards cancer initiation and progression.

Folk medicines have been using plant extracts for therapeutic use for centuries, based on common knowledge and observation of effects (Tapsell et al. 2006). Today, several ongoing studies aim to clarify the mechanisms of action of phytochemicals and to identify the molecular targets they interact with. The results reveal remarkably complex actions and interactions. In particular, diet and specific diet-derived compounds and their combination may represent therapeutic and preventive approaches for the future, with an impact on global health.

To identify the beneficial compounds housed in the plant kingdom, specimens were processed and extracts obtained and sequentially purified. Several molecules endowed with pharmaceutical activity have been isolated.

Attention was initially focused on natural extracts, as happened with willow extract, the parent of salicylic acid, and then moved to the design of new synthetic molecules whose chemical structure mimics the naturally existing ones.

This approach gave birth to families of analogs and derived compounds that share the same backbone but differ in some functional groups. One significant example is aspirin, acetyl-salicyclic acid, and in the cancer field the taxanes, based on molecules derived from yew.

In the cancer prevention field some of the most promising plant and dietary derivatives (Araldi et al. 2008) are genistein from soy beans, daidzein from red clover, silybinin from *Sylibum*, quercetin from apples, resveratrol from red grapes, xanthohumol from hop (Dell'Eva et al. 2007) epigallocathechin gallate (EGCG) from *Camelia Sinensis* (whose leaves are used for green tea), lycopene from tomatoes, β-carotene from apricots, capsaicin from chilli pepper, vitamin E from corn, hyperforin from St John's Worth (Lorusso et al. 2009), isothiocyanates and indoles from cruciferous vegetables and triterpenoids from citrus fruits (Vannini et al. 2007). Many of these compounds have already been studied in vitro, corroborated preclinically in vivo and some tested on humans, both as monotherapy and in combined administration (Liby 2008).

Needless to say that dietary habits themselves have profound effects on health. Epidemiological data and clinical investigations confirm the Feuerbach's phylosophical concept *'We are what we eat'*. Nutrition guidelines from health agencies suggests consumption of vegetables and fruits between three and five times a day and to be physically active. The 'cookbook' for diet related health involves aspects other than just food choice or a healthy lifestyle. In fact, the food quality also depends on the methods of culture (cultivation), processing, preparation, cooking and storage of food. Some molecules are present in an inactive form and need to be heated to reach the optimal condition to be effective. This is the case, for example, of lycopene, the carotenoid of tomatoes whose molecular structure is modified when heated making it more active. Lycopene is considered to be protective against prostate cancer (Unlu et al. 2007). Other vitamins are inactivated by heat and need to be stored and consumed without heating (Tena et al. 2009). The difference in the antioxidant properties between green tea and black tea are due to the differences in processing of the tea leaves (Lin et al. 2008). When the leaves are fermented for black tea, they loose up to two thirds of their content in polyphenols, their major anti-oxidant cancer-preventive moieties. Also the texture and physical properties of food can play a role, for instance fiber is protective towards colorectal cancer. Furthermore, not all methods of preparation are healthy: grilled, barbequed and fried meat are likely to favor colon and rectal cancer, due to the formation of carcinogenic aromatic structures (Anderson et al. 2002). Meat in general should be consumed in restricted quantities. Alcoholic beverages increase the risk of cancer. Alcohol and 'empty' calories, such as sweets, should be avoided or consumed with attention.

The trend of cancer incidence and mortality indicated by the WHO suggests that our own choices in dietary habits and life style have an impact to our health, disease risk and longevity. To fight cancer, as well as obesity, diabetes and metabolic syndrome, it is not always necessary to make use of drugs when we can decrease the incidence of such disorders by adopting a healthy and preventive lifestyle.

The book series 'Diet and cancer' has the aim to explore the therapeutic and preventive properties of foods, beverages, spices and their derivatives as well as to evaluate the scientific basis of the impact of food and food derived molecules in the prevention of cancer.

Acknowledgements I would like to thank Dr Ilaria Sogno (MultiMedica Milan) for her invaluable contribution. Our studies on diet and cancer are supported by AIRC Associazione Italiana Ricerca sul Cancro), Compagnia di San Paolo and Fondazione Berlucchi. I am grateful to Alessandra Panvini for assistance and Paola Corradino for helping with the bibliography.

References

Anderson KE, Sinha R, Kulldorff M, Gross M, Lang NP, Barber C, Harnack L, DiMagno E, Bliss R, Kadlubar FF (2002) Meat intake and cooking techniques: associations with pancreatic cancer. Mutat Res 506–507:225–231

Araldi EM, Dell'aica I, Sogno I, Lorusso G, Garbisa S, Albini A (2008) Natural and synthetic agents targeting inflammation and angiogenesis for chemoprevention of prostate cancer. Curr Cancer Drug Targets 8:146–155. Review

Berrino F, De Angelis R, Sant M, Rosso S, Bielska-Lasota M, Coebergh JW, Santaquilani M (2007) EUROCARE Working group. Survival for eight major cancers and all cancers combined for European adults diagnosed in 1995–1999: results of the EUROCARE-4 study. Lancet Oncol 8:773–783

Coleman MP, Quaresma M, Berrino F, Lutz JM, De Angelis R, Capocaccia R, Baili P, Rachet B, Gatta G, Hakulinen T, Micheli A, Sant M, Weir HK, Elwood JM, Tsukuma H, Koifman S, E Silva GA, Francisci S, Santaquilani M, Verdecchia A, Storm HH, Young JL (2008) CONCORD working group. Cancer survival in five continents: a worldwide population-based study (CONCORD). Lancet Oncol 9:730–756

Dell'Eva R, Ambrosini C, Vannini N, Piaggio G, Albini A, Ferrari N (2007) AKT/NF-kappaB inhibitor xanthohumol targets cell growth and angiogenesis in hematologic malignancies. Cancer 110:2007–2011

Doll R, Peto R (1981) The causes of cancer: quantitative estimates of avoidable risks of cancer in the United States today. J Natl Cancer Inst 66:1191–1308. Review

Ewertz M, Gill C (1990) Dietary factors and breast-cancer risk in Denmark. Int J Cancer 46: 779–784

Liby K, Risingsong R, Royce DB, Williams CR, Yore MM, Honda T, Gribble GW, Lamph WW, Vannini N, Sogno I, Albini A, Sporn MB (2008) Prevention and treatment of experimental estrogen receptor-negative mammary carcinogenesis by the synthetic triterpenoid CDDO-methyl Ester and the rexinoid LG100268. Clin Cancer Res 14:4556–4563

Lin LZ, Chen P, Harnly JM (2008) New phenolic components and chromatographic profiles of green and fermented teas. J Agric Food Chem 56:8130–8140

Lorusso G, Vannini N, Sogno I, Generoso L, Garbisa S, Noonan DM, Albini A (2009) Mechanisms of Hyperforin as an anti-angiogenic angioprevention agent. Eur J Cancer 45:1474–1484

Nomura AM, Marchand LL, Kolonel LN, Hankin JH (1991) The effect of dietary fat on breast cancer survival among Caucasian and Japanese women in Hawaii. Breast Cancer Res Treat 18:S135–S141

Parkin DM (2004) International variation. Oncogene 23:6329–6340. Review

Riboli E (1992) Nutrition and cancer: background and rationale of the European Prospective Investigation into Cancer and Nutrition (EPIC). Ann Oncol 3:783–791. Review

Sugimura T, Terada M, Yokota J, Hirohashi S, Wakabayashi K (1992) Multiple genetic alterations in human carcinogenesis. Environ Health Perspect 98:5–12

Tapsell LC, Hemphill I, Cobiac L, Patch CS, Sullivan DR, Fenech M, Roodenrys S, Keogh JB, Clifton PM, Williams PG, Fazio VA, Inge KE (2006) Health benefits of herbs and spices: the past, the present, the future. Med J Aust 185:S4–S24. Review

Tena N, García-González DL, Aparicio R (2009) Evaluation of virgin olive oil thermal deterioration by fluorescence spectroscopy. J Agric Food Chem 57:10505–10511

Unlu NZ, Bohn T, Francis DM, Nagaraja HN, Clinton SK, Schwartz SJ (2007) Lycopene from heat-induced cis-isomer-rich tomato sauce is more bioavailable than from all-trans-rich tomato sauce in human subjects. Br J Nutr 98:140–146

Vannini N, Lorusso G, Cammarota R, Barberis M, Noonan DM, Sporn MB, Albini A (2007) The synthetic oleanane triterpenoid, CDDO-methyl ester, is a potent antiangiogenic agent. Mol Cancer Ther 6:3139–3146

Wu AH, Ursin G, Koh WP, Wang R, Yuan JM, Khoo KS, Yu MC (2008) Green tea, soy, and mammographic density in Singapore Chinese women. Cancer Epidemiol Biomarkers Prev 17:3358–3365

Chapter 1
Cruciferous Vegetables – and Biological Activity of Isothiocyanates and Indoles

Richard Mithen, Charlotte Armah, and Maria Traka

Abstract Epidemiological studies correlate diets that are relatively rich in cruciferous vegetables with a reduction in the incidence and progression of cancer at various sites. These vegetables are characterised by their accumulation of sulphur-containing glycoisdes know as glucosinolates. In this chapter, we initially review the epidemiological evidence and comment upon the potential interaction between diet and polymorphisms at GST loci. We then discuss the biological activity of isothiocyanates and indoles that are derived from glucosinolates following ingestion of cruciferous vegetables, and which may underlie their protective effects.

Keywords Cruciferous vegetables · Chemoprevention · Isothiocyanates · Indoles

Contents

R. Mithen (✉)
Institute of Food Research, Colney Lane, Norwich, NR4 7UA, UK
e-mail: Richard.mithen@bbsrc.ac.uk

M. Mutanen, A.-M. Pajari (eds.), *Vegetables, Whole Grains, and Their Derivatives in Cancer Prevention*, Diet and Cancer 2, DOI 10.1007/978-90-481-9800-9_1,
© Springer Science+Business Media B.V. 2011

1.1 Introduction

Cruciferous vegetables belong to the Brassicaceae within the Capparales – a plant order characterised by the synthesis of a group of sulphur containing glycosides commonly known as glucosinolates. These vegetables are widely consumed throughout the world within most societies, and are important parts of both large scale commercial agriculture and subsistence farming. Traditionally, forms of *Brassica oleracea*, such as cabbages, cauliflowers, broccoli, Brussels sprouts and kales, have been of particularly importance in westernised countries and sub Sahara Africa, and forms of *Brassica rapa*, such as Chinese cabbage or Bok Choi, have been a major part of the diet of Asiatic countries. Glucosinolates accumulate in all tissues within these vegetables, and following degradation produce a range of products of which isothiocyanates and indole derivatives are the most prominent (Figs. 1.1 and 1.2).

The evidence that diets relatively rich in cruciferous vegetables can reduce the risk of incidence or progression of cancer is largely based upon a large body of epidemiological evidence that has been accumulated over the previous three decades. This evidence is complemented by experimental studies with cell and animal models. These experimental studies have focussed on the bioactivity of either the vegetables themselves and relatively crude extracts or individual bioactive components, and have sought to not only provide evidence for anti-carcinogenic activity but also to elucidate the underlying molecular processes that mediate chemoprotection. There is also a small number of acute or longer term human intervention studies that have assessed the effect of cruciferous vegetables on potential biomarkers associated with cancer risk.

While cruciferous vegetables contain a range of potential bioactive compounds that may mediate these health effects, by far the greatest attention has been paid to the bioactivity of glucosinolates and their degradation products. These sulphur-containing glycosides are uniquely found in this group of vegetable crops and it is likely that isothiocyanates and indoles that are derived from these compounds are of considerable importance in mediating anticarcinogenic activity. However, it is also likely that the health benefits of cruciferous vegetables arise from the

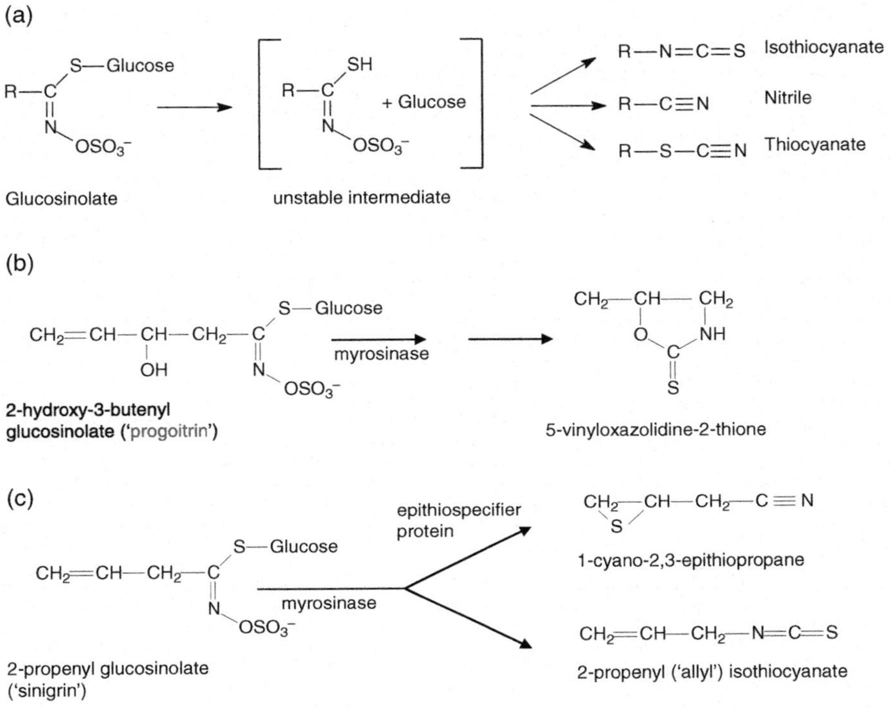

(a)

(b)

(c)

Fig. 1.1 (a) Structure of glucosinolates and enzymic degradation to isothiocyanates and nitriles and, more rarely, thiocyanantes. Examples of side chains of glucosinolates occurring in cruciferous vegetables, R, are shown in Fig. 1.3. (b) Glucosinolates that have a β-hydroxy group form unstable isothiocyanates that cyclise to produce oxazolidine-2-thiones. (c) Glucosinolates with alkenyl side chains may degrade to produce either isothiocyanates or, in the presence of epithiospecifier protein, epithionitriles

complex mixture of plant secondary metabolites, vitamins, minerals and fibre that they contain. In this review, we initially summarise the recent epidemiological data, and then discuss the bioactivity of glucosinolates and other compounds that may be of importance in mediating the health benefits of these vegetables.

1.2 Epidemiological Evidence for the Chemoprotective Effect of Cruciferous Vegetables

The evidence for the heath benefits of any group of fruit and vegetables is largely based upon epidemiological studies that correlate diet with health, but cannot provide any causative association. The majority of reported studies are case control studies, within which diet is assessed retrospectively and comparisons made between individuals who have cancer and matched controls who are healthy. These studies are relatively inexpensive, typically involve several hundred but not

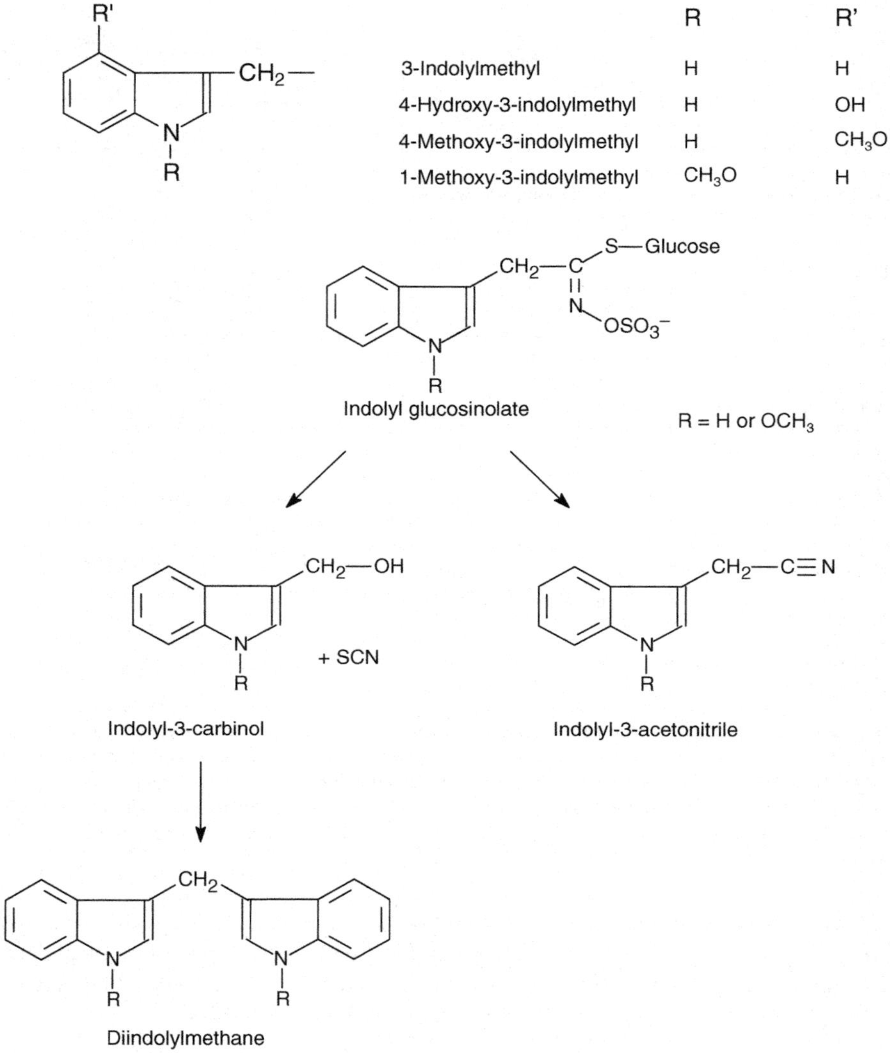

Fig. 1.2 Indole glucosinolates derived from tryptophan. These occur in all cruciferous vegetables. Indole-3-carbinol dimerises under acidic conditions to give diindolylmethane

thousands of individuals, and frequently provide evidence for the positive or negative effects of dietary components. However, case control studies suffer from two major problems. Firstly, they do not give any indication of absolute risk, and thus can give a misleading impression of the extent of protection. Secondly, selection of the control group is complex and challenging, particularly as diets rich in fruits and vegetables are often highly correlated with other lifestyle attributes and socioeconomic status. Furthermore, due to the large number of studies there is likely to be bias in the reporting of studies that have a positive outcome, as opposed to those that find no association between diet and health. More recently, several long term prospective studies involving many thousands of volunteers have provided further evidence for the associations between diet and health. These studies themselves also suffer from problems as their large size may prevent important regional variations in diet-health interactions being evident, and may not identify health benefits within specific subgroups of the population defined by, for example, age, genotype or lifestyle.

In general, and acknowledging that there are several exceptions, while a large number of case control studies have provided evidence for the potential protective effect against cancer of several groups of fruits and vegetables, less support has been obtained following longer term and larger prospective cohort studies. An exception to this has been the relatively consistent evidence that diets rich in cruciferous vegetables can reduce risk of cancer at several sites. These have provided an association between reduction in risk of the four most prevalent cancers – lung, breast, colon and prostate, briefly summarised below – with diets rich in cruciferous vegetables. In addition a reduction in risk of cancers at other sites, including kidney (Moore et al. 2007) bladder (Tang et al. 2008) gastric (Moy et al. 2009) thyroid (Dal Maso et al. 2009) and pancreatic have been reported.

1.2.1 Cruciferous Vegetables and Genetic Polymorphisms at GST Loci

A potential complicating factor in the analyses of epidemiological data is the likely interaction between cruciferous vegetables and genetic polymorphisms at glutathione S-transferase loci, mainly those at GSTT1, GSTM1 and GSTP1, which have been reported in several studies. Polymorphisms at these genetic loci may influence cancer risk, and may also interact with diet to further influence risk. The GST gene family comprises 16 genes in six subfamilies – alpha (GSTA), mu (GSTM), omega (GSTO), pi (GSTP), theta (GSTT) and zeta (GSTZ) (Nebert and Vasiliou 2004). Polymorphisms have been described in many genes of this family, including null mutations in GSTM1 and GSTT1, resulting in the absence of a functional gene product. The frequency of the homozygous null genotype of GSTM1 varies between 39 and 63%, while homozygous null frequencies of GSTT1 are 10–21% for Caucasians, but can be as high as 64% within some Asian populations (Cotton et al. 2000). It has been widely assumed, without experimental evidence, that expression of a functional GSTM1 or GSTT1 allele will lead to more rapid excretion of isothiocyanates derived from glucosinolates, and thus reduce the potential health benefits of cruciferous vegetables. However, the epidemiological data suggests that the interactions between a cruciferous rich diet, GST polymorphisms and health benefits is complex, and often appears paradoxical. Several epidemiological studies based in the US have concluded that GSTM1 positive individuals gain greater cancer protection from either broccoli consumption or total cruciferous vegetable consumption than GSTM1 nulls (Spitz et al. 2000b;

Joseph et al. 2004; Wang et al. 2004b). Additional support for this thesis comes from the study of Lin et al. (1998), in which there was a significant reduction in colorectal adenomas only in GSTM1 positive individuals in subjects who consumed a single portion of broccoli per week, although both GSTM1 positives and nulls had reduced incidence of adenomas with higher levels of broccoli consumption. In contrast, studies based in Asia conclude that GSTM1 nulls and GSTT1 nulls may gain greater protection than GSTM1 and GSTT1 positives from crucifer consumption (which would comprise mainly Chinese cabbage as opposed to broccoli) estimated either by food frequency questionnaires (Zhao et al. 2001a) or by quantification of isothiocyanates in urine (London et al. 2000; Fowke et al 2003; Moy et al. 2009), which has been correlated with crucifer intake (Chung et al. 1998; Seow et al. 1998). A potential explanation for this apparent paradox, although one that requires testing, may be the contrasting patterns of crucifer consumption within these different locations. In the US, about 40% of crucifer consumption is broccoli, whereas consumption of *B. rapa*, either as turnips or Chinese cabbage is very low (Lin et al. 1998; Slattery et al. 2000; Ambrosone et al. 2004; Wang et al. 2004b). Conversely, in Singapore and Shanghai, the majority of *Brassica* vegetable consumption is Chinese cabbage and other forms of *B. rapa* (Seow et al. 2002b; Fowke et al. 2003). These differences may be critical in interpreting the effect of GST genotype. Within the US, the most prevalent isothiocyanate in the diet will be sulforaphane, obtained from broccoli and some other forms of *B. oleracea*, whereas in the Shanghai and Singapore the most prevalent isothiocyanates will be 3-butenyl and 4-pentenyl isothiocyanates, obtained from *B. rapa*. The enzymology of isothiocyanates and 2-propenyl isothiocyanates with GST isozymes are different (Zhang et al. 1995). Assuming that the biochemistry of 2-propenyl isothiocyanate is similar to that of 3-butenyl and 4-pentenyl isothiocyanates, we can expect that GSTM1 deletion will have contrasting effects on the metabolism of isothiocyanates and alkenyl isothiocyanates.

In addition to studies on the potential modifying effect of GSTT1 and GSTM1, there is some data that diets rich in cruciferous vegetables may also interact with allelic polymorphisms at GSTA1 and GSTP1 to influence risk of breast cancer. In both cases, there was evidence that cruciferous vegetables could ameliorate the enhanced risk associated with the GSTA1*B/*B and GSTP1 Val/Val genotypes (Ahn et al. 2006; Lee et al. 2008).

1.2.2 Lung Cancer

Lam et al. (2009) report a systematic review and meta analysis of all the data associated with cruciferous vegetables and lung cancer risk up until 2007 (Lam et al. 2009), involving the analyses of 8,227 cases of lung cancer in Europe (Agudo et al. 1997; Nyberg et al. 1998; Brennan et al. 2000, 2005; Voorrips et al. 2000; Caicoya 2002; Lewis et al. 2002; Miller et al. 2004), United States (Chow et al. 1992; Feskanich et al. 2000; Spitz et al. 2000a; Neuhouser et al. 2003; Wang et al. 2004b), Asia (Koo 1988; Zhao et al. 2001b), Canada (Hu et al. 2002) and Australia

(Pierce et al. 1989), from six prospective cohort studies and 12 case control studies. The risk for those in the highest categories of total cruciferous vegetable consumption was 22% less in case control studies and 17% lower in cohort studies. They concluded that half the number of prospective cohort studies and eight of the 12 case control studies, showed an inverse association between cruciferous vegetable consumption and lung cancer risk in a dose response manner. Several of the case control studies (Spitz et al. 2000a; Zhao et al. 2001b; Lewis et al. 2002; Wang et al. 2004b; Brennan et al. 2005) reported a greater reduction in risk in individuals that were either GSTM1 null and/or GSTT1 null.

1.2.3 Colorectal Cancer

Case control studies have reported a reduction in risk of colorectal cancer with cruciferous vegetable consumption. For example, Seow and colleagues report the results of a prospective epidemiological study based in Singapore in which individuals who lacked both GSTM1 and GSTT1 and were the highest consumers of cruciferous vegetables had a 57% reduction in risk compared to low consumers (Seow et al. 2002a). Similar data has also been reported by Yang et al. (2010) for the reduction in risk of colorectal cancer within the Shanghai Women's Health study, in which an inverse association between colorectal cancer risk and urinary isothiocyanates was only found amongst individuals who were either GSTT1 or GSTM1 null (Yang et al. 2010).

1.2.4 Breast Cancer

Case controlled studies conducted in the US, Sweden and China suggested that women diagnosed with breast cancer consumed significantly less cruciferous vegetables than those not diagnosed (Terry et al. 2001; Fowke et al. 2003; Ambrosone et al. 2004). However when the results of several large cohort studies were examined, no link could be found between breast cancer and cruciferous vegetables consumption (Smith-Warner et al. 2001). As with cancer at other sites, interactions with GST polymorphisms maybe of importance, as discussed above (Ahn et al. 2006; Lee et al. 2008)

1.2.5 Prostate Cancer

A large cohort study involving over 29,000 men has provided good evidence that consumption of cruciferous vegetables, and broccoli in particular, can significantly reduce the risk of the occurrence of aggressive prostate cancer (Kirsh et al. 2007). These data complement other cohort and case control studies that have, in general, supported a negative association between cruciferous vegetable consumption and either the incidence or progression of prostate cancer (Cohen et al. 2000; Kristal and Lampe 2002; Giovannucci et al. 2003). Analyses of these data are confounded by the extent of screening for PSA amongst the study subjects that can introduce bias into the data (Kristal and Stanford 2004).

1.3 Organosulphur Compounds in Cruciferous Vegetables

Organo-sulphur compounds are of particular importance in cruciferous vegetables in mediating plant-herbivore and plant-pathogen interactions, in influencing flavour and consumer acceptability and in health promoting and anticarcinogenic activity. There are two significant sulphur pools within secondary metabolism, glucosinolates and S-methyl cysteine sulphoxide (SMCSO). Glucosinolate degradation products such as isothiocyanates and indoles have been widely implicated in the health benefits of cruciferous vegetable consumption, as discussed below, while SMCSO and its derivatives have been much less explored. SMCSO has largely been considered an undesirable compound as its enzymic or thermal degradation following storage or cooking gives rise to methanethiol, dimethyl disulphide and other sulphides that are responsible for the 'off flavours' of cruciferous vegetables that reduces consumer acceptability and market value (Marks et al. 1992; Stoewsand 1995). However, a small number of studies suggest that SMCSO and related sulphur compounds may be of importance in mediating health benefits (Marks et al. 1993), and further studies are warranted.

The glucosinolate molecule consists of a β-thioglucose moiety, a sulfonated oxime moiety and a variable side chain, derived from an amino acid. While glucosinolates with more than 120 side chain structures have been described (Fahey et al. 2001), only about 16 of these are commonly found within cruciferous vegetables (Fig. 1.3). Seven of these 120 side chain structures correspond directly to a protein amino acid (alanine, valine, leucine, isoleucine, phenylalanine, tyrosine and tryptophan). The remaining glucosinolates have side chain structures which arise in three ways. Firstly, many glucosinolates are derived from chain-elongated forms of protein amino acids, notably from methionine, but also from phenylalanine and branch chain amino acids. Secondly, the structure of the side chain may be modified after amino acid elongation and glucosinolate biosynthesis by, for example, the oxidation of the methionine sulfur to sulfinyl and sulfonyl, and by the subsequent loss of the ω-methylsulfinyl group to produce a terminal double bond. Subsequent modifications may also involve hydroxylation and methoxylation of the side chain. Chain elongation and modification interact to result in several homologous series of glucosinolates, such as those with methylthioalkyl side chains ranging from CH_3S $(CH_2)_3-$ to $CH_3(CH_2)_8-$, and methylsulfinylalkyl side chains ranging from $CH_3SO(CH_2)_3-$ to $CH_3SO(CH_2)_{11}-$. Thirdly, some glucosinolates occur which contain relatively complex side chains such as o-(α-L-rhamnopylransoyloxy)-benzyl glucosinolate in *Reseda odorata* and glucosinolates containing a sinapoyl moiety in *Raphanus sativus*. Several comprehensive reviews of glucosinolate structure and biosynthesis have recently been published (Mithen et al. 2000; Mithen, 2001a, b; Halkier and Gershenzon 2006; Yan and Chen 2007).

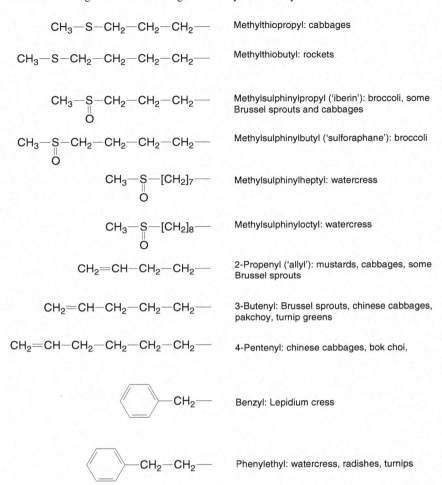

Fig. 1.3 Glucosinolate side chains found within frequently consumed cruciferous vegetables and salad crops. Most crops would contain between 2 and 5 methionine-derived glucosinolates along with tryptophan derived glucosinolates (see Fig. 1.2)

Despite the potential large number of glucosinolates, the major cruciferous crops have a restricted range of glucosinolates. All of these have a mixture of indolylmethyl and *N*-methoxyindolylmethyl glucosinolates, derived from tryptophan, and either a small number of methionine-derived or phenylalanine-derived glucosinolates. The greatest diversity within a species is found in *B. oleracea*, which includes such crops as broccoli, cabbages, Brussels sprouts and kales. These contain indolyl glucosinolates combined with a small number of methionine-derived glucosinolates. For example, broccoli (*B. oleracea* var. *italica*) accumulates 3-methylsuphinylpropyl and 4-methylsulfinylbutyl glucosinolates, while other botanical forms of *B. oleracea* have mixtures of 2-propenyl, 3-butenyl and

2-hydroxy-3-butenyl. Some cultivars of cabbage and Brussels sprouts also contain significant amounts of methylthiopropyl and methylthiobutyl glucosinolates. *B. rapa* (Chinese cabbage, Bok Choi, turnips etc) and *B. napus* (Swedes) contains 3-butenyl and sometimes 4-pentenyl glucosinolates and often their hydroxylated homologues. In addition to methionine-derived glucosinolates, phenylethyl glucosinolate usually occurs in low levels in many vegetables. Several surveys of glucosinolate variation between cultivars of *Brassica* species have been reported, for example *B. rapa* (Carlson et al. 1987a; Hill et al. 1987) and *B. oleracea* (Carlson et al. 1987b; Kushad et al. 1999).

The distinctive taste of many minor horticultural cruciferous crops is due to their glucosinolate content. For example, watercress accumulates large amounts of phenylethyl glucosinolate, combined with low levels of 7-methylsulfinylheptyl and 8-methylsulfinyloctyl glucosinolates, rockets (*Eruca* and *Diplotaxis* species) possess 4-methylthiobutyl glucosinolate, and cress (*Lepidium spp*) contains benzyl glucosinolate. Glucosinolates are also the precursors of flavour compounds in condiments derived from crucifers. For example, *p*-hydroxybenzyl glucosinolate accumulates in seeds of white (or English) mustard (*Sinapis alba*), 2-propenyl and 3-butenyl glucosinolates in seeds of brown mustard (*B. juncea*). 2-Propenyl and other glucosinolates occur in roots of horseradish (*Armoracia rustica*) and wasabi (*Wasabia japonica*). Despite widespread assumptions, the contribution of glucosinolate degradation products to the flavour and aroma of cooked cruciferous vegetables remains to be fully explored. In a study of 19 broccoli cultivars it was found that there was no relationship between glucosinolates and flavour (Baik et al. 2003), and it is likely that the greatest contribution to flavour is from dimethyl disulphide and related compounds derived from the thermal degradation of SMCSO.

1.4 Biological Activity of Isothiocyanates

1.4.1 Glucosinolate Degradation

In the intact plant, glucosinolates are probably located in the vacuole of many cells and are also concentrated within specialized cells. Following tissue disruption, glucosinolates are hydrolysed by thioglucosidases, known as myrosinases. Myrosinase activity results in the cleavage of the thio-glucose bond to give rise to unstable thiohydroximate-*O*-sulfonate. This aglycone spontaneously rearranges to produce several products (Bones and Rossiter 1996). Most frequently, it undergoes a Lossen rearrangement to produce an isothiocyanate (Fig. 1.1a). Aglycones from glucosinolates which contain β-hydroxylated side chains, such as 2-hydroxy-3-butenyl ('progoitrin') found in the seeds of oilseed rape and some horticultural brassicas, such as Brussels sprouts and Chinese cabbage, spontaneously cyclise to form the corresponding oxazolidine-2-thiones (Fig. 1.1b). If the isothiocyanate contains a double bond, in the presence of an epithiospecifier protein (ESP), the isothiocyanate may rearrange to produce an epithionitrile (Foo et al. 2000; Lambrix et al. 2001) (Fig. 1.1c). ESP is also likely to be involved in the production of nitriles from glucosinolates such as methylsulfinylalkyls (Matusheski et al. 2006). Cooking can denature both ESP and myrosinase (Sarikamis et al. 2006), in which case intact glucosinolates can be metabolized by microbial thioglucosidases in the colon to generate isothiocyanates (Rouzaud et al. 2003). Tryptophan derived glucosinolates do not form isothiocyanates but a range of indole compounds (Fig. 1.2). Following ingestion of cruciferous vegetables with intact myrosinase, isothiocyanates will be formed in the mouth and rapidly absorbed in the upper GI tract and subsequently metabolized (Conaway et al. 2000b; Gasper et al. 2005). When myrosinases in the plant tissue are deactivated, such as by cooking or blanching prior to freezing, glucosinolates are hydrolysed in the distal gut by microbial activity, and the resulting isothiocyanates are absorbed from the lower GI tract (Conaway et al. 2000b).

1.4.2 Human Metabolism of Isothiocyanates and Indoles

Following absorption into the epithelial cells of the GI tract, isothiocyanates spontaneously conjugate with glutathione although this may be further promoted by glutathione transferases. The glutathione conjugate is then exported to the systemic circulation via the multidrug resistance associated protein-1 (MRP1), MRP2 and P-glycoprotein-1 (Pgp-1) (Payen et al. 2001; Zhang and Callaway 2002). The isothiocyanate-glutathione conjugate is metabolised via the mercapturic acid pathway in which the glutathione conjugate undergoes further enzymatic modifications including cleavage of glutamine, which yields cysteine-glycine-conjugates, cleavage of glycine, yielding cysteine-conjugates and finally acetylation to produce *N*-acetylcysteine (NAC)-conjugates that are excreted in urine (Brusewitz et al. 1977). However, it has been shown that 45% of ingested sulforaphane (the major isothiocyanate derived from 4-methylsulphinylbutyl glucosinolate that accumulates in broccoli) in the plasma occurs as the free isothiocyanate, as opposed to thiol conjugates, and it has been speculated that the isothiocyanate-glutathione conjugate may be cleaved in the plasma to release the free, and biologically active isothiocyanate, possibly through GSTM1 activity (Gasper et al. 2005) (Fig. 1.4). The peak concentration of isothiocyanates and its thiol conjugates following consumption of a standard portion of broccoli is less than 2 μM, falling to low (nM) levels within a few hours (Gasper et al. 2005). The amount of ingested sulforaphane from broccoli excreted is dependent upon GSTM1 genotype, with individuals with at least one functional GSTM1 allele excreting less isothiocyanate-thiol conjugates than those who have a homozygous deletion (Gasper et al. 2005; Steck et al. 2007), contrary to previous assumptions. This suggests that there may be other metabolic fates for isothiocyanates than mercapturic acid metabolism, such as interaction with a variety of proteins that may have physiological consequences.

The human metabolism of indole glucosinolate derivatives has not been adequately investigated. In the acid environment of the stomach indole-3-carbinol (I3C)

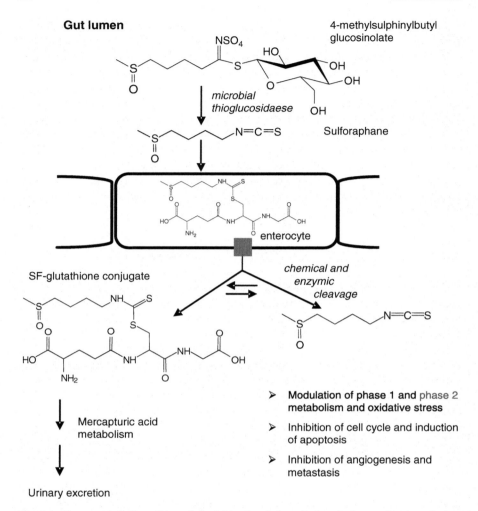

Fig. 1.4 Human metabolism of 4-methylsulphinylbutyl glucosinolate. In the gut, the glucosinolate is converted to the corresponding isothiocyanate (sulforaphane) via microbial thioglucosidases. The isothiocyanate conjugates with glutathione within enterocytes, and is then pumped into the systemic circulation, and metabolised through the mercapturic acid pathway. The presence of unconjugated isothiocyanates in the plasma suggests that the glutathione conjugate is cleaved, whether this is through the action of glutathione transferase is yet to be investigated

will dimerise to form diindolylmethane (DIM), and may form additional conjugates. While pharmacokinetic studies in mice were able to detect both I3C and DIM in plasma and several tissues (Anderton et al. 2004), in a study in women, only DIM was detectable in plasma (Reed et al. 2005, 2006). It should also be noted that the doses used in these studies were significantly higher than those which would be obtained through the consumption of cruciferous vegetables.

1.5 Anticarcinogenic Activity of Isothiocyanates and Indoles in Cancer Rodent Models

Many studies with rodent models have provided evidence that isothiocynates and indoles can reduce the incidence and progression of cancer at multiple sites. These studies have suggested that these compounds can suppress carcinogen-induced tumorigenesis in rodents, and also suppress carcinogenesis induced by knockout of tumor suppressor genes such as APC and PTEN. A summary of some of these studies is provided below.

Extracts of 3-day-old broccoli sprouts were highly effective in reducing the incidence, multiplicity, and rate of development of mammary tumors in dimethyl-benz(a)anthracene (DMBA)-treated rats (Fahey et al. 1997). Isothiocyanates alone also prevented DMBA-induced preneoplastic lesions in mouse mammary glands (Gerhauser et al. 1997) and rat mammary tumors (Zhang et al. 1994) and blocked benzo[*a*]pyrene (BaP)-evoked forestomach tumors in ICR mice (Fahey et al. 2002). Isothiocyanates have been shown to decrease incidence of atypical hyper-plasias in pancreatic ducts of hamsters and the incidence and multiplicity of *N*-nitrosobis(2-oxopropyl)amine (BOP) initiated adenocarcinomas (Kuroiwa et al. 2006). Isothiocyanates effectively reduced the formation of colonic aberrant crypt foci in azoxymethane (AOM)-treated rats (Chung et al. 2000). Recently, isothiocyanates have also been shown to inhibit skin tumorigenesis acting prior to the initiation stage in mice (Xu et al. 2006a) and retard the growth of PC-3 human prostate cancer xenografts in nude mice (Singh et al. 2004a). Together with their NAC conjugates, isothiocyanates inhibited the growth of lung carcinomas from benign tumors by reducing cell proliferation and inducing apoptosis in the tobacco carcinogen–treated A/J mice [a mixture of 3 μmol BaP and 3 μmol 4-(methylnitrosamino)-1-(3-pyridyl)-1-butanone (NNK)] (Conaway et al. 2005).

In addition to chemically induced cancer models, there have been a relatively small number of studies with genetic models of human cancers in rodents. It has been shown that supplementing the diet with isothiocyanates can reduce the incidence and rate of development of tumours in the APCMin/+ model of intestinal cancer (Hu et al. 2006; Khor et al. 2006; Shen et al. 2007), and also in the TRAMP model of prostate cancer (Keum et al. 2009; Singh et al. 2009).

The chemopreventive effects of isothiocyanates and indoles probably involve multiple mechanisms that are likely to interact to reduce the risk of carcinogenesis and cancer progression. These include:

- Inhibition of phase 1 cytochrome *P*450 enzymes
- Induction of phase 2 metabolism enzymes,
- Antioxidant functions through increased tissue GSH levels
- Apoptosis-inducing properties
- Induction of cell cycle arrest
- Anti-inflammatory properties
- Inhibition of angiogenesis and
- Modulation of hormone receptor signalling

1.5.1 Inhibition of Phase 1 Enzymes and DNA-Adducts

Virtually all the dietary and environmental carcinogens are subjected to metabolism once they enter the human body. This enzymatic process occurs mainly through the oxidation as well as, to a lesser extent, reduction and hydrolysis, which transforms the chemical molecules to become more hydrophilic. This physiological event is called phase 1 metabolism, which is primarily catalyzed by the cytochrome P450 enzymes (CYPs). As a consequence, procarcinogens are usually converted into highly reactive intermediates that can bind to critical macromolecules such as DNA, RNA and protein. So far, 57 CYPs have been identified in humans based on their similarity of DNA sequence and some protein functions (Nelson et al. 1993). Phase 1 enzymes typically carry out oxidation and reduction reactions that make carcinogens more water soluble, but at the same time are capable of activating compounds to electrophilic species, which can damage DNA. A large body of data is available, which demonstrates that isothiocyanates may inhibit DNA-adduct and chemical carcinogenesis through alteration of the level of certain CYP isoforms in rodents via a competitive mechanism as well as by a direct covalent modification (Yang et al. 1994; Zhang and Talalay 1994). For example isothiocyanates decreased enzyme activities in rat hepatocytes associated with CYPs 1A1 and 2B1/2, namely ethoxyresorufin-O-deethylase and pentoxyresorufin-O-dealkylase, in a dose-dependent manner (Maheo et al. 1997). Isothiocyanates (0.1–10 μM) gave a marked inhibition of CYP2E1 and CYP1A2-mediated DNA strand breakage by the carcinogens NDMA and 2-amino-3-methylimidazo[4,5-*f*]quinoline (IQ) (Barcelo et al. 1998). In isothiocyanate-treated human hepatocytes, although the expression of CYP1A2 was unaffected, the expression of CYP3A4, the major CYP in human liver, was markedly decreased at both mRNA and activity levels (Maheo et al. 1997). These observations demonstrate that in intact human and rat hepatocytes, isothiocyanates may cause enzyme inhibition of some but not all CYPs and, in the case of CYP3A4, inhibit both its enzyme activity and its expression, probably mediated by the steroid and xenobiotic receptor (Gross-Steinmeyer et al. 2005; Zhou et al. 2006). Associated with the ability of isothiocyanates to inhibit phase 1 enzymes, is its ability to inhibit the formation of carcinogen-induced DNA adducts. In vitro antimutagenicity studies strongly suggest that isothiocyanates are potent inhibitors of the mutagenicity induced by heterocyclic amines (HCA) (Shishu and Kaur 2003). Treatment with isothiocyanates (1–10 μM) significantly reduced the level of PhIP-DNA adducts in human HepG2 cells and human hepatocytes in a dose-dependent manner.

1.5.2 Induction of Phase 2 Detoxification Enzymes

One important process in chemoprotection by isothiocyanates involves modulation of the activity of the so-called phase 2 enzymes, which convert carcinogens to inactive metabolites that are readily excreted from the body, thus preventing their reaction with DNA. Although phase 2 enzymes have been traditionally recognized as those catalyzing the conjugation of endogenous ligands, glutathione (GSH) and glucuronic acid, to endo- and xenobiotic substrates, this classification is expanding to include proteins that catalyze a wide variety of reactions that confer cytoprotection against the toxicity of electrophiles and reactive oxygen species. Isothiocyanates have received much attention over the past decade as they were found to be potent inducers of phase 2 enzymes in mammals (Prochaska et al. 1992; Zhang et al. 1992; Talalay 2000), such as quinone reductase (NAD[P]H:quinone oxidoreductase, NQO1, EC 1.6.99.2), glutathione S-transferases (GST, EC 2.5.1.18) and UDP-glucuronosyltransferase (UGT, EC 2.4.1.17) amongst others. The modulation of phase 2 gene expression and enzyme activity by isothiocyanates has been determined in a number of model cell lines of different origin, derived from liver hepatoma, human HepG2 and mouse Hepa1c1c7. For example, isothiocyanates and its GSH conjugate increased significantly both UGT1A1 and GSTA1 mRNA levels in HepG2 and HT29 cells (Basten et al. 2002). When Hepa1c1c7 cells were exposed to increasing levels of isothiocyanates for 24 h, NQO1 showed a 3-fold maximal induction over control at 2.5 μM isothiocyanates (Matusheski and Jeffery 2001). The effect of isothiocyanates on phase 2 enzyme modulation has also been studied extensively in prostate cancer, where isothiocyanates were shown to significantly induce phase 2 enzyme expression and activity in the human prostate cell lines LNCaP, MDA PCa 2a, MDA PCa 2b, PC-3, and TSU-Pr1 treated with 0.1–15 μM isothiocyanates (Brooks et al. 2001; Jiang et al. 2003). Induction of GST and NQO1 has also been reported in cultured bladder cells (Zhang et al. 2006). Isothiocyanates have also shown to be effective at inducing phase 2 enzymes in vivo. Rats and mice given isothiocyanates for 4–5 days at high dose levels (up to 1,000 μmol/kg/d), increased phase 2 enzyme activities in the liver, lung, mammary gland, pancreas, stomach, small intestine, and colon of the animals (Zhang et al. 1992; Posner et al. 1994; Gerhauser et al. 1997; Matusheski and Jeffery 2001; Keck et al. 2002). At low dose (40 μmol/kg/d), isothiocyanates increased GST and NQO1 activities in the duodenum, forestomach, and/or the urinary bladder of the animals, with the greatest effects being seen in the urinary bladder (Munday and Munday 2004; Zhang et al. 2006). Similarly, isothiocyanates produced modest but significant increases in the enzymatic activities of NQO1, total GST and GST-mu in prostate tissue of rats compared to control animals (Jones and Brooks 2006). Thus, isothiocyanates can modulate the xenobiotic-metabolising enzyme systems, shifting the balance of carcinogen metabolism towards detoxification, and this may be an important mechanism of its chemopreventive activity.

1.5.3 Isothiocyanates and Oxidative Stress

Although isothiocyanates are not direct-acting antioxidants or prooxidants (Zhang et al. 2005), there is substantial evidence that isothiocyanates act indirectly to increase the antioxidant capacity of animal cells, and their abilities to cope with oxidative stress (Fahey and Talalay 1999). Induction of phase 2 enzymes is one means by which isothiocyanates enhance the cellular antioxidant capacity. Enzymes induced by isothiocyanates such as GSTs and NQO1 can function as protectors against oxidative stress (Yanaka et al. 2005). Isothiocyanates are also very potent inducers of HO-1 that catalyses the conversion of heme to biliverdin which in turn is reduced enzymatically to bilirubin (Prestera and Talalay 1995; Jeong et al. 2005; Keum et al. 2006). Among the various genes encoding proteins that possess anti-oxidant characteristics, HO-1 has attracted particular interest as it is finely up-regulated by stress conditions and generates products that might have important biological activities. HO-1 displays antioxidant, antiapoptotic, and anti-inflammatory effects and appears to have a complex role in angiogenesis (reviewed in (Prawan et al. 2005; Ryter et al. 2006)). To protect themselves from oxidative stress, cells are equipped with reducing buffer systems including the GSH and thioredoxin (Trx) reductase. GSH is an important tripeptide thiol which in addition to being the substrate for GSTs, maintains cellular oxidation–reduction balance and protects cells against free radical species. ITCs rapidly accumulate in cells as a result of conjugation with intracellular thiols, especially GSH, to levels reaching 100- to 200-fold over the extracellular concentrations (Zhang 2000, 2001; Callaway et al. 2004). Exposure of cells to ITCs such as isothiocyanates leads, at least transiently, to a decrease in the pool of cellular – SH groups, which will undoubtedly render cells more susceptible to oxidative stress and stress-induced damage (Kim et al. 2003a). Both GSH loss and oxidation have been associated with an increased expression of the rate-limiting enzyme of GSH synthesis GCS (also known as glutamine-L-cysteine ligase, GLCL) and several other detoxification systems including GSTs and NQO1, in response to the stimulation of the Nrf2–ARE signalling pathway by ITCs (Scharf et al. 2003). When HepG2 cells were incubated with 5 μM isothiocyanates for 24 h, significant elevations of GSH content (4.3 fold), NQO1 and GST activity were observed and these elevations were closely related with the total intracellular accumulation (Ye and Zhang 2001). GR also plays a critical role by regenerating reduced GSH from the oxidized form. Surprisingly, GR activities were inhibited consistently by isothiocyanates in six out of seven cell lines, Hepa1c1c7, HepG2, MCF7, MDA-MB-231, LNCaP, and HT-29 cells, except HeLa cells where only a slight induction was observed (Jiang et al. 2003). Isothiocyanates also induce glutathione peroxidase (Gpx), an enzyme that catalyzes the reduction of organic hydroperoxide and hydrogen peroxide, in human Caco-2 cells (Banning et al. 2005) and mouse Hepa1c1c7 cells (Keck and Finley 2006).

The other major ubiquitous factor responsible for maintaining proteins in their reduced state is Trx, which is reduced by electrons from NADPH via thioredoxin reductase (TrxR) (reviewed in (Nakamura 2005). Functions of some transcription factors, such as nuclear factor-κB (NF-κB), AP-1 and p53, are mediated by Trx. TrxR can directly remove apoptotic inducers such as H_2O_2 and indirectly activate anti-apoptotic activity of NF-κB and reduced Trx (reviewed in (Burke-Gaffney et al. 2005)). The predominant cytoplasmic/nuclear form, Trx-1, and the mitochondrial form, Trx-2, both protect against oxidative stress. Isothiocyanates up-regulated the expression of the inducible form, TrxR1, in a dose-dependent manner in HepG2 cells (Hintze et al. 2003; Zhang et al. 2003), Hepa1c1c7 mouse hepatoma cells (Hintze et al. 2005; Keck and Finley 2006), MCF-7 cells (Wang et al. 2005),

EAhy926 endothelial cells (Campbell et al. 2007) and in LNCaP human cell cultures (unpublished results). Isothiocyanates accounted for most of the ARE-activated transcriptional induction of these antioxidant genes by broccoli (Hintze et al. 2005). Together, the changes induced by isothiocyanates promote cellular defences against carcinogens by increasing the reductive capacity of the cell. The overall indirect antioxidant role of isothiocyanates can be attributed to (a) increased tissue GSH levels, (b) effects on phase 2 enzyme regulation (antioxidant role of GSTs, NQO1 and HO-1) and (c) effects on redox enzymes/proteins regulation (TrxR, GCS), although the cytoprotection as a result of an initial induction of oxidative stress by isothiocyanates should not be dismissed, as recently reviewed and discussed by Zhang et al. (2005).

1.5.4 Apoptosis Mediated by Isothiocyanates

Apoptosis, or programmed cell death, is a highly regulated process that occurs under a range of physiological and pathological conditions as part of the cellular mechanism. Apoptosis plays important roles in the development and maintenance of homeostasis and in the elimination of cells that are damaged or no longer necessary for the organism. Inappropriate regulation of apoptosis may cause serious disorders, such as neural degeneration, autoimmune diseases and cancers. The classical hallmarks of apoptosis such as chromatin condensation, translocation of phosphatidylserine across the plasma membrane, and DNA fragmentation have been shown to be induced by isothiocyanates in a variety of colon (Gamet-Payrastre et al. 2000), prostate (Singh et al. 2004a; Choi et al. 2006), medulloblastoma (Gingras et al. 2004) and mammary cell lines (Jackson and Singletary 2004b). The mechanisms by which isothiocyanates induce apoptosis has been extensively explored with cell models, and several key processes within the apoptotic pathways have been shown to be affected by isothiocyanates, such as induction of caspases (Yu et al. 1998; Xu and Thornalley 2000; Gingras et al. 2004), disruption of mitochondrial integrity (Singh et al. 2005; Tang and Zhang 2005) through induction of the proapoptotic members of the Bcl-2 family and release of mitochondrial proteins cytochrome c, Smac/DIABLO and AIF (Gamet-Payrastre et al. 2000; Choi and Singh 2005; Singh et al. 2005; Karmakar et al. 2006). Isothiocyanates may also induce apoptosis via the JNK/MAPK signaling pathway (Hu et al. 2003; Xiao and Singh 2002; Xu et al. 2006b)

1.5.5 Cell Cycle Regulation by Isothiocyanates

Isothiocyanates may exert their anticarcinogenic effect through arresting the cell cycle at different stages of its progression. This arrest has been documented in colon, prostate, breast, bladder and T-cells and resulted in both G_0/G1 and G2/M phase block depending on the cell type. Additionally, S-phase block as a result of isothiocyanate treatment has been reported in human UM-UC-3 bladder cells (Tang and Zhang 2004). Consistent with inhibition of cell cycle in response to isothiocyanates, transcriptome analysis performed on Caco-2 cells revealed that isothiocyanates induce expression of several cell cycle related genes, including p21$^{\text{waf1/cip1}}$ and GADD45β (Traka et al. 2005). Additionally, isothiocyanates enhanced the expression of KLF4, PC3$^{\text{TIS21/BTG2}}$, SMAR1 and CKSHS2, all of which have been associated with regulation of the cell cycle, and decreased expression of members of the minichromosome maintenance family (MCM4 and MCM7) associated with DNA synthesis (Traka et al. 2005). Consistent with a block in the G$_0$/G1 phase of the cell cycle isothiocyanates down-regulated expression of the Cyclin D1 protein in prostate and colon cells (Chiao et al. 2002; Shen et al. 2006) and additionally reduced levels of its associated kinase cdk4 in DU-145 prostate cells (Wang et al. 2004a). Significant reduction in the levels of Cyclin D3 and slight reduction in Cyclin D2 and associated CDK4 and Cdk6 were also reported in non-transformed T lymphocytes (Fimognari et al. 2002). Arrest at the G$_0$/G1 phase of the cell cycle in response to isothiocyanates in prostate cells was associated with reduced phosphorylation of the Rb tumor suppressor protein that activates the transition from G(1)- to S-phase (Wang et al. 2004a). Isothiocyanates also induce cell cycle arrest at the G2/M phase by regulating expression of Cyclin B1. In human colon and breast cells 15 μM isothiocyanates for up to 48 h increased Cyclin B1 protein expression (Gamet-Payrastre et al. 2000; Jackson and Singletary 2004a). In HT29 cells this G2/M phase arrest was achieved by maintaining the cdc2 kinase in its active dephosphorylated form, and was associated with phosphorylation/activation of the Rb protein (Parnaud et al. 2004). In contrast, isothiocyanate treatment on prostate PC-3 and bladder UM-UC-3 cells resulted in reduced expression of Cyclin B1 (Singh et al. 2004b; Tang and Zhang 2004). The G2/M phase arrest in PC-3 cells activated the DNA damage checkpoint pathway through activation of checkpoint kinase 2 (Chk2) and subsequent phosphorylation of cell division cycle 25C (Singh et al. 2004b). Finally, S-phase arrest reported in UM-UC-3 cells in response to isothiocyanates treatment was also associated with reduced levels of Cyclin A (Tang and Zhang 2004).

1.5.6 Microtubule Disruption by Isothiocyanates

Another possible mechanism for the arrest in cell cycle progression by isothiocyanates was described by Jackson and colleagues and involved disruption of microtubules by inhibition of tubulin polymerization (Jackson and Singletary 2004b, a). A microtubule is a polymer of globular tubulin subunits, consisting of a- and b-tubulins, essential for mitosis, cell motility and transport (Nogales 1999). The dynamic character of microtubules is expressed through the ability of its subunits to move through the polymer as a result of polymerization at one end and depolymerization at the other. Disruption of tubulin polymerization interferes with mitosis with a catastrophic outcome for the cell, a process that is targeted by many anticancer drugs, e.g. paclitaxel and taxotere (Bhalla 2003). The first evidence that isothiocyanates inhibits tubulin polymerization was observed in the mouse mammary carcinoma cell line F3II (Jackson and Singletary 2004b). In these cells low concentrations of isothiocyanates (15 μM) caused mitotic cells to display aberrant and mildly depolymerized spindles, whereas high doses of isothiocyanates (100–300 μM) inhibited tubulin polymerization. Similar effects were also obtained in bovine endothelial cells (Jackson et al. 2006) and the human breast adenocarcinoma cells MCF-7, where the inhibition of tubulin polymerization was specifically attributed to the ITC group of the isothiocyanate molecule (Jackson and Singletary 2004a).

1.5.7 Histone Modification by Isothiocyanates

Recently, isothiocyanates have been implicated in the modification of histone acetylation, a highly dynamic process that exerts profound control on gene expression by altering chromatin structure. In vivo, histone acetylation depends on the balance between the enzymes with histone acetylase activity and enzymes that deacetylate histones (histone deacetylase, HDAC) (Struhl 1998). Histone acetylation is associated with an open chromatin conformation, allowing for gene transcription, whereas HDACs maintain the chromatin in the closed, nontranscribed state. HDACs are recognized as promising targets for the development of anticancer drugs as they are usually over-expressed in several tumor cells and tissues (Kim et al. 2003b). The first report on the effect of isothiocyanates on histone modification comes from human embryonic kidney 293 cells and colon HCT116 cells, where treatment with 15 μM isothiocyanates decreased HDAC activity and increased acetylated histones H3 and H4 in both cell lines (Myzak et al. 2004). Interestingly, HDAC inhibition was attributed to the isothiocyanate metabolites, isothiocyanate-cysteine and isothiocyanate-NAC, rather than the parent compound. Treatment of 15 μM isothiocyanate also inhibited HDAC activity in BPH-1, LnCaP and PC-3 prostate cells and increased acetylated levels of H3 and H4 (Myzak et al. 2006b). Additionally, one of the potential mechanisms that isothiocyanates increase expression of $p21^{waf1/cip1}$ was found to be increased binding of acetylated H4 to the promoter of $p21^{waf1/cip1}$ (Myzak et al. 2004, 2006b). Finally, the results of in vitro studies were complemented with in vivo work on the APC^{min} mouse model of intestinal carcinogenesis albeit with small group sizes. Six hours post gavage with 10 μmol isothiocyanate or its metabolite isothiocyanate-NAC, HDAC activity in the colonic mucosa was reduced and acetylated H3 and H4 was increased (Myzak et al. 2006a). Ten-week long feeding with 6 μmol/day isothiocyanate also resulted in increased acetylated H4 in colonic polyps and to a lesser extent in adjacent normal-looking mucosa (Myzak et al. 2006a).

1.5.8 Inhibition of Angiogenesis and Metastasis by Isothiocyanates

Angiogenesis is a prerequisite for the growth of solid tumors and metastasis. Without new blood vessel formation leading to the development of intratumoral capillary networks, tumor progression is severely limited. Several studies suggest that isothiocyanates can interfere with all essential steps of neovascularization from proangiogenic signalling and basement membrane integrity to endothelial cell proliferation, migration, and tube formation. Metastatic cells in the circulation have to perform a series of events to reach a distant site for establishing a new colony. The effect of isothiocyanates on the inhibition of B16F-10 melanoma cells-induced metastasis has been studied in C57BL/6 mice (Thejass and Kuttan 2006). B16F-10 melanoma cells are highly metastatic and form colonies of tumor nodules in the lungs when administered through tail vein, which in turn promote lung fibrosis and collagen deposition. Metastasis is a multi-step process, which involves a series of steps, adhesion of the cancer cells to the basement membrane, invasion through the basement membrane, circulation, extravasation and proliferation at a new distant site. These findings suggest that isothiocyanates reduced the invasion of B16F-10 melanoma cells by the inhibition of activation of MMPs, thereby inhibiting lung metastasis (Thejass and Kuttan 2006).

1.6 Anticarcinogenic Activity of Indoles: Modulation of Hormone Receptor Signalling

As discussed above, tryptophan derived glucosinolates are hydrolysed to indole-3-carbinol (I3C) and related compounds. Within the acid environment of the stomach, indole-3-carbinol dimerises to produce 3-3'-diindolymethane (DIM). These two compounds have been shown to have a wide range of biological activity in both animal and cell models, much of it similar to that observed with isothiocyanates, although different in detail (Weng et al. 2008). These effects include modulation of phase 1 metabolism (Ebert et al. 2005), induction of cell cycle arrest and apoptosis (Chinni et al. 2001; Garikapaty et al. 2006) and inhibition of angiogenesis and metastasis (Meng et al. 2000a; Aggarwal and Ichikawa 2005). One important feature of these compounds is their ability to modulate several cell signalling pathways, including the estrogen and androgen receptor pathways (Firestone and Sundar 2009). Of particular interest is the ability of I3C and DIM to disrupt estrogen receptor pathways which are of importance in driving cellular prolfiferation in hormone sensitive cancers, such as those of the breast and cervix. Estrogens mediate their cellular response through two distinct intracellular receptors that are encoded by separate genes, ER-α and ER-β. After activation through ligand binding, each ER regulates the downstream gene transcription. The ratio of ER-α to ER-β activation is of importance in determining the rate of proliferation of cancer cells: a high ER-α to ER-β ratio correlates with enhanced proliferation, whereas the converse is associated with lower levels of proliferation. Several studies have shown that treating cells with I3C leads to the activation of ER-β, and the down regulation of ER-α, leading to enhancement of antiproliferation signalling (Meng et al. 2000b; Riby et al. 2000a, b; Wang et al. 2006; Mulvey et al. 2007) . I3C and DIM also mediate their effect by acting as ligands for the AhR receptor.

1.7 Human Intervention Studies

In contrast to the multitude of studies with cell and animal models, there has been relatively few human intervention studies to investigate whether diets rich in cruciferous vegetables can affect biomarkers associated with a reduction in cancer risk, and whether any of the mechanisms observed in model systems also occur in humans. A particular concern is that the range of concentrations that are frequently used with cell and animal models are far higher than that which is obtained in the plasma from normal dietary practice, and frequently cells are exposed to the plant derived bioactive compound as opposed to the corresponding human metabolites, so care must be taken in interpreting results from model systems and extrapolation to humans. With regard to isothiocyanates, cell cultures are frequently exposed to concentrations between 10 and 100 μM for up to 24 h, whereas following consumption of cruciferous vegetables the concentration of isothiocyanates and their thiol conjugates in the plasma is likely to be less than 1 μM for maybe 30 min prior to accumulation in the bladder. Likewise, cells are often exposed to indole-3-carbinol, whereas this compound undergoes extensive metabolism in the stomach prior to absorption. It is conceivable, that these compounds may accumulate in certain tissues enhancing their effective concentration and increasing the duration of their exposure.

Human intervention studies with cruciferous vegetables have largely been of two types. Firstly, a series of studies have been undertaken to quantify the pharmacokinetics of isothiocyanates and their thiol metabolites from either raw or processed cruciferous vegetables (Conaway et al. 2000a; Vermeulen et al. 2008) and the effect of GST genotype (Gasper et al. 2005; Steck et al. 2007). Studies on the human metabolism of indole glucosinolate derivatives are still required. Secondly, there have been a series of studies that have sought to investigate changes in gene and protein expression or enzyme activity following a crucifer rich diet. In a series of studies Lampe and colleagues have shown that diets rich in cruciferous vegetables interact with GSTT1 and GSTM1 genotypes to affect the levels or activity of serum CYP1A2, GSTA1/2 and bilirubin (a marker of UGT1A1 activity) (Peterson et al. 2005, 2009; Navarro et al. 2009), consistent with cellular studies on the effect of isothiocyanates and indoles on modulation of phase 1 and phase 2 metabolism. Likewise, ingesting broccoli sprouts – a rich source of sulforaphane – has been shown to induce phase 2 enzyme expression in nasal lavage cells (Riedl et al. 2009). Induction of certain phase 2 genes was also demonstrated to occur after a single meal of broccoli that had enhanced levels of glucosinolates in gastric mucosa, although consuming standard broccoli did not result in induction of phase 2 genes, or genes associated with, for example cell cycle arrest (Gasper et al. 2007). In a longer term intervention, the effect of a 12 month broccoli-rich diet on changes in gene expression in prostate biopsy samples obtained from men who were deemed to be at risk of prostate cancer was investigated, and it was suggested that diet interacted with GSTM1 genotype to perturb several cell signalling pathways that have been associated with carcinogenesis (Traka et al. 2008).

1.8 Conclusions

In conclusion, the evidence for the protective effects of cruciferous vegetables in the diet, and the potential role of glucosinolate degradation products has grown considerably over the last decade. The challenge that lies ahead is to extend the extensive work on cell and animal models into well designed human studies with well established biomarkers of cancer risk, and to translate our existing knowledge into good quality dietary advice and, potentially, the development of novel food products.

References

Aggarwal BB, Ichikawa H (2005) Molecular targets and anticancer potential of indole-3-carbinol and its derivatives. Cell Cycle 4:1201–1215

Agudo A, Esteve MG, Pallares C et al (1997) Vegetable and fruit intake and the risk of lung cancer in women in Barcelona, Spain. Eur J Cancer 33:1256–1261

Ahn J, Gammon MD, Santella RM et al (2006) Effects of glutathione S-transferase A1 (GSTA1) genotype and potential modifiers on breast cancer risk. Carcinogenesis 27:1876–1882

Ambrosone CB, McCann SE, Freudenheim JL et al (2004) Breast cancer risk in premenopausal women is inversely associated with consumption of broccoli, a source of isothiocyanates, but is not modified by GST genotype. J Nutr 134:1134–1138

Anderton MJ, Manson MM, Verschoyle RD et al (2004). Pharmacokinetics and tissue disposition of indole-3-carbinol and its acid condensation products after oral administration to mice. Clin Cancer Res 10:5233–5241.

Baik HY, Juvik J, Jeffery EH et al (2003) Relating glucosinolate content and flavor of broccoli cultivars. J Food Sci 68:1043–1050

Banning A, Deubel S, Kluth D et al (2005) The GI-GPx gene is a target for Nrf2. Mol Cell Biol 25:4914–4923

Barcelo S, Mace K, Pfeifer AM et al (1998) Production of DNA strand breaks by N-nitrosodimethylamine and 2-amino-3-methylimidazo[4,5-f]quinoline in THLE cells expressing human CYP isoenzymes and inhibition by sulforaphane. Mutat Res 402:111–120

Basten GP, Bao Y, Williamson G (2002) Sulforaphane and its glutathione conjugate but not sulforaphane nitrile induce UDP-glucuronosyl transferase (UGT1A1) and glutathione transferase (GSTA1) in cultured cells. Carcinogenesis 23:1399–1404

Bhalla KN (2003) Microtubule-targeted anticancer agents and apoptosis. Oncogene 22:9075–9086

Bones AM, Rossiter JT (1996) The myrosinase-glucosinolate system, its organisation and biochemistry. Physiologia Plantarum 97:194–208

Brennan P, Fortes C, Butler J et al (2000) A multicenter case-control study of diet and lung cancer among non-smokers. Cancer Causes Control 11:49–58

Brennan P, Hsu CC, Moullan N et al (2005) Effect of cruciferous vegetables on lung cancer in patients stratified by genetic status: a mendelian randomisation approach. Lancet 366:1558–1560

Brooks JD, Paton VG, Vidanes G (2001) Potent induction of phase 2 enzymes in human prostate cells by sulforaphane. Cancer Epidemiol Biomarkers Prev 10:949–954

Brusewitz G, Cameron BD, Chasseaud LF et al (1977) The metabolism of benzyl isothiocyanate and its cysteine conjugate. Biochem J 162:99–107

Burke-Gaffney A, Callister ME, Nakamura H (2005) Thioredoxin: friend or foe in human disease? Trends Pharmacol Sci 26:398–404

Caicoya M (2002) Lung cancer and vegetable consumption in Asturias, Spain. A case control study. Med Clin 119:206–210

Callaway EC, Zhang Y, Chew W et al (2004) Cellular accumulation of dietary anticarcinogenic isothiocyanates is followed by transporter-mediated export as dithiocarbamates. Cancer Lett 204:23–31

Campbell L, Howie F, Arthur JR et al (2007) Selenium and sulforaphane modify the expression of selenoenzymes in the human endothelial cell line EAhy926 and protect cells from oxidative damage. Nutrition 23:138–144

Carlson DG, Daxenbichler ME, Tookey HL et al (1987a) Glucosinolates in turnip tops and roots – cultivars grown for greens and or roots. J Am Soc Hortic Sci 112:179–183

Carlson DG, Daxenbichler ME, Vanetten CH et al (1987b) Glucosinolates in crucifer vegetables – broccoli, Brussels- sprouts, cauliflower, collards, kale, mustard greens, and kohlrabi. J Am Soc Hortic Sci 112:173–178

Chiao JW, Chung FL, Kancherla R et al (2002) Sulforaphane and its metabolite mediate growth arrest and apoptosis in human prostate cancer cells. Int J Oncol 20:631–636

Chinni SR, Li Y, Upadhyay S et al (2001) Indole-3-carbinol (I3C) induced cell growth inhibition, G1 cell cycle arrest and apoptosis in prostate cancer cells. Oncogene 20:2927–2936

Choi S, Singh SV (2005) Bax and Bak are required for apoptosis induction by sulforaphane, a cruciferous vegetable-derived cancer chemopreventive agent. Cancer Res 65:2035–2043

Choi S, Lew KL, Xiao H et al (2006) D,L-Sulforaphane-induced cell death in human prostate cancer cells is regulated by inhibitor of apoptosis family proteins and Apaf-1. Carcinogenesis 28:151–162

Chow WH, Schuman LM, McLaughlin JK et al (1992) A cohort study of tobacco use, diet, occupation, and lung cancer mortality. Cancer Causes Control 3:247–254

Chung FL, Conaway CC, Rao CV et al (2000) Chemoprevention of colonic aberrant crypt foci in Fischer rats by sulforaphane and phenethyl isothiocyanate. Carcinogenesis 21:2287–2291

Chung FL, Jiao D, Getahun SM et al (1998) A urinary biomarker for uptake of dietary isothiocyanates in humans. Cancer Epidemiol Biomarkers Prev 7:103–108

Cohen JH, Kristal AR, Stanford JL (2000) Fruit and vegetable intakes and prostate cancer risk. J Natl Cancer Inst 92:61–68

Conaway CC, Getahun SM, Liebes LL et al (2000a) Disposition of glucosinolates and sulforaphane in humans after ingestion of steamed and fresh broccoli. Nutr Cancer Int J 38:168–178

Conaway CC, Getahun SM, Liebes LL et al (2000b) Disposition of glucosinolates and sulforaphane in humans after ingestion of steamed and fresh broccoli. Nutr Cancer 38:168–178

Conaway CC, Wang CX, Pittman B et al (2005) Phenethyl isothiocyanate and sulforaphane and their N-acetylcysteine conjugates inhibit malignant progression of lung adenomas induced by tobacco carcinogens in A/J mice. Cancer Res 65:8548–8557

Cotton SC, Sharp L, Little J et al (2000) Glutathione S-transferase polymorphisms and colorectal cancer: a HuGE review. Am J Epidemiol 151:7–32

Dal Maso L, Bosetti C, La Vecchia C et al (2009) Risk factors for thyroid cancer: an epidemiological review focused on nutritional factors. Cancer Causes Control 20:75–86

Ebert B, Seidel A, Lampen A (2005) Induction of phase-1 metabolizing enzymes by oltipraz, flavone and indole-3-carbinol enhance the formation and transport of benzo[a]pyrene sulfate conjugates in intestinal Caco-2 cells. Toxicol Lett 158:140–151

Fahey JW, Talalay P (1999) Antioxidant functions of sulforaphane: a potent inducer of Phase II detoxication enzymes. Food Chem Toxicol 37:973–979

Fahey JW, Zhang Y, Talalay P (1997) Broccoli sprouts: an exceptionally rich source of inducers of enzymes that protect against chemical carcinogens. Proc Natl Acad Sci USA 94:10367–10372

Fahey JW, Zalcmann AT, Talalay P (2001) The chemical diversity and distribution of glucosinolates and isothiocyanates among plants. Phytochemistry 56:5–51

Fahey JW, Haristoy X, Dolan PM et al (2002). Sulforaphane inhibits extracellular, intracellular, and antibiotic-resistant strains of Helicobacter pylori and prevents benzo[a]pyrene-induced stomach tumors. Proc Natl Acad Sci USA 99:7610–7615

Feskanich D, Ziegler RG, Michaud DS et al (2000) Prospective study of fruit and vegetable consumption and risk of lung cancer among men and women. J Natl Cancer Inst 92:1812–1823

Fimognari C, Nusse M, Berti F et al (2002) Cyclin D3 and p53 mediate sulforaphane-induced cell cycle delay and apoptosis in non-transformed human T lymphocytes. Cell Mol Life Sci 59:2004–2012

Firestone GL, Sundar SN (2009) Minireview: modulation of hormone receptor signaling by dietary anticancer indoles. Mol Endocrinol 23:1940–1947

Foo HL, Gronning LM, Goodenough L et al (2000) Purification and characterisation of epithiospecifier protein from *Brassica napus*: enzymic intramolecular sulphur addition within alkenyl thiohydroximates derived from alkenyl glucosinolate hydrolysis. FEBS Lett 468: 243–246

Fowke JH, Chung FL, Jin F et al (2003) Urinary isothiocyanate levels, brassica, and human breast cancer. Cancer Res 63:3980–3986

Gamet-Payrastre L, Li P, Lumeau S et al (2000) Sulforaphane, a naturally occurring isothiocyanate, induces cell cycle arrest and apoptosis in HT29 human colon cancer cells. Cancer Res 60: 1426–1433

Garikapaty VP, Ashok BT, Tadi K et al (2006) 3,3′-Diindolylmethane downregulates pro-survival pathway in hormone independent prostate cancer. Biochem Biophys Res Commun 340: 718–725

Gasper AV, Al-Janobi A, Smith JA et al (2005) Glutathione S-transferase M1 polymorphism and metabolism of sulforaphane from standard and high-glucosinolate broccoli. Am J Clin Nutr 82:1283–1291

Gasper AV, Traka M, Bacon JR et al (2007) Consuming broccoli does not induce genes associated with xenobiotic metabolism and cell cycle control in human gastric mucosa. J Nutr 137: 1718–1724

Gerhauser C, You M, Liu J et al (1997) Cancer chemopreventive potential of sulforamate, a novel analogue of sulforaphane that induces phase 2 drug-metabolizing enzymes. Cancer Res 57:272–278

Gingras D, Gendron M, Boivin D et al (2004) Induction of medulloblastoma cell apoptosis by sulforaphane, a dietary anticarcinogen from Brassica vegetables. Cancer Lett 203: 35–43

Giovannucci E, Rimm EB, Liu Y et al (2003) A prospective study of cruciferous vegetables and prostate cancer. Cancer Epidemiol Biomarkers Prev 12:1403–1409

Gross-Steinmeyer K, Stapleton PL, Tracy JH et al (2005) Influence of Matrigel-overlay on constitutive and inducible expression of nine genes encoding drug-metabolizing enzymes in primary human hepatocytes. Xenobiotica 35:419–438

Halkier BA, Gershenzon J (2006) Biology and biochemistry of glucosinolates. Annu Rev Plant Biol 57:303–333

Hill CB, Williams PH, Carlson DG et al (1987) Variation in glucosinolates in oriental brassica vegetables. J Am Soc Hortic Sci 112:309–313

Hintze KJ, Wald K, Finley JW (2005) Phytochemicals in broccoli transcriptionally induce thioredoxin reductase. J Agric Food Chem 53:5535–5540

Hintze KJ, Wald KA, Zeng H et al (2003) Thioredoxin reductase in human hepatoma cells is transcriptionally regulated by sulforaphane and other electrophiles via an antioxidant response element. J Nutr 133:2721–2727

Hu J, Mao Y, Dryer D et al (2002) Risk factors for lung cancer among Canadian women who have never smoked. Cancer Detect Prev 26:129–138

Hu R, Kim BR, Chen C et al (2003) The roles of JNK and apoptotic signaling pathways in PEITC-mediated responses in human HT-29 colon adenocarcinoma cells. Carcinogenesis 24: 1361–1367

Hu R, Khor TO, Shen G et al (2006) Cancer chemoprevention of intestinal polyposis in ApcMin/+ mice by sulforaphane, a natural product derived from cruciferous vegetable. Carcinogenesis 27:2038–2046

Jackson SJ, Singletary KW (2004a) Sulforaphane inhibits human MCF-7 mammary cancer cell mitotic progression and tubulin polymerization. J Nutr 134:2229–2236

Jackson SJ, Singletary KW (2004b) Sulforaphane: a naturally occurring mammary carcinoma mitotic inhibitor, which disrupts tubulin polymerization. Carcinogenesis 25:219–227

Jackson SJ, Singletary KW, Venema RC (2006) Sulforaphane suppresses angiogenesis and disrupts endothelial mitotic progression and microtubule polymerization. Vascul Pharmacol 46:77–84

Jeong WS, Keum YS, Chen C et al (2005) Differential expression and stability of endogenous nuclear factor E2-related factor 2 (Nrf2) by natural chemopreventive compounds in HepG2 human hepatoma cells. J Biochem Mol Biol 38:167–176.

Jiang ZQ, Chen C, Yang B et al (2003) Differential responses from seven mammalian cell lines to the treatments of detoxifying enzyme inducers. Life Sci 72:2243–2253

Jones SB, Brooks JD (2006) Modest induction of phase 2 enzyme activity in the F-344 rat prostate. BMC Cancer 6:62

Joseph MA, Moysich KB, Freudenheim JL et al (2004) Cruciferous vegetables, genetic polymorphisms in glutathione s-transferases m1 and t1, and prostate cancer risk. Nutr Cancer 50:206–213

Karmakar S, Weinberg MS, Banik NL et al (2006) Activation of multiple molecular mechanisms for apoptosis in human malignant glioblastoma T98G and U87MG cells treated with sulforaphane. Neuroscience 141:1265–1280

Keck AS, Finley JW (2006) Aqueous extracts of selenium-fertilized broccoli increase selenoprotein activity and inhibit DNA single-strand breaks, but decrease the activity of quinone reductase in Hepa 1c1c7 cells. Food Chem Toxicol 44:695–703

Keck AS, Staack R, Jeffery EH (2002) The cruciferous nitrile crambene has bioactivity similar to sulforaphane when administered to Fischer 344 rats but is far less potent in cell culture. Nutr Cancer 42:233–240

Keum YS, Khor TO, Lin W et al (2009) Pharmacokinetics and pharmacodynamics of broccoli sprouts on the suppression of prostate cancer in transgenic adenocarcinoma of mouse prostate (TRAMP) mice: implication of induction of Nrf2, HO-1 and apoptosis and the suppression of Akt-dependent kinase pathway. Pharm Res 26:2324–2331

Keum YS, Yu S, Chang PP et al (2006) Mechanism of action of sulforaphane: inhibition of p38 mitogen-activated protein kinase isoforms contributing to the induction of antioxidant response element-mediated heme oxygenase-1 in human hepatoma HepG2 cells. Cancer Res 66: 8804–8813

Khor TO, Hu R, Shen G et al (2006) Pharmacogenomics of cancer chemopreventive isothiocyanate compound sulforaphane in the intestinal polyps of ApcMin/+ mice. Biopharm Drug Dispos 27:407–420

Kim BR, Hu R, Keum YS et al (2003a) Effects of glutathione on antioxidant response elementmediated gene expression and apoptosis elicited by sulforaphane. Cancer Res 63:7520–7525

Kim DH, Kim M, Kwon HJ (2003b) Histone deacetylase in carcinogenesis and its inhibitors as anti-cancer agents. J Biochem Mol Biol 36:110–119

Kirsh VA, Peters U, Mayne ST et al (2007) Prospective study of fruit and vegetable intake and risk of prostate cancer. J Natl Cancer Inst 99:1200–1209

Koo LC (1988) Dietary habits and lung cancer risk among Chinese females in Hong Kong who never smoked. Nutr Cancer 11:155–172

Kristal AR, Lampe JW (2002) Brassica vegetables and prostate cancer risk: a review of the epidemiological evidence. Nutr Cancer 42:1–9

Kristal AR, Stanford JL (2004) Cruciferous vegetables and prostate cancer risk: confounding by PSA screening. Cancer Epidemiol Biomarkers Prev 13:1265

Kuroiwa Y, Nishikawa A, Kitamura Y et al (2006) Protective effects of benzyl isothiocyanate and sulforaphane but not resveratrol against initiation of pancreatic carcinogenesis in hamsters. Cancer Lett 241:275–280

Kushad MM, Brown AF, Kurilich AC et al (1999) Variation of glucosinolates in vegetable crops of Brassica oleracea. J Agric Food Chem 47:1541–1548

Lam TK, Gallicchio L, Lindsley K et al (2009) Cruciferous vegetable consumption and lung cancer risk: a systematic review. Cancer Epidemiol Biomarkers Prev 18:184–195

Lambrix V, Reichelt M, Mitchell-Olds T et al (2001) The Arabidopsis epithiospecifier protein promotes the hydrolysis of glucosinolates to nitriles and influences Trichoplusia ni herbivory. Plant Cell 13:2793–2807

Lee SA, Fowke JH, Lu W et al (2008) Cruciferous vegetables, the GSTP1 Ile105Val genetic polymorphism, and breast cancer risk. Am J Clin Nutr 87:753–760

Lewis S, Brennan P, Nyberg F et al (2002) Cruciferous vegetable intake, GSTM1 genotype and lung cancer risk in a non-smoking population. IARC Sci Publ 156:507–508

Lin HJ, Probst-Hensch NM, Louie AD et al (1998) Glutathione transferase null genotype, broccoli, and lower prevalence of colorectal adenomas. Cancer Epidemiol Biomarkers Prev 7:647–652

London SJ, Yuan JM, Chung FL et al (2000) Isothiocyanates, glutathione S-transferase M1 and T1 polymorphisms, and lung-cancer risk: a prospective study of men in Shanghai, China. Lancet 356:724–729

Maheo K, Morel F, Langouet S et al (1997) Inhibition of cytochromes P-450 and induction of glutathione S-transferases by sulforaphane in primary human and rat hepatocytes. Cancer Res 57:3649–3652

Marks HS, Anderson JA, Stoewsand GS (1993) Effect of S-methyl cysteine sulfoxide and its metabolite methyl methane thiosulfinate, both occurring naturally in brassica vegetables, on mouse genotoxicity. Food Chem Toxicol 31:491–495

Marks HS, Hilson JA, Leichtweis HC et al (1992) S-methylcysteine sulfoxide in brassica vegetables and formation of methyl methanethiosulfinate from Brussels-sprouts. J Agric Food Chem 40:2098–2101

Matusheski NV, Jeffery EH (2001) Comparison of the bioactivity of two glucoraphanin hydrolysis products found in broccoli, sulforaphane and sulforaphane nitrile. J Agric Food Chem 49:5743–5749

Matusheski NV, Swarup R, Juvik JA et al (2006) Epithiospecifier protein from broccoli (*Brassica oleracea* L. ssp. italica) inhibits formation of the anticancer agent sulforaphane. J Agric Food Chem 54:2069–2076

Meng Q, Goldberg ID, Rosen EM et al (2000a) Inhibitory effects of Indole-3-carbinol on invasion and migration in human breast cancer cells. Breast Cancer Res Treat 63:147–152

Meng Q, Yuan F, Goldberg ID et al (2000b) Indole-3-carbinol is a negative regulator of estrogen receptor-alpha signaling in human tumor cells. J Nutr 130:2927–2931

Miller AB, Altenburg HP, Bueno-de-Mesquita B et al (2004) Fruits and vegetables and lung cancer: findings from the European prospective investigation into cancer and nutrition. Int J Cancer 108:269–276

Mithen R (2001a) Glucosinolates and their degradation products. Adv Bot Res 35:214–262

Mithen RF (2001b) Glucosinolates and their degradation products. Adv Bot Res 35:213–262.

Mithen RF, Dekker M, Verkerk R et al (2000) The nutritional significance, biosynthesis and bioavailability of glucosinolates in human foods. J Sci Food Agric 80:967–984

Moore L, Brennan P, Karami S et al (2007) Glutathione S-transferase polymorphisms, cruciferous vegetable intake, and cancer risk in the Central and Eastern European Kidney Cancer Study. Carcinogenesis 28:1960–1964

Moy KA, Yuan JM, Chung FL et al (2009) Isothiocyanates, glutathione S-transferase M1 and T1 polymorphisms and gastric cancer risk: a prospective study of men in Shanghai, China. Int J Cancer 125:2652–2659

Mulvey L, Chandrasekaran A, Liu K et al (2007) Interplay of genes regulated by estrogen and diindolylmethane in breast cancer cell lines. Mol Med 13:69–78

Munday R, Munday CM (2004) Induction of phase II detoxification enzymes in rats by plant-derived isothiocyanates: comparison of allyl isothiocyanate with sulforaphane and related compounds. J Agric Food Chem 52:1867–1871

Myzak MC, Karplus PA, Chung FL et al (2004) A novel mechanism of chemoprotection by sulforaphane: inhibition of histone deacetylase. Cancer Res 64:5767–5774

Myzak MC, Dashwood WM, Orner GA et al (2006a) Sulforaphane inhibits histone deacetylase in vivo and suppresses tumorigenesis in Apc-minus mice. FASEB J 20:506–508

Myzak MC, Hardin K, Wang R et al (2006b) Sulforaphane inhibits histone deacetylase activity in BPH-1, LnCaP and PC-3 prostate epithelial cells. Carcinogenesis 27:811–819

Nakamura H (2005) Thioredoxin and its related molecules: update 2005. Antioxid Redox Signal 7:823–828

Navarro SL, Chang JL, Peterson S et al (2009) Modulation of human serum glutathione S-transferase A1/2 concentration by cruciferous vegetables in a controlled feeding study is influenced by GSTM1 and GSTT1 genotypes. Cancer Epidemiol Biomarkers Prev 18: 2974–2978

Nebert DW, Vasiliou V (2004) Analysis of the glutathione S-transferase (GST) gene family. Hum Genomics 1:460–464

Nelson DR, Kamataki T, Waxman DJ et al (1993) The P450 superfamily: update on new sequences, gene mapping, accession numbers, early trivial names of enzymes, and nomenclature. DNA Cell Biol 12:1–51

Neuhouser ML, Patterson RE, Thornquist MD et al (2003) Fruits and vegetables are associated with lower lung cancer risk only in the placebo arm of the beta-carotene and retinol efficacy trial (CARET). Cancer Epidemiol Biomarkers Prev 12:350–358

Nogales E (1999) A structural view of microtubule dynamics. Cell Mol Life Sci 56:133–142

Nyberg F, Agrenius V, Svartengren K et al (1998) Dietary factors and risk of lung cancer in never-smokers. Int J Cancer 78:430–436

Parnaud G, Li P, Cassar G et al (2004) Mechanism of sulforaphane-induced cell cycle arrest and apoptosis in human colon cancer cells. Nutr Cancer 48:198–206

Payen L, Courtois A, Loewert M et al (2001) Reactive oxygen species-related induction of multidrug resistance-associated protein 2 expression in primary hepatocytes exposed to sulforaphane. Biochem Biophys Res Commun 282:257–263

Peterson S, Bigler J, Horner NK et al (2005) Cruciferae interact with the UGT1A1*28 polymorphism to determine serum bilirubin levels in humans. J Nutr 135:1051–1055

Peterson S, Schwarz Y, Li SS et al (2009) CYP1A2, GSTM1, and GSTT1 polymorphisms and diet effects on CYP1A2 activity in a crossover feeding trial. Cancer Epidemiol Biomarkers Prev 18:3118–3125

Pierce RJ, Kune GA, Kune S et al (1989) Dietary and alcohol intake, smoking pattern, occupational risk, and family history in lung cancer patients: results of a case-control study in males. Nutr Cancer 12:237–248

Posner GH, Cho CG, Green JV et al (1994) Design and synthesis of bifunctional isothiocyanate analogs of sulforaphane: correlation between structure and potency as inducers of anticarcinogenic detoxication enzymes. J Med Chem 37:170–176

Prawan A, Kundu JK, Surh YJ (2005) Molecular basis of heme oxygenase-1 induction: implications for chemoprevention and chemoprotection. Antioxid Redox Signal 7:1688–1703

Prestera T, Talalay P (1995) Electrophile and antioxidant regulation of enzymes that detoxify carcinogens. Proc Natl Acad Sci USA 92:8965–8969

Prochaska HJ, Santamaria AB, Talalay P (1992) Rapid detection of inducers of enzymes that protect against carcinogens. Proc Natl Acad Sci USA 89:2394–2398

Reed GA, Peterson KS, Smith HJ et al (2005) A phase I study of indole-3-carbinol in women: tolerability and effects. Cancer Epidemiol Biomarkers Prev 14:1953–1960

Reed GA, Arneson DW, Putnam WC et al (2006) Single-dose and multiple-dose administration of indole-3-carbinol to women: pharmacokinetics based on 3,3′-diindolylmethane. Cancer Epidemiol Biomarkers Prev 15:2477–2481

Riby JE, Chang GH, Firestone GL et al (2000a) Ligand-independent activation of estrogen receptor function by 3, 3′-diindolylmethane in human breast cancer cells. Biochem Pharmacol 60: 167–177

Riby JE, Feng C, Chang YC et al (2000b) The major cyclic trimeric product of indole-3-carbinol is a strong agonist of the estrogen receptor signaling pathway. Biochemistry 39:910–918

Riedl MA, Saxon A, Diaz-Sanchez D (2009) Oral sulforaphane increases Phase II antioxidant enzymes in the human upper airway. Clin Immunol 130:244–251

Rouzaud G, Rabot S, Ratcliffe B et al (2003) Influence of plant and bacterial myrosinase activity on the metabolic fate of glucosinolates in gnotobiotic rats. Br J Nutr 90:395–404

Ryter SW, Alam J, Choi AM (2006) Heme oxygenase-1/carbon monoxide: from basic science to therapeutic applications. Physiol Rev 86:583–650

Sarikamis G, Marquez J, MacCormack R et al (2006) High glucosinolate broccoli: a delivery system for sulforaphane. Mol Breed 18:219–228

Scharf G, Prustomersky S, Knasmuller S et al (2003) Enhancement of glutathione and g-glutamylcysteine synthetase, the rate limiting enzyme of glutathione synthesis, by chemoprotective plant-derived food and beverage components in the human hepatoma cell line HepG2. Nutr Cancer 45:74–83

Seow A, Yuan JM, Sun CL et al (2002a) Dietary isothiocyanates, glutathione S-transferase polymorphisms and colorectal cancer risk in the Singapore Chinese Health Study. Carcinogenesis 23:2055–2061

Seow A, Shi CY, Chung FL et al (1998) Urinary total isothiocyanate (ITC) in a population-based sample of middle-aged and older Chinese in Singapore: relationship with dietary total ITC and glutathione S-transferase M1/T1/P1 genotypes. Cancer Epidemiol Biomarkers Prev 7: 775–781

Seow A, Poh WT, Teh M et al (2002a) Diet, reproductive factors and lung cancer risk among Chinese women in Singapore: evidence for a protective effect of soy in nonsmokers. Int J Cancer 97:365–371

Seow A, Yuan JM, Sun CL et al (2002b) Dietary isothiocyanates, glutathione S-transferase polymorphisms and colorectal cancer risk in the Singapore Chinese Health Study. Carcinogenesis 23:2055–2061

Shen G, Xu C, Chen C et al (2006) p53-independent G1 cell cycle arrest of human colon carcinoma cells HT-29 by sulforaphane is associated with induction of p21CIP1 and inhibition of expression of cyclin D1. Cancer Chemother Pharmacol 57:317–327

Shen G, Khor TO, Hu R et al (2007) Chemoprevention of familial adenomatous polyposis by natural dietary compounds sulforaphane and dibenzoylmethane alone and in combination in ApcMin/+ mouse. Cancer Res 67:9937–9944

Shishu, Kaur IP (2003) Inhibition of mutagenicity of food-derived heterocyclic amines by sulforaphane – a constituent of broccoli. Indian J Exp Biol 41:216–219

Singh AV, Xiao D, Lew KL et al (2004a) Sulforaphane induces caspase-mediated apoptosis in cultured PC-3 human prostate cancer cells and retards growth of PC-3 xenografts in vivo. Carcinogenesis 25:83–90

Singh SV, Herman-Antosiewicz A, Singh AV et al (2004b). Sulforaphane-induced G2/M phase cell cycle arrest involves checkpoint kinase 2-mediated phosphorylation of cell division cycle 25C. J Biol Chem 279:25813–25822

Singh SV, Srivastava SK, Choi S et al (2005) Sulforaphane-induced cell death in human prostate cancer cells is initiated by reactive oxygen species. J Biol Chem 280: 19911–19924

Singh SV, Warin R, Xiao D et al (2009) Sulforaphane inhibits prostate carcinogenesis and pulmonary metastasis in TRAMP mice in association with increased cytotoxicity of natural killer cells. Cancer Res 69:2117–2125

Slattery ML, Kampman E, Samowitz W et al (2000) Interplay between dietary inducers of GST and the GSTM-1 genotype in colon cancer. Int J Cancer 87:728–733

Smith-Warner SA, Spiegelman D, Yaun SS et al (2001) Intake of fruits and vegetables and risk of breast cancer: a pooled analysis of cohort studies. JAMA 285:769–776

Spitz MR, Duphorne CM, Detry MA et al (2000a) Dietary intake of isothiocyanates: evidence of a joint effect with glutathione S-transferase polymorphisms in lung cancer risk. Cancer Epidemiol Biomarkers Prev 9:1017–1020

Spitz MR, Duphorne CM, Detry MA et al (2000b) Dietary intake of isothiocyanates: Evidence of a joint effect with glutathione S-transferase polymorphisms in lung cancer risk. Cancer Epidemiol Biomarkers Prev 9:1017–1020

Steck SE, Gammon MD, Hebert JR et al (2007) GSTM1, GSTT1, GSTP1, and GSTA1 polymorphisms and urinary isothiocyanate metabolites following broccoli consumption in humans. J Nutr 137:904–909

Stoewsand GS (1995) Bioactive organosulfur phytochemicals in brassica-oleracea vegetables – a review. Food Chem Toxicol 33:537–543

Struhl K (1998) Histone acetylation and transcriptional regulatory mechanisms. Genes Dev 12:599–606

Talalay P (2000) Chemoprotection against cancer by induction of phase 2 enzymes. Biofactors 12:5–11

Tang L, Zhang Y (2004) Dietary isothiocyanates inhibit the growth of human bladder carcinoma cells. J Nutr 134:2004–2010

Tang L, Zhang Y (2005) Mitochondria are the primary target in isothiocyanate-induced apoptosis in human bladder cancer cells. Mol Cancer Ther 4:1250–1259

Tang L, Zirpoli GR, Guru K et al (2008) Consumption of raw cruciferous vegetables is inversely associated with bladder cancer risk. Cancer Epidemiol Biomarkers Prev 17:938–944

Terry P, Wolk A, Persson I et al (2001) Brassica vegetables and breast cancer risk. JAMA 285:2975–2977

Thejass P, Kuttan G (2006) Antimetastatic activity of sulforaphane. Life Sci 78:3043–3050

Traka M, Gasper AV, Smith JA et al (2005) Transcriptome analysis of human colon Caco-2 cells exposed to sulforaphane. J Nutr 135:1865–1872

Traka M, Gasper AV, Melchini A et al (2008) Broccoli consumption interacts with GSTM1 to perturb oncogenic signalling pathways in the prostate. PLoS One 3:e2568

Vermeulen M, Klopping-Ketelaars IW, van den Berg R et al (2008) Bioavailability and kinetics of sulforaphane in humans after consumption of cooked versus raw broccoli. J Agric Food Chem 56:10505–10509

Voorrips LE, Goldbohm RA, van Poppel G et al (2000) Vegetable and fruit consumption and risks of colon and rectal cancer in a prospective cohort study: The Netherlands Cohort Study on Diet and Cancer. Am J Epidemiol 152:1081–1092

Wang L, Liu D, Ahmed T et al (2004a) Targeting cell cycle machinery as a molecular mechanism of sulforaphane in prostate cancer prevention. Int J Oncol 24:187–192

Wang LI, Giovannucci EL, Hunter D et al (2004b) Dietary intake of cruciferous vegetables, glutathione S-transferase (GST) polymorphisms and lung cancer risk in a Caucasian population. Cancer Causes Control 15:977–985

Wang TT, Milner MJ, Milner JA et al (2006) Estrogen receptor alpha as a target for indole-3-carbinol. J Nutr Biochem 17:659–664

Wang W, Wang S, Howie AF et al (2005) Sulforaphane, erucin, and iberin up-regulate thioredoxin reductase 1 expression in human MCF-7 cells. J Agric Food Chem 53:1417–1421

Weng JR, Tsai CH, Kulp SK et al (2008) Indole-3-carbinol as a chemopreventive and anti-cancer agent. Cancer Lett 262:153–163

Xiao D, Singh SV (2002) Phenethyl isothiocyanate-induced apoptosis in p53-deficient PC-3 human prostate cancer cell line is mediated by extracellular signal-regulated kinases. Cancer Res 62:3615–3619

Xu C, Huang MT, Shen G et al (2006a) Inhibition of 7,12-Dimethylbenz(a)anthracene-Induced Skin Tumorigenesis in C57BL/6 Mice by Sulforaphane Is Mediated by Nuclear Factor E2-Related Factor 2. Cancer Res 66:8293–8296

Xu C, Shen G, Yuan X et al (2006b) ERK and JNK signaling pathways are involved in the regulation of activator protein 1 and cell death elicited by three isothiocyanates in human prostate cancer PC-3 cells. Carcinogenesis 27:437–445

Xu K, Thornalley PJ (2000) Studies on the mechanism of the inhibition of human leukaemia cell growth by dietary isothiocyanates and their cysteine adducts in vitro. Biochem Pharmacol 60:221–231

Yan X, Chen S (2007) Regulation of plant glucosinolate metabolism. Planta 226: 1343–1352

Yanaka A, Zhang S, Tauchi M et al (2005) Role of the nrf-2 gene in protection and repair of gastric mucosa against oxidative stress. Inflammopharmacology 13:83–90

Yang CS, Smith TJ, Hong JY (1994) Cytochrome P-450 enzymes as targets for chemoprevention against chemical carcinogenesis and toxicity: opportunities and limitations. Cancer Res 54:1982s–1986s.

Yang G, Gao YT, Shu XO et al (2010) Isothiocyanate exposure, glutathione S-transferase polymorphisms, and colorectal cancer risk. Am J Clin Nutr 91:704–711

Ye L, Zhang Y (2001) Total intracellular accumulation levels of dietary isothiocyanates determine their activity in elevation of cellular glutathione and induction of Phase 2 detoxification enzymes. Carcinogenesis 22:1987–1992

Yu R, Mandlekar S, Harvey KJ et al (1998) Chemopreventive isothiocyanates induce apoptosis and caspase-3-like protease activity. Cancer Res 58:402–408

Zhang J, Svehlikova V, Bao Y et al (2003) Synergy between sulforaphane and selenium in the induction of thioredoxin reductase 1 requires both transcriptional and translational modulation. Carcinogenesis 24:497–503

Zhang Y (2000) Role of glutathione in the accumulation of anticarcinogenic isothiocyanates and their glutathione conjugates by murine hepatoma cells. Carcinogenesis 21:1175–1182

Zhang Y (2001) Molecular mechanism of rapid cellular accumulation of anticarcinogenic isothiocyanates. Carcinogenesis 22:425–431

Zhang Y, Callaway EC (2002) High cellular accumulation of sulphoraphane, a dietary anticarcinogen, is followed by rapid transporter-mediated export as a glutathione conjugate. Biochem J 364:301–307

Zhang Y, Talalay P (1994) Anticarcinogenic activities of organic isothiocyanates: chemistry and mechanisms. Cancer Res 54:1976s–1981s

Zhang Y, Kensler TW, Cho CG et al (1994) Anticarcinogenic activities of sulforaphane and structurally related synthetic norbornyl isothiocyanates. Proc Natl Acad Sci USA 91:3147–3150

Zhang Y, Kolm RH, Mannervik B et al (1995) Reversible conjugation of isothiocyanates with glutathione catalyzed by human glutathione transferases. Biochem Biophys Res Commun 206:748–755

Zhang Y, Li J, Tang L (2005) Cancer-preventive isothiocyanates: dichotomous modulators of oxidative stress. Free Radic Biol Med 38:70–77

Zhang Y, Munday R, Jobson HE et al (2006) Induction of GST and NQO1 in cultured bladder cells and in the urinary bladders of rats by an extract of broccoli (*Brassica oleracea* italica) Sprouts. J Agric Food Chem 54:9370–9376

Zhang Y, Talalay P, Cho CG et al (1992) A major inducer of anticarcinogenic protective enzymes from broccoli: isolation and elucidation of structure. Proc Natl Acad Sci USA 89:2399–2403

Zhao B, Seow A, Lee EJD et al (2001a) Dietary isothiocyanates, glutathione S-transferase-M1,-T1 polymorphisms and lung cancer risk among Chinese women in Singapore. Cancer Epidemiol Biomarkers Prev 10:1063–1067

Zhao B, Seow A, Lee EJ et al (2001b) Dietary isothiocyanates, glutathione S-transferase -M1, -T1 polymorphisms and lung cancer risk among Chinese women in Singapore. Cancer Epidemiol Biomarkers Prev 10:1063–1067

Zhou C, Poulton EJ, Grun F et al (2006) The dietary isothiocyanate, sulforaphane is an antagonist of the human steroid and xenobiotic nuclear receptor (SXR). Mol Pharmacol 71:220–229

Chapter 2
Green Leafy Vegetables in Cancer Prevention

Marja Mutanen, Mikael Niku, and Seija Oikarinen

Abstract Green leafy vegetables contain a wealth of potential chemopreventive compounds. Chlorophyll and its derivatives can trap aflatoxin and other mutagens by complex formation and appear protective against carcinogens in various animal and human models. They also have antioxidative and immunomodulatory properties. Folate is essential in DNA synthesis and methylation, and is required especially by rapidly proliferating tissues. For cancer prevention, dietary folate may be preferable to the much more stable folic acid used in fortification. Of the various green vegetables, spinach and perilla have been widely studied. Spinach has high antioxidant content, and its glycolipid fractions inhibit cancer cell proliferation and suppress tumours in murine models. Luteolin, rosmarinic acid and triterpenes extracted from perilla leaves are potent antitumourigenic and anti-inflammatory agents.

Keywords Spinach · Perilla · Chlorophyll · Folate · Luteolin · Rosmarinic acid · Triterpenes · Chemoprevention

Contents

M. Mutanen (✉)
Department of Food and Environmental Sciences, (Nutrition), University of Helsinki, Helsinki, Finland
e-mail: marja.mutanen@helsinki.fi

M. Mutanen, A.-M. Pajari (eds.), *Vegetables, Whole Grains, and Their Derivatives in Cancer Prevention*, Diet and Cancer 2, DOI 10.1007/978-90-481-9800-9_2,
© Springer Science+Business Media B.V. 2011

2.1 Introduction

Green leafy vegetables are good sources of for example chlorophyll, folates, flavonoids, polyphenols, glycolipids, and antioxidants, all of which are potential chemopreventive agents. The experimental work with different types of vegetables indicate that certain vegetables may either as such or through their specific pattern of compounds possess anticarcinogenic effects in humans and different animal models. The anticarcinogenic mechanisms have also been established in vitro for some of these compounds. The epidemiological studies have not been able to answer the question how different types of fruits and vegetables or their constituents modulate the risk of different cancers. Vegetables (sometimes with fruits) are often used as a single dietary constituent in epidemiological study approach and thus the possibility for specific vegetables to be detected as cancer preventive substance is not possible. In addition, genetic variation in genes such as cytochrome P450 family that are involved in metabolism of vegetable components potentially modify relationships between vegetable intake and cancer risk. In this chapter we concentrate on two main chemopreventive compound found in green leafy vegetables, chlorophyll and folates. In addition, two leafy vegetables commonly used in different parts of the world, spinach and perilla leaves and their constituents are discussed.

2.2 Green Leafy Vegetables as Sources of Chemopreventive Compounds

2.2.1 Chlorophylls and Chlorophyllins

Chlorophylls and chlorophyllins (Fig. 2.1) are ubiquitous pigments with reported chemopreventive properties. Chlorophylls are the principal photoreceptors in green plants, responsible for their colour. Common green vegetables contain 20–2,000 micrograms of chlorophylls per gram of fresh tissue (Khachik et al. 1986). Chlorophyllins are semi-synthetic water-soluble chlorophyll derivatives commonly used as food additives. For practical reasons, commercially available chlorophyllins are used in most experimental studies. Food processing and digestion produce a multitude of further chlorophyll derivatives, the absorption and bioavailability of which is incompletely understood (for a review, see Ferruzzi and Blakeslee 2007).

Chlorophyll derivatives have shown potential chemopreventive activity in various in vitro and in vivo models. Best documented is their ability to trap mutagens

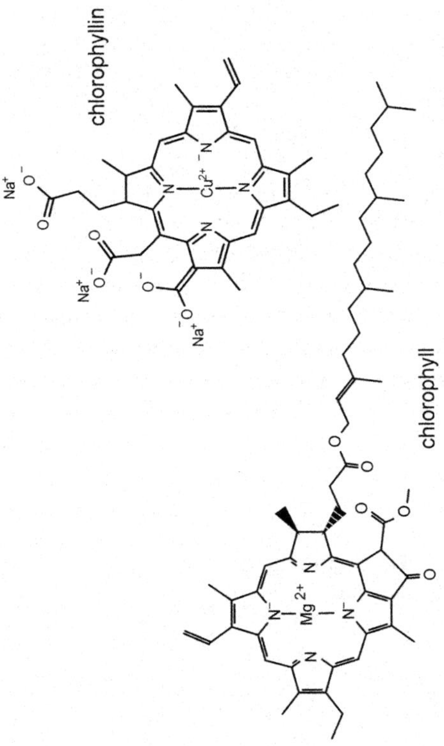

Fig. 2.1 Chemical structures of chlorophyll and clorophyllin. Source: The PubChem: http://www.ncbi.nlm.nih.gov/About/disclaimer.html

by complex formation. Chlorophyllin binds mutagens such as acridine orange, quinacrine mustard, doxorubicin, dibenzopyrene and aflatoxin, and appears to decrease mutagen binding to DNA in vitro (Pietrzak et al. 2006, 2008; Simonich et al. 2007, 2008). In animal models, chlorophyllins reduce aflatoxin intestinal absorption, tissue concentration and hepatic carcinogenesis if given together with the carcinogen (Breinholt et al. 1995, 1999; Hayashi et al. 1999). Chlorophyll protects rats from heme-induced mucosal damage; interestingly, chrolophyllin is not protective (de Vogel et al. 2005a). An epidemiological study suggest that high dietary heme/chlorophyll ratio may elevate colon cancer risk (Balder et al. 2006). A clinical intervention study with humans exposed to dietary aflatoxins showed that chlorophyllin (100 mg three times daily) can effectively reduce urinary concentrations of an excreted DNA adduct biomarker (Egner et al. 2001).

Other chemopreventive mechanisms are possible, as chlorophyllin metabolites actually are absorbed from the intestine (Egner et al. 2000). Chlorophyllin is known as a potent antioxidant, and it has been shown to protect against oxidative damage in vitro and ex vivo, after injection or dietary administration in mice (Kamat et al. 2000; Kumar et al. 2004; Kwang Kyun Park et al. 2003). It also induces phase II detoxification activity in liver (Dingley et al. 2003; Fahey et al. 2005). Immunomodulatory effects have been reported with murine macrophages in vitro (Cho et al. 2000; Yun et al. 2005, 2006). In various cancer cell lines, chlorophyllin reduces ERK activation, cyclin D1 and β-catenin and induces differentiation and apoptosis (Chiu et al. 2005; Díaz et al. 2003; Carter et al. 2004). In vivo, effects on colonic carcinogenesis appear complex and depend on dosage and the use of natural chrolophyll versus chlorophyllins (Blum et al. 2003).

2.2.2 Folate

Vitamins such as B2, B6, B12 and folate that are related to one carbon metabolism are of interest in carcinogenesis since they take part in DNA syntheses and methylation reactions in the cell. Folate is in the centre of these metabolic reactions and has been in a focus of cancer prevention during the last decade. Since green leafy vegetables and plant kingdom in general are considerable sources of folate in human diet, the evidence behind folate and carcinogenesis is discussed in this chapter.

From the green leafy vegetables especially nettle, parsley and kale are good sources of folate (190–120 μg/100 g). In addition to green leafy vegetables, also some beans contain much: brown and white beans 390 μg/100 g, soybean 370 μg/100 g, and green beans 145 μg/100 g. Similarly asparagus, beet, broccoli, Brussels sprout, cauliflower, and kohlrabi are good sources of folate (180–80 μg/100 g).

Folate is a generic name for a food-based group of B vitamins containing an aromatic pteridine ring linked to p-aminobenzoic acid and a glutamate residude. Humans get folate either as this natural form or in supplements or through food fortification as pharmaceutical totally oxidized form of folate, i.e folic acid (FA). Food folate is very unstable and rapidly loses its activity during storage and food preparation. FA, on the contrary, is highly stable over months. Both folate and FA are absorbed in the intestine as carrier mediated processes, and bioavailability of FA is twice as high than natural folates. During absorption folate undergo hydrolyses to methyltetrahydrofolate (methylTHF), which is a predominant form of folate in circulation. Also FA is converted to methylTHF to some extent. It has been shown that the process becomes saturated at doses of 270 μg and at higher levels FA is transported to circulation as FA. From the carcinogenesis point of view the role of free FA has raised some concern (see below). Commonly used amount of FA in supplement is 400 μg meaning that a regular use of FA as supplement produces a sustain level of FA in plasma.

There are several extensive reviews on folate metabolism and reader is referred to them (Kim 2007) and only schematic representation of folate metabolism is illustrated here. Figure 2.2 (Hubner and Houlston 2009) shows the essential role of methylTHF for the synthesis of nucleotides and for the provision of methyl groups for the maintenance of DNA methylation in dividing cells.

The recommendation of folate intake is 400 μg/d and in several populations this is not achieved. Strong evidence behind low folate status and neural tube defect has in several countries lead to recommendations of FA supplements to women of

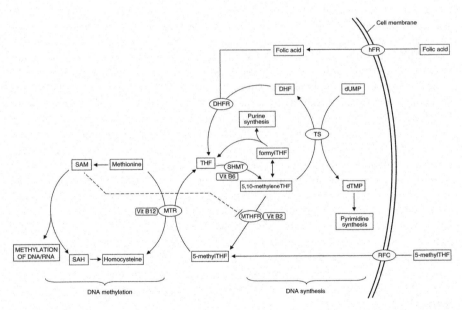

Fig. 2.2 Schematic representation of folate metabolism illustrating the entry of natural folates and folic acid into the pathway, and flow of methyl group towards either DNA synthesis or DNA methylation. RFC, reduced folate carrier; hFR, human folate receptor; MTR, methionine synthase; MTHFR, methylenetetrahydrofolate reductase; SHMT, serine hydroxymethyltransferase; TS, thymidylate synthase; THF, tetrahydrofolate; DHF, dihydrofolate; SAM, *S*-adenosylmethionine; SAH, *S*-adenosylhomocysteine; dUMP, deoxyuridine monophosphate; dTMP, deoxythymidine monophosphate. (Hubner and Houlston 2009)

reproductive age. In addition, food fortification with FA to increase folate status of the population is used in the US since 1998 and some other countries. The purpose of these fortifications has been to provide an average an additional 100 μg FA/d. Since epidemiological evidence has for long shown inverse relationship between the consumption of vegetables and fruits and the incidence of several cancers, several secondary prevention trials in humans with FA has been carried out lately. The outcome of these trials has shown the complexity in folate in cancer prevention and supported the evidence, which was got from the animal experiments, notably that the efficacy of folate in cancer prevention is time and dose dependent and supplemental FA may not always by beneficial. These aspects of folate and FA are discussed below.

Low folate status has been associated with increased risk of cancers of the colon, esophageal, gastric, pancreatic, and breast and the evidence has been recently discussed in the following articles: Kim (2007), Larsson et al. (2006), and Ulrich (2007). In his recent comprehensive review on folate and colorectal cancer (CRC) Kim (2007) comes to the conclusion that even if the overall evidence from epidemiologic, animal, and intervention studies supports the inverse association between folate status and the risk of colorectal cancer the effect of folate is bimodal. Rapidly proliferating tissues, including tumour tissue, have greater requirement for folate. Tumor tissues over express folate receptors to meet their increased need for increased demand for DNA synthesis and proliferation. In precancerous colon tissue and already established tumours folate deficiency below requirements seem to have inhibitory effect whereas folate supplementation above requirements promotes the process by supporting cell divisions. This may explain the disappointing results, which have been obtained lately in human supplementation trials. All of them were secondary preventions trials, with subjects with established primary colon cancer. In addition, FA was used in supplements indicating that there was free FA present in circulation. Since tumor tissue has much higher affinity for FA than methylTHF the demand for methylation reactions of the transformed tissue is easily achieved. In addition, unmetabolized FA in plasma has been shown to be associated with reduced natural killer cell cytotoxicity in humans (Troen et al. 2006). Natural killer cells are effector lymphocytes of the innate immune system that control several types of tumors and microbiological infection (Vivier et al. 2008). The situation is different for normal mucosa tissue. Then folate deficiency appears to predispose the tissue to neoplastic transformation and folate supplementation within physiological range prevents transformation. Also in this situation pharmacological supplemental doses of FA enhance the transformation of normal colon mucosa to precancerous tissue. The dual modulatory role of folate in carcinogenesis is illustrated in Fig. 2.3 (Kim 2007).

Meta-analysis for case-control and cohort studies on folate and esophageal, gastric, and pancreatic cancer risk showed inverse relation of dietary folate intake and risk of for esophageal and pancreatic cancers. The results for gastric cancer were inconsistent. In most studies the MTHFR 677TT genotype, which is associated with reduced enzyme activity (and lower conversion of dietary folate into methylTHF) was associated into higher risk of all three cancers (Larsson et al. 2006). It was

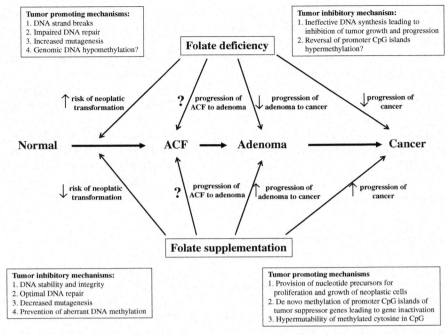

Fig. 2.3 Dual modulatory role of folate in carcinogenesis: cancer develops over decades, if not lifetime, through different stages of premalignant lesions in the target organ. Folate deficiency in normal tissues predispose them to neoplastic transformation, and modest supplemental levels suppress, whereas supraphysiologic doses of supplementation enhances, the development of tumors in normal tissues. In contrast, folate deficiency has an inhibitory effect whereas folate supplementation has a promoting effect on the progression of established neoplasms. It is unknown at present the effect of folate deficiency and supplementation on the progression of early precursor or preneoplastic lesions of CRC (e. g., aberrant crypt foci, ACF) to adenoma and to frank cancer. The mechanisms by which folate exerts dual modulatory effects on carcinogenesis depending on the timing and dose of folate intervention relate to its essential role in one-carbon transfer reactions involved in DNA synthesis and biological methylation reactions (Kim 2007)

suggested that aberrant DNA methylation may play a role in the development of these cancers. DNA methylation has been shown to be significantly lower in individuals with the TT genotype than those carrying CC genotype and TT genotype is directly correlated with folate status (Friso et al. 2002). Three prospective studies on supplemental FA and risk of pancreatic cancer support the picture that was noticed with colon cancer. An inverse association was found between dietary folate intake and pancreatic cancer risk, but none indicated an inverse relation with supplemental FA intake.

The recent epidemiological evidence on folate and the risk of breast cancer follows the picture already suggested in connection with colon carcinogenesis (Ulrich 2007). There exist a nonlinear relation between folate status and breast cancer risk. Higher folate status may be needed to protect postmenopausal women with very low folate intake. However, those having adequate intake do not benefit increased intake of folate and high supplemental FA may actually increase cancer risk (Stolzenberg-Solomon et al. 2006).

Due the low stability it is not possible to do clinical prospective trials or mechanistic studies in animals with natural dietary folate. Also studies using foods with high folate concentration are complicated with accompanying compounds ingested, which also may have a role in cancer susceptible. The accumulating data, however, support natural folate over the supplemental FA in cancer prevention. Absorption and movement of folate through cell membranes differs between folate and FA and physiological consequences of unmetabolized FA in still largely unknown. The adequate folate status should be sustained throughout the lifespan and very high intakes (at least through FA) should be avoided. This is best achieved through diet that contains good folate sources.

2.3 Spinach (*Spinacia oleracea*)

Spinach is composed of various active compounds, such as flavonoids and other polyphenolic active ingredients acting synergistically as anti-inflammatory, antioxidative, and anticancer agents. Spinach leaves contain approximately 1,000 mg of total flavonoids per kilogram fresh weight, of which main are patuletin (3,5,7,3',4'-penthahydroxy-6-methoxyflavone) and spinacetin (3,5,7, 4'-tetrahydroxy-6,3'-dimethoxyflavone). In addition, spinach contains several flavonol and flavonoid glycosides. These are glucuronides and acylated di-and triglycosides of methylated and methylene dioxide derivatives of 6-oxygenated flavonols. Glucuronides are more water-soluble than glycosides and acylated compounds (Lomnitski et al. 2003). Furthermore spinach contains several glycolipids (Murakami et al. 2003) as well as considerable amounts of chlorofyll. Spinach is one of the most important antioxidative vegetables, usually consumed after boiling either fresh or frozen leaves.

2.3.1 Glycolipids Fraction from Spinach

The major glycolipids fraction from spinach consists mainly of three glycolipids; monogalactosyl diacylglycerol (MGDG), digalactosyl diacylglycerol (DGDG), and sulfoquinovosyl diacylglycerol (SQDG) with slightly different effects in in vitro (Murakami et al. 2003). Glycolipids fraction, especially SQDG, inhibits DNA polymerase activity and cancer cell growth in vitro (Kuriyama 2005; Maeda et al. 2007). Injection of SQDG also suppressed tumour growth significantly in nude mice bearing solid tumors of HeLa cells (Maeda et al. 2007). Oral administration of three main glycolipids (20 mg/kg) in BALB/c mice in a colon-26 tumor graft study induced about 56% decrease in the solid tumor volume. This decrement was accompanied with an inhibition of angiogenesis and the expression of cell proliferation marker proteins such as Ki-67, proliferating cell nuclear antigen (PCNA), and Cyclin E in the tumor tissue (Maeda et al. 2008). SQDG, but not other glycolipids, binds to Cdt1 and inhibits Cdt1-geminin interaction in vitro, with 50% inhibition observed at concentration of 2 μg/ml. Cdt1, a human replication initiation protein, regulates DNA replication and geminin modulates Cdt1 action by direct binding (Mizushina et al. 2008). Similarly, only SQDG fraction inhibited in vitro the double-stranded DNA (dsDNA) binding activity of human p53 DNA binding domain DBD indicating that SQDG might regulate the activity of p53 for cell division, cell cycle checkpoint and tumor suppression (Iijima et al. 2007). Both MGDG and SQDG have been shown to suppress microvessel growth in an ex vivo angiogenesis model using a rat aortic ring (Matsubara et al. 2005).

2.3.2 A Water-Soluble Natural Antioxidant (NAO)

Water-soluble extract isolated from spinach leaves, so called a natural antioxidant mixture of spinach (NAO) is an effective free-radical scavenger and inhibits the lipoxygenase enzyme activity. The main active compounds of NAO are polyphenols, which include flavonoid and p-coumaric acid derivatives (Bergman et al. 2001). The antioxidative activity of NAO in vitro and in vivo exceeds to that of other known antioxidants such as N-acetylcysteine, butylated hydroxytoluene, and vitamin E. Furthermore, NAO is stable at high temperature and it lacks toxicity (Lomnitski et al. 2003). At the level of 200 mg/kg NAO reduced plasma peroxide levels and significantly reduced hyperplasia in dorsal and lateral lobes in the TRAMP mice, a model of prostate cancer, and also dose-dependently inhibited cellular proliferation in prostatic carcinoma cell lines (Nyska et al. 2003; Bakshi et al. 2004). Topically or orally administered NAO reduced dermally induced skin papilloma multiplicity in the v-Ha-*ras* transgenic mouse model (Nyska et al. 2001).

2.3.3 Neoxanthin, a Major Carotenoid in Green Leafy Vegetables

Green leafy vegetables including spinach leaves contain carotenoids called epoxy-xantophylls (epoxide-containing xanthophylls). The main epoxyxanthophyll in spinach is neoxanthin that is partially converted during digestion into neochrome-isomers. The ability of neoxanthin and (R/S)-neochrome to inhibit PC-3 human prostate cancer cells proliferation in vitro has been shown (Asai et al. 2004). To evaluate the relevance of the in vitro studies in humans, estimate the intestinal absorption of neoxanthin were evaluated by measuring the plasma concentrations of epoxyxanthophyll and their metabolites before and after 1 week of spinach intake (3.0 mg neoxanthin/d). The plasma concentrations of neoxanthin and its metabolites (neochrome stereoisomers) remained very low (about 1 nmol/l), whereas those of beta-carotene and lutein were markedly increased. These results indicated that the plasma response to dietary epoxyxanthophylls was very low in humans even after 1-week intake of epoxyxanthophyll-rich diets (Asai et al. 2008).

2.4 Perilla (*Perilla frutescens*)

2.4.1 Perilla Leaf Extracts (PLEs)

Perilla (*Perilla frutescens* (L.) Britton, Lamiaceae, also known as the mint family) is
an annual herb native to Asia. Perilla leaves are used as vegetables and spicy herbs
or medical purposes, and perilla seed oil, a rich source of the omega-3 fatty acid
alpha-linolenic acid, is used as edible oil. Anticarcinogenic effect of PLE and its
affecting components have been tested in a murine, two-stage skin carcinogenesis
model where cancer is initiated by application of 7,12-dimethylbenz[*a*]anthracene
(DMBA) and promoting by application of 12-tetradecanoylphorbol 13-asetate
(TPA). TPA induces inflammation and is a skin tumour-promoting agent. Another
mouse model for skin cancer is the Tg.AC mouse carrying the v-Ha-*ras* structural
gene linked to a ζ-globulin promoter. Mice carrying this oncogene exhibit epithelial
proliferation and formation of papillomas when treated with tumour promoters such
as TPA.

Topical application twice a week with 1 mg of PLE to DMBA/TPA-treated
mice resulted in a significant reduction in tumour incidence and multiplicity.
When DMBA/TPA-treated mice ingested PLE ad libitum, no significant effect
was observed in tumour incidence or average number of tumours, but treatment
resulted in a significant reduction in the papilloma weight (Ueda et al. 2003). The
same authors (Ueda et al. 2002) have previously shown that PLE suppressed the
tumour necrosis factor-alpha (TNF-alpha) production in vivo. Mechanistically, PLE
has been shown to dose-dependently induced apoptosis through the combinations
of mitochondrial, death receptor-mediated, and endoplasmic reticulum pathways
and suppressed the cell proliferation via p21-mediated G1 phase arrest in human
leukemia HL-60 cells (Kwak et al. 2009). PLE induced also apoptosis on human
hepatoma HepG2 cells (Lin et al. 2007).

Various PLEs were further fractionated to find out the affecting anti-carcinogenic
components. So far, luteolin (3′,4′,5,7-tetrahydroxyflavone) (Ueda et al. 2002,
2003), rosmarinic acid (Osakabe et al. 2004; Lin et al. 2007) and triterpene acids
(Banno et al. 2004) isolated from perilla has been shown to be the most promising
chemopreventive molecules.

2.4.2 Luteolin, a Flavonoid

Luteolin is a flavone, a subclass of flavonoids, that exists a part from perilla in vegetables and (medicinal) herbs e.g. artichoke, celery, green pepper, spinach, parsley,
sage and, thyme (Anonymous 2007). Daily intake of luteolin has been estimated to
be less than 1 mg/d (Seelinger et al. 2008; Somerset and Johannot 2008). The anti-
carcinogenic mechanism of luteolin has been widely studied in vitro and in vivo,
and its anticancer property is associated with the induction of apoptosis, and inhibition of cell proliferation, metastasis and angiogenesis (Lim do et al. 2007; Lin et al.
2008; Seelinger et al. 2008). Furthermore, it suppresses cell survival pathways such

as phosphatidylinositol 3′-kinase (PI3K)/Akt, nuclear factor kappa B (NF-kappaB) and X-linked inhibitor of apoptosis protein (XIAP) pathways (Lin et al. 2008). Ueda et al. (2003) suggested that luteolin was the chemopreventive component in PLE, and luteolin treatment with a dose 1 mg/mouse/application inhibited mouse skin tumour promotion. In addition, some epidemiological studies suggest an inverse correlation between dietary flavone (including apigenin and luteolin) intake and the risk of some cancer types (see Seelinger et al. 2008).

2.4.3 *Rosmarinic Acid (RA), a Polyphenol*

An anticarcinogenic effect of *Perilla frutescens* leaf extracts containing rosmarinic acid (RA), caffeic acid and luteolin were tested in the DMBA/TPA-induced murine skin cancer model (Osakabe et al. 2004). All fractions reduced significantly the tumour incidence and tumour multiplicity. The fraction containing 40% (w/w) of RA was the most efficient in preventing tumour progression. Therefore, the authors prepared a new fraction from perilla that contained 68% (w/w) of RA, while the level of luteolin and caffeic acid was negligible. Short-term experiments (1–5 h to 24 h) showed that RA containing fraction or an equivalent amount of pure RA had significant anti-inflammatory properties such as ear histology of TPA-treated mice, myeloperoxidase activity, chemokine expression, eicosanoid concentration, and cyclooxygenase-2 expression. Furthermore, both the high RA fraction and RA were able to decrease the levels of oxidative stress markers and the levels of 8OH-dG adducts. Lin et al. (2007) have reported that PLE (containing RA) induced apoptosis and regulated the expression of several apoptosis-related genes in human hepatoma HepG2 in vitro. Pure RA (10 µg/ml; a dose equivalent to 105 µg/ml of PLE) had similar, but less potent effect. In human leukemia U937 cells RA inhibits TNF-alpha-induced ROS generation and NF-kappaB activation, and enhances TNF-alpha-induced apoptosis (Moon et al. 2010). In two human colon carcinoma-derived cell lines, HCT15 and CO115, RA induces apoptosis in both cell lines, whereas cell proliferation was inhibited only in HCT15. RA inhibited ERK phosphorylation in HCT15 and had no effects on Akt phosphorylation in CO115 cells (Xavier et al. 2009).

2.4.4 *Tormentic Acid, a Triterpene*

Nine triterpene carboxylic acids isolated from ethanol extracts of the leaves of green and red perilla and eight of them were tested for their anti-inflammatory properties on TPA-induced ear edema inflammation in mice (Banno et al. 2004). All the compounds tested inhibited TPA - induced inflammation at 0.03–0.3 mg/ear of the 50% inhibitory dose. One of these compounds, tormentic acid, exhibited the strongest inhibitory effect, quite comparable with that of a commercial drug hydrocortisone. Topical application of tormentic acid resulted in a significant reduction in tumours with DMBA/TPA-treated mice. The average number of papillomas was 4.8 and 8.6/mouse in the control group after 10 and 18 weeks experimental period, and 1.4 and 4.5/mouse in the tormentic acid-treated group at the same time points.

2.5 Conclusions

Based on animal and in vitro cell culture studies it can be concluded that at least some type green leafy vegetables and their constituents may have stronger potential in cancer prevention than so far realized. Epidemiological evidence is difficult to obtain due to the complex nature of diet and difficulties to separate different types of green leafy vegetables consumed. Human studies with well-established biomarkers are needed to show the efficacy of certain type of green leafy vegetables or their specific compounds on cancer prevention.

References

Anonymous (2007) USDA database for the flavonoid content of selected foods. Release 2.1.

Asai A, Terasaki M, Nagao A (2004) An epoxide-furanoid rearrangement of spinach neoxanthin occurs in the gastrointestinal tract of mice and in vitro: formation and cytostatic activity of neochrome stereoisomers. J Nutr 134:2237–2243

Asai A, Yonekura L, Nagao A (2008) Low bioavailability of dietary epoxyxanthophylls in humans. Br J Nutr 100:273–277

Bakshi S, Bergman M, Dovrat S et al (2004) Unique natural antioxidants (NAOs) and derived purified components inhibit cell cycle progression by downregulation of ppRb and E2F in human PC3 prostate cancer cells. FEBS Lett 573:31–37

Banno N, Akishisa T, Tokuda H et al (2004) Triterpene acids from the leaves of *Perilla frutescens* and their anti-inflammatory and antitumor-promoting effects. Biosci Biotechnol Biochem 68:85–90

Balder HF, Vogel J, Jansen MCJF et al (2006) Heme and chlorophyll intake and risk of colorectal cancer in the Netherlands cohort study. Cancer Epidemiol Biomarkers Prev 15:717–725

Bergman M, Varshavsky L, Gottlieb HE et al (2001) The antioxidant activity of aqueous spinach extract: chemical identification of active fractions. Phytochemistry 58:143–152

Blum CA, Xu M, Orner GA et al (2003) Promotion versus suppression of rat colon carcinogenesis by chlorophyllin and chlorophyll: modulation of apoptosis, cell proliferation, and beta-catenin/Tcf signaling. Mutat Res 523–524:217–223

Breinholt V, Arbogast D, Loveland P et al (1999) Chlorophyllin chemoprevention in trout initiated by aflatoxin B(1) bath treatment: an evaluation of reduced bioavailability vs. target organ protective mechanisms. Toxicol Appl Pharmacol 158:141–151

Breinholt V, Hendricks J, Pereira C et al (1995) Dietary chlorophyllin is a potent inhibitor of aflatoxin B1 hepatocarcinogenesis in rainbow trout. Cancer Res 55:57–62

Carter O, Bailey GS, Dashwood RH (2004) The dietary phytochemical chlorophyllin alters E-cadherin and beta-catenin expression in human colon cancer cells. J Nutr 134:3441S–3444S

Chiu LC, Kong CK, Ooi VE (2005) The chlorophyllin-induced cell cycle arrest and apoptosis in human breast cancer MCF-7 cells is associated with ERK deactivation and Cyclin D1 depletion. Int J Mol Med 16:735–740

Cho KJ, Han SH, Kim BY et al (2000) Chlorophyllin suppression of lipopolysaccharide-induced nitric oxide production in RAW 264.7 cells. Toxicol Appl Pharmacol 166:120–127

de Vogel J, Jonker-Termont DSML, Katan MB et al (2005a) Natural chlorophyll but not chlorophyllin prevents heme-induced cytotoxic and hyperproliferative effects in rat colon. J Nutr 135:1995–2000 de Vogel J, Jonker-Termont DSML, van Lieshout EMM et al (2005b) Green vegetables, red meat and colon cancer: chlorophyll prevents the cytotoxic and hyperproliferative effects of haem in rat colon. Carcinogenesis 26:387–393

Díaz GD, Li Q, Dashwood RH (2003) Caspase-8 and apoptosis-inducing factor mediate a cytochrome c-independent pathway of apoptosis in human colon cancer cells induced by the dietary phytochemical chlorophyllin. Cancer Res 63:1254–1261

Dingley KH, Ubick EA, Chiarappa-Zucca ML et al (2003) Effect of dietary constituents with chemopreventive potential on adduct formation of a low dose of the heterocyclic amines PhIP and IQ and phase II hepatic enzymes. Nutr Cancer 46:212–221

Egner PA, Stansbury KH, Snyder EP et al (2000) Identification and characterization of chlorin e(4) ethyl ester in sera of individuals participating in the chlorophyllin chemoprevention trial. Chem Res Toxicol 13:900–906

Egner PA, Wang JB, Zhu YR et al (2001) Chlorophyllin intervention reduces aflatoxin-DNA adducts in individuals at high risk for liver cancer. Proc Natl Acad Sci USA 98:14601–14606

Fahey JW, Stephenson KK, Dinkova-Kostova AT et al (2005) Chlorophyll, chlorophyllin and related tetrapyrroles are significant inducers of mammalian phase 2 cytoprotective genes. Carcinogenesis 26:1247–1255

Ferruzzi M, Blakeslee J (2007) Digestion, absorption, and cancer preventative activity of dietary chlorophyll derivatives. Nutr Res 27:1–12

Friso S, Girelli D, Trabetti E (2002) A1298C methylenetetrahydrofolate reductase mutation and coronary artery disease: relationships with C677T polymorphism and homocysteine/folate metabolism. Clin Exp Med 2:7–12

Hayashi T, Schimerlik M, Bailey G (1999) Mechanisms of chlorophyllin anticarcinogenesis: dose-responsive inhibition of aflatoxin uptake and biodistribution following oral co-administration in rainbow trout. Toxicol Appl Pharmacol 158:132–140

Hubner RA, Houlston RS (2009) Folate and colorectal cancer prevention. Br J Cancer 100:233–239

Iijima H, Kasai N, Chiku H (2007) Structure-activity relationship of a glycolipid, sulfoquinovosyl diacylglycerol, with the DNA binding activity of p53. Int J Mol Med 19:41–48

Kamat JP, Boloor KK, Devasagayam TPA (2000) Chlorophyllin as an effective antioxidant against membrane damage in vitro and ex vivo. Biochim Biophys Acta 1487:113–127

Khachik F, Beecher GR, Whittaker NF (1986) Separation, identification, and quantification of the major carotenoid and chlorophyll constituents in extracts of several green vegetables by liquid chromatography. J Agric Food Chem 34:603–616

Kim Y-I (2007) Folate and colorectal cancer: an evidence-based critical review. Mol Nutr Food Res 51:267–292

Kumar SS, Shankar B, Sainis KB (2004) Effect of chlorophyllin against oxidative stress in splenic lymphocytes in vitro and in vivo. Biochim Biophys Acta 1672:100–111

Kuriyama I, Musumi K, Yonezawa Y et al (2005) Inhibitory effects of glycolipids fraction from spinach on mammalian DNA polymerase activity and human cancer cell proliferation. J Nutr Biochem 16:594–601

Kwak CS, Yeo EJ, Moon SC et al (2009) Perilla leaf, Perilla frutescens, induces apoptosis and G1 phase arrest in human leukemia HL-60 cells through the combinations of death receptor-mediated, mitochondrial, and endoplasmic reticulum stress-induced pathways. J Med Food 12:508–17

Lin C-S, Kuo C-L, Wang J-P et al (2007) Growth inhibitory and apoptosis inducing effect of *Perilla frutescens* extract on human hepatoma HepG2 cells. J Ethnopharmacol 112: 557–567

Lin Y, Shi R, Wang X et al (2008) Luteolin, a flavonoid with potential for cancer prevention and therapy. Curr Cancer Drug Targets 8:634–646

Lim do Y, Jeong Y, Tyner AL et al (2007) Induction of cell cycle arrest and apoptosis in HT-29 human colon cancer cells by the dietary compound luteolin. Am J Physiol Gastrointest Liver Physiol 292:G66–G75

Lomnitski L, Bergman M, Nyska A (2003) Composition, efficacy, and safety of spinach extracts. Nutr Cancer 46:222–231

Maeda N, Hada T, Yoshida H et al (2007) Inhibitory effect on replicative DNA polymerases, human cancer cell proliferation, and in vivo anti-tumor activity by glycolipids from spinach. Curr Med Chem 14:955–967

Maeda N, Kokai Y, Ohtani S et al (2008) Anti-tumor effect of orally administered spinach glycolipid fraction on implanted cancer cells, colon-26, in mice. Lipids 43:741–748

Matsubara K, Matsumoto H, Mizushina Y, Mori M, Nakajima N, Fuchigami M, Yoshida H, Hada T. Inhibitory effect of glycolipids from spinach on in vitro and ex vivo angiogenesis. Oncol Rep 2005;14:157–160.

Mizushina Y, Takeuchi T, Hada T et al (2008) The inhibitory action of SQDG (sulfoquinovosyl diacylglycerol) from spinach on Cdt1-geminin interaction. Biochimie 90:947–956

Moon DO, Kim MO, Lee JD et al (2010) Rosmarinic acid sensitizes cell death through suppression of TNF-alpha-induced NF-kappaB activation and ROS generation in human leukemia U937 cells. Cancer Lett 288:183–191

Murakami C, Kumagai T, Hada T et al (2003) Effects of glycolipids from spinach on mammalian DNA polymerases. Biochem Pharmacol 65:259–267

Nyska A, Lomnitski L, Spalding J et al (2001) Topical and oral administration of the natural water-soluble antioxidant from spinach reduces the multiplicity of papillomas in the Tg.AC mouse model. Toxicol Lett 122:33–44

Nyska A, Suttie A, Bakshi S et al (2003) Slowing tumorigenic progression in TRAMP mice and prostatic carcinoma cell lines using natural anti-oxidant from spinach, NAO – a comparative study of three anti-oxidants. Toxicol Pathol 31:39–51

Larsson SC, Giovannucci E, Wolk A (2006) Folate intake, *MTHFR* polymorphisms, and risk of esophageal, gastric, and pancreatic cancer: a Meta-analysis. Gastroeneterology 131: 1271–1283

Osakabe N, Yasuda A, Natsume M et al (2004) Rosmarinic acid inhibits epidermal inflammatory responses: anticarcinogenic effect of *Perilla frutescens* extract in the murine two-stage skin model. Carcinogenesis 25:549–57

Park KK, Park JH, Jung YJ et al (2003) Inhibitory effects of chlorophyllin, hemin and tetrakis (4-benzoic acid)porphyrin on oxidative DNA damage and mouse skin inflammation induced by 12-O-tetradecanoylphorbol-13-acetate as a possible anti-tumor promoting mechanism. Mutat Res 542:89–97

Pietrzak M, Halicka HD, Wieczorek Z et al (2008) Attenuation of acridine mutagen ICR-191 – DNA interactions and DNA damage by the mutagen interceptor chlorophyllin. Biophys Chem 135:69–75

Pietrzak M, Wieczorek Z, Wieczorek J (2006) The "interceptor" properties of chlorophyllin measured within the three-component system: intercalator-DNA-chlorophyllin. Biophys Chem 123:11–19

Seelinger G, Merfort I, Wölfle U et al (2008) Anti-carcinogenic effects of the flavonoid luteolin. Molecules 13:2628–2651

Simonich MT, Egner PA, Roebuck BD et al (2007) Natural chlorophyll inhibits aflatoxin B1-induced multi-organ carcinogenesis in the rat. Carcinogenesis 28:1294–1302

Simonich MT, McQuistan T, Jubert C et al (2008) Low-dose dietary chlorophyll inhibits multi-organ carcinogenesis in the rainbow trout. Food Chem Toxicol 46:1014–1024

Somerset SM, Johannot L (2008) Dietary flavonoid sources in Australian adults. Nutr Cancer 60:442–449

Stolzenberg-Solomon RZ, Chang S-C, Leitzmann MF et al (2006) Folate intake, alcohol use, and postmenopausal breast cancer risk in the Prostate, Lung, Colorectal, and Ovarian Cancer Screening Trial. Am J Clin Nutr 83:895–904

Troen AM, Mitchell B, Sorensen B et al (2006) Unmetabolized folic acid in plasma is associated with reduced natural killer cell cytotoxicity among postmenopausal women. J Nutr 136: 189–194

Ueda H, Yamazaki C, Yamazaki M (2002) Luteolin as an anti-inflammatory and anti-allergic constituent of *Perilla frutescens*. Biol Pharm Bull 25:1197–2002

Ueda H, Yamazaki C, Yamazaki M (2003) Inhibitory effect of Perilla leaf extract and luteolin on mouse skin tumor promotion. Biol Pharm Bull 26:560–563

Ulrich CM (2007) Folate and cancer prevention: a closer look at a complex picture. Am J Clin Nutr 86:271–273

Vivier E, Tomasello E, Baratin M et al (2008) Functions of natural killer cells. Nat Immunol 9: 503–510

Xavier CP, Lima CF, Fernandes-Ferreira M (2009) Salvia fruticosa, Salvia officinalis, and rosmarinic acid induce apoptosis and inhibit proliferation of human colorectal cell lines: the role in MAPK/ERK pathway. Nutr Cancer 61:564–571

Yun C, Jeon YJ, Yang Y et al (2006) Chlorophyllin suppresses interleukin-1 beta expression in lipopolysaccharide-activated RAW 264.7 cells. Int Immunopharmacol 6:252–259

Yun C, Son CG, Chung DK (2005) Chlorophyllin attenuates IFN-gamma expression in lipopolysaccharide-stimulated murine splenic mononuclear cells via suppressing IL-12 production. Int Immunopharmacol 5:1926–1935

Chapter 3
The Role of Tomato Lycopene in Cancer Prevention

Joseph Levy, Shlomo Walfisch, Andrea Atzmon, Keren Hirsch, Marina Khanin, Karin Linnewiel, Yael Morag, Hagar Salman, Anna Veprik, Michael Danilenko, and Yoav Sharoni

Abstract The role of the tomato carotenoid lycopene in cancer prevention has gained considerable interest in recent years. Most studies reported an inverse association between tomato intake or blood lycopene level and the risk of various types of cancer. This is supported by mechanistic studies with various cell culture and animal models. The biochemical processes involved in the chemoprotective effects of lycopene and other carotenoids are not completely understood. In this review we will primarily address the mechanisms proposed for the cancer preventive activity of tomato lycopene, focusing on the induction of phase II enzymes and the inhibition of growth factors, such as insulin-like growth factor, and sex hormones such as estrogens and androgens.

Keywords Tomato lycopene · Phase II enzymes · Growth factors · Sex hormones · Chemoprevention

Contents

J. Levy (✉)
Department of Clinical Biochemistry, Faculty of Health Sciences, Ben-Gurion University and Soroka Medical Center of Kupat Holim, Beer-Sheva, Israel
e-mail: lyossi@bgu.ac.il

M. Mutanen, A.-M. Pajari (eds.), *Vegetables, Whole Grains, and Their Derivatives in Cancer Prevention*, Diet and Cancer 2, DOI 10.1007/978-90-481-9800-9_3,
© Springer Science+Business Media B.V. 2011

3.1 Introduction

Cancer chemoprevention involves the use of natural or synthetic compounds to reduce the risk of developing cancer. There is considerable epidemiologic evidence suggesting an association between the consumption of fruits and vegetables and reduced incidence of cancer (Riboli and Norat 2003; Temple and Gladwin 2003). In particular, carotenoids have been implicated as cancer-preventive agents (van Poppel 1993). β-Carotene has received the most attention because of its provitamin A activity and its prevalence in many foods. However, findings from intervention studies with β-carotene were disappointing (Heinonen et al. 1994; Omenn et al. 1996), and thus other carotenoids such as lycopene, the main tomato carotenoid, became the subject of more intensive investigation (Krinsky and Johnson 2005). Giovannucci (1999, 2005) has published comprehensive analysis of the epidemiologic literature on the relation of tomato consumption and cancer prevention. He found that most of the reviewed studies reported an inverse association between tomato intake or blood lycopene level and the risk of various types of cancer. Giovannucci suggested that lycopene may contribute to these beneficial effects of tomato-containing foods but that the anticancer properties could also be explained by interactions among multiple components found in tomatoes such as phytoene, phytofluene, and β-carotene. Additional support for the anticancer effects of these and other carotenoids was found with diverse cancer cells in vitro (Amir et al. 1999; Levy et al. 1995; Pastori et al. 1998; Prakash et al. 2001). For example, we have shown that lycopene inhibits mammary, endometrial, lung, and leukemic cancer cell growth in a dose-dependent manner (IC_{50} 2 μmol/l) (Amir et al. 1999; Levy et al. 1995; Nahum et al. 2001).

The biochemical processes involved in the chemoprotective effects of fruits and vegetables are not completely understood. In this review we will primarily address the mechanisms proposed for the cancer preventive activity of tomato lycopene, focusing on the induction of phase II enzymes and the inhibition of growth factor and sex hormone activity.

3.2 Dietary Sources and Bioavailability of Lycopene

Lycopene is chemically defined as an acyclic carotene with 11 conjugated double bonds, normally in the all-trans configuration. The double bonds are subject to isomerization, and various cis isomers (mainly Astorg et al. 1994; Bohm and Bitsch 1999; Campbell et al. 1993 or Carroll et al. 2000) are found in plants and also in blood. Since the human body is unable to synthesize carotenoids the body is totally dependent on dietary supply of these compounds. In general, tomato fruit and tomato-based food products provide at least 85% of dietary lycopene in humans. The remaining 15% are usually obtained from other fruits and vegetables that contain lycopene, such as watermelon, pink grapefruit, guava, and papaya, although at much lower levels than tomatoes.

Tomato juice, tomato soup, ketchup, pizza, and spaghetti sauce are the major contributing tomato products in the diet. Uptake of carotenoids from the diet has been studied for many years. The bioavailability of dietary lycopene appears to depend upon several factors. It is absorbed better from lipid-rich diets and from cooked, rather than raw foods (Bohm and Bitsch 1999; Stahl and Sies 1992). Once ingested, lycopene appears in plasma, initially in the chylomicrons and VLDL (very low-density lipoprotein) fractions and later in LDL (low density lipoproteins, the so-called 'bad' cholesterol) and HDL (high-density lipoproteins, often called 'good' cholesterol). The highest levels are found in LDL. Serum concentrations of lycopene are ranging between approximately 0.1–1.0 μM with large interpersonal variations.

Genetic variation may affect circulating levels of carotenoids. For instance, a polymorphism in the β-carotene 15,15'-Monooxygenase 1 gene was found to affect plasma carotenoid levels (Ferrucci et al. 2009). A specific G allele near the β-carotene 15,15'-monooxygenase 1 (BCMO1) gene, was associated with higher β-carotene and α-carotene levels and lower lycopene, zeaxanthin, and lutein levels. This finding may explain the data showing that dietary intake of these lipid-soluble antioxidant vitamins is only moderately correlated with their plasma levels (Talegawkar et al. 2008).

Lycopene is found in most human tissues but is not accumulated uniformly (Khachik et al. 2002). There is a preferential accumulation of lycopene in the adrenals and testes. The confirmed ability to increase lycopene levels in tissues is one prerequisite for using it as a dietary supplement to improve health. Indeed, we reported that supplementation of tomato lycopene oleoresin in volunteers undergoing elective surgery produced a significant increase in carotenoids in plasma, skin, and adipose tissues (Walfisch et al. 2003). Little is known about the metabolism or degradation of lycopene in mammals. A number of oxygenated metabolites have been found in plasma and tissues (Hu et al. 2006; Lian et al. 2007; Ziouzenkova et al. 2007) but more studies are needed in order to estimate their physiological roles, if any.

3.3 Mechanism of Action of Lycopene

3.3.1 Activation of the Antioxidant Response Element (ARE) Transcription System and the Induction of Phase II Enzymes

In recent years, evidence has accumulated indicating that the cancer preventive action of dietary ingredients in general and tomato lycopene in particular is, at least in part, due to the induction of phase II detoxifying and antioxidant enzymes (Talalay 2000). This is a major mechanism for chemical protection against carcinogenesis, mutagenesis, and other forms of toxicity. Indeed, induction of phase II enzymes can be achieved in many target tissues by administering any of a diverse array of naturally occurring and synthetic chemical agents (Astorg et al. 1994; Dingley et al. 2003; Iqbal et al. 2003; Prochaska and Talalay 1988). The phase II cytoprotective enzymes include detoxifying and antioxidant enzymes such as glutathione S-transferase, NAD(P)H:quinone oxidoreductase 1, superoxide dismutase, and heme oxygenase-1. The promoter regions of the inducible genes encoding phase II enzymes contain the antioxidant response element (ARE), which upon binding of the transcription factor nuclear factor E2-related factor 2 (Nrf2) leads to increased expression of these genes. Nrf2 is a basic leucine zipper redox-sensitive transcription factor that under normal unstimulated conditions remains sequestered in the cytosol by Kelch-like ECH-associated protein 1 (Keap1). Putative chemopreventive agents disrupt the Nrf2-Keap1 association, thereby releasing Nrf2 which then translocates to the nucleus and drives the gene expression of phase II enzymes and other redox regulators such as thioredoxin and thioredoxin reductase.

Several studies have shown that dietary antioxidants, such as 1,2-dithiole-3-thiones (Kwak et al. 2001), phenolic flavonoids (Kong et al. 2001; Martin et al. 2004), curcuminoids (Balogun et al. 2003), and isothiocyanates (Talalay and Fahey 2001), may function as anticancer agents by activating the Nrf2/ARE transcription system. We hypothesized that carotenoids also activate this transcription system, because several carotenoids have been found to induce phase II enzymes (Breinholt et al. 2000; Gradelet et al. 1996). Indeed, we have shown that different tomato carotenoids (lycopene, phytoene, phytofluene, and β-carotene) as well as the algal xantophyl astaxanthin, transactivate ARE and induce the expression of phase II enzymes (Ben-Dor et al. 2005).

Various electrophilic phytonutrients have been shown to induce the ARE system via interaction with Keap1 (Dinkova-Kostova et al. 2002). However, hydrophobic carotenoids such as lycopene lack any electrophilic group and thus are unlikely to directly interact with Keap1. Thus, we suggested that carotenoid oxidation products and not the intact carotenoids stimulate the ARE system. Indeed, our recent study (Linnewiel et al. 2009) supported this hypothesis by two lines of evidence: (a) Oxidized derivatives, extracted by ethanol from partially oxidized lycopene, transactivated ARE with a similar potency to that of the unextracted lycopene mixture, whereas the intact carotenoid showed a non-significant effect. (b) Using a series of characterized apo-carotenals and diapo-carotenals that potentially can be derived from in vivo metabolism of carotenoids we defined a structure-activity relationship which suggests that the reactivity of the carbon-carbon double bond adjacent to the terminal aldehyde group is a major factor in activation of ARE.

3.3.2 Interference with the Insulin Like Growth Factor (IGF) System

Growth factor activity is a well-documented target for many anticancer drugs. Tumor cell growth is regulated by endocrine, paracrine and, probably the most important, autocrine growth factor production. These factors are crucial for the uncontrolled, rapid cell proliferation which is the hallmark of cancer development and metastasis. Thus, down regulation of oncogenic growth factor signaling by phyto-nutrients in general and tomato carotenoids in particular, were widely studied. Among myriad of growth factors, the IGF system has received the main attention. However, the involvement of other growth factor systems, such as the platelet-derived growth factor (PDGF) and vascular endothelial growth factor (VEGF) systems, which are important for tumor development and vascularization, were also reported.

The interest in the role of the IGF system in cancer prevention stems from two basic observations. First, IGF-I is an important risk factor for several major cancers (Chan et al. 1998; Giovannucci 2003); and second, the activity of this complex growth factor system can be modulated by various dietary regimes including tomato carotenoids (Levy et al. 2008). Two possible mechanisms can account for the lowering of IGF-related cancer risk by tomato lycopene. This carotenoid may decrease IGF-I plasma levels, thereby diminishing the risk associated with its elevation, and/or it can interfere with IGF-I activity in the cancer cell. Evidence for the successful intervention in the IGF system by tomato carotenoids, using these two strategies in model systems and in humans, will be presented in this review.

The IGF system is comprised of the IGF ligands (IGF-I and IGF-II), cell surface receptors that mediate the biological effects of the IGFs, including the IGF-I receptor (IGF-IR), the IGF-II receptor (IGF-IIR), and the insulin receptor (IR), as well as a family of IGF-binding proteins (IGFBPs). These binding proteins (IGFBP-1 to -6) affect the half-lives and availability of the IGFs in the circulation and in extra-cellular fluids. Thus, IGF action is determined by the availability of IGF-I to interact with the IGF-I receptor, which is regulated by the relative concentrations of the IGFBPs (LeRoith and Roberts 2003). For example, a high concentration of IGFBP-3, the main IGF binding protein in plasma, reduces IGF-I action. IGF-IR is a transmembrane protein tyrosine kinase, which mediates the biological effects of IGF-I and most of the actions of IGF-II. Binding of IGF-I to the IGF-IR results in receptor autophosphorylation, phosphorylation of intracellular substrates, and activation of specific signaling processes, which promote growth (LeRoith and Roberts 2003).

Several epidemiological studies addressed an association between tomato products or lycopene consumption and components of the IGF system (Signorello et al. 2000; Vrieling et al. 2004), but only one found a possible positive association between lycopene intake and IGFBP-3 (Holmes et al. 2002). In other studies, tomato consumption was inversely associated with IGF-I levels and/or its molar ratio with IGFBP-3 in disease-free men (Gunnell et al. 2003; Mucci et al. 2001). Mucci et al. suggested that the mechanism by which tomato lycopene prevents prostate cancer may be related to its ability to decrease IGF-I blood levels (Mucci et al. 2001). A more recent study (Tran et al. 2006) investigated whether intakes of fruit, vegetables, and antioxidants (β-carotene, lycopene, and vitamin C) are associated with plasma IGF-I and IGFBP-3 concentrations. Although higher intake of citrus fruit and vitamin C were associated with higher concentrations of IGF-I and with lower concentrations of IGFBP-3, total intakes of β-carotene and lycopene were not related to either IGF-I or IGFBP-3 concentrations.

At the cellular level, we have previously demonstrated that lycopene inhibits the growth of breast, endometrial, lung cancer (Levy et al. 1995) and leukemic (Amir et al. 1999) cells. Furthermore, growth stimulation of MCF-7 human breast cancer cells by IGF-I was markedly reduced by lycopene (Karas et al. 1995, 2000).

Interestingly, these effects were not accompanied by either necrotic or apoptotic cell death but were associated with a marked inhibition of serum- and IGF-I-stimulated cell cycle transition from G1 to S phase (Amir et al. 1999; Karas et al. 2000; Nahum et al. 2001, 2006). Lycopene treatment markedly reduced the IGF-I stimulation of tyrosine phosphorylation of insulin receptor substrate 1 (IRS-1). These effects were not associated with changes in the number or affinity of IGF-I receptors, but with an increase in membrane-associated IGFBPs. Inhibition of cell cycle progression was evident also by other carotenoids such as β-carotene (Murakoshi et al. 1989) and fucoxanthin, a carotenoid prepared from brown algae (Okuzumi et al. 1990).

3.3.2.1 Carotenoids and Regulation of the Cell Cycle

Deregulated cell cycle is one of the major hallmarks of the cancer cell. Thus, elucidation of the mode by which carotenoids inhibit cell cycle progression would provide a mechanistic basis for the anti-cancer effect of these micronutrients. Cell cycle progression is activated by growth factors primarily during G1 phase. The main components of the cell cycle machinery, which acts as growth factor sensors are the D type cyclins (Sherr 1995). Cyclin D1 is an oncogene that is overexpressed in many breast cancer cell lines as well as in primary tumors (Buckley et al. 1993). Interestingly, many anticancer agents, including those used for breast cancer therapy, convey their inhibitory effect in G1 phase primarily by reducing cyclin D1 levels, for example, pure antiestrogens (Carroll et al. 2000; Watts et al. 1994), tamoxifen (Planas Silva et al. 1997), retinoids (Teixeira and Pratt 1997; Zhou et al. 1997) and progestins (Musgrove et al. 1998). We have demonstrated that the lycopene inhibition of serum-stimulated cell cycle traverse from G1 to S phase correlates with reduction in cyclin D1 levels, resulting in inhibition of both cdk4 and cdk2 kinase activity (Nahum et al. 2001). Inhibition of cdk4 was directly related to lower amount of cyclin D1-cdk4 complexes while inhibition of cdk2 was related to retention of p27 molecules in cyclin E-cdk2 complexes due to the reduction in cyclin D1 level. These results together with the fact that neither cyclin E nor cdk2 or cdk4 levels were changed by lycopene treatment, suggest that the inhibitory effect of this carotenoid on cell cycle progression is mediated primarily by downregulation of cyclin D1. To further support this suggestion we determined the effect of lycopene on IGF-I-stimulated cell cycle progression in a clone of MCF-7 cells capable of exogenously controlling cyclin D1 expression. This study demonstrated that ectopic expression of cyclin D1 can overcome cell cycle inhibition caused by lycopene and all-trans retinoic acid suggesting that attenuation of cyclin D1 levels by these compounds impairs the mitogenic action of IGF-I (Nahum et al. 2006).

3.3.2.2 Lycopene and the IGF System in Prostate Cancer

More recently (Kanagaraj et al. 2007), the action of lycopene on components of the IGF system was examined in PC-3 androgen-independent prostate cancer cells. Cells treated with lycopene showed a significant decrease in proliferation which was accompanied by increased level of IGFBP-3 and a decrease in the IGF-IR expression. These changes were associated with increased apoptotic cell death. In prostate stromal cells, which are androgen-dependent, lycopene was found to reverse dihydrotestosterone (DHT) stimulation of IGF-I production by reducing nuclear localization of androgen receptor and β-catenin (Liu et al. 2008). Moreover, lycopene inhibited IGF-I-stimulated prostate epithelial cell growth, perhaps by attenuating IGF-I effects on serine phosphorylation of Akt and GSK3β and tyrosine phosphorylation of GSK3β (Liu et al. 2008). The inhibition of IGF-I activity in non-cancerous prostate cells suggests that in addition to prevention of prostate cancer, lycopene may prevent the non-malignant growth of prostate tissue which is evident in benign prostate hyperplasia (BPH). The effect of lycopene on normal prostate tissue was also examined in an animal model to gain insight into the mechanisms by which lycopene can contribute to primary prostate cancer prevention (Herzog et al. 2005; Siler et al. 2004). Young rats were supplemented with lycopene for up to 8 week. Lycopene accumulated predominantly in the lateral prostate lobe which is primarily affected by malignancy. Transcriptomics analysis revealed that lycopene treatment mildly but significantly reduced gene expression of androgen-metabolizing enzymes and androgen targets. In addition, local expression of IGF-I was decreased in the lateral lobe (Herzog et al. 2005).

Higher intake of lycopene is related to a lower risk of lung cancer (Giovannucci 1999). Liu et al. (2003) examined the effect of lycopene on the IGF system in a smoking ferret model. Lycopene supplementation at low and high doses which are equivalent to an intake of 15 and 60 mg/d in humans, respectively, was tested. Ferrets supplemented with lycopene and exposed to smoke had significantly higher plasma IGFBP-3 levels and a lower IGF-I/IGFBP-3 ratio than ferrets exposed to smoke alone. Both low- and high-dose lycopene supplementations substantially inhibited smoke-induced squamous metaplasia and PCNA expression in the lungs of the ferrets. The authors concluded that lycopene may mediate its protective effects against smoke-induced lung carcinogenesis in ferrets through up-regulating IGFBP-3 which promotes apoptosis and inhibits cell proliferation.

As mentioned above, among several growth factors which may be regulated by lycopene in tumor cells, the IGF system has received the main attention. However, the involvement of other growth factor systems, such as the platelet-derived growth factor (PDGF) and vascular endothelial growth factor (VEGF) systems, which are important for tumor development and vascularization, were also examined. For example, oral supplementation with lycopene or β-carotene has been found to markedly decrease plasma levels of VEGF and matrix metalloproteinase (MMP)-2, which contribute to tumor metastasis, in human hepatoma SK-Hep-1 xenograft mouse model (Huang et al. 2008). This was associated with attenuation of tumor proliferation, invasion, and angiogenesis, indicating that lycopene and β-carotene supplementation can reduce experimental tumor metastasis in vivo. Lycopene was reported to inhibit PDGF-BB-induced signaling and cell migration in human cultured skin fibroblasts through a novel mechanism of action, i.e. direct binding to PDGF-BB (Chiang et al. 2007; Wu et al. 2007).

3.3.2.3 Human Intervention Studies

Probably the most interesting data on lycopene interference with the IGF system were obtained in human intervention studies. To determine whether short intervention with dietary tomato lycopene extract will affect serum levels of the IGF system components, a double-blind, randomized, placebo-controlled study was conducted in colon cancer patients (Walfisch et al. 2007). Patients, candidates for colectomy ($n = 56$), were supplemented with tomato lycopene extract for a period from a few days to a few weeks prior surgery, which resulted in an increase in plasma lycopene levels by about two-fold. A small, non-significant increase in lycopene plasma levels was also detected in the placebo group. The plasma concentration of IGF-I decreased significantly by about 25% after tomato lycopene extract supplementation, as compared to the placebo group. No significant change was observed in IGFBP-3 or IGF-II levels, whereas the IGF-I/IGFBP-3 molar ratio decreased significantly. These results support the hypothesis that tomato lycopene has a role in the prevention of colon and, possibly, other types of cancer by modulating the plasma levels of IGF-I which has been suggested as a risk factor for those malignancies. In another, randomized double-blind, placebo-controlled study in healthy male volunteers, plasma levels of lycopene, IGF-I and IGFBP-3 were analyzed before and after a four-week lycopene supplementation (Graydon et al. 2007). Median change in lycopene was higher in subjects who received lycopene than in those on placebo. There was no difference in median changes in IGF-I or IGFBP-3 concentrations between the intervention and placebo groups. However, in the intervention group the change in lycopene concentration was associated with the change in IGFBP-3. The authors concluded that this association suggests a potential effect of lycopene supplementation on IGFBP-3.

Riso et al. (2006) supplemented twenty healthy subjects with a tomato-based drink in a double-blind, cross-over study. Subjects consumed a tomato drink or a placebo for 26 days separated by 26 days wash-out. The tomato drink intake increased plasma lycopene, phytoene, phytofluene, and β-carotene concentrations without a significant effect on IGF-I levels. However, changes in lycopene before and after each experimental period were inversely and significantly correlated with those of IGF-I. No such correlation was found with the other carotenoids.

Voskuil and coworkers (Voskuil et al. 2008) examined the effects of lycopene on the IGF system in a randomized, placebo-controlled, double-blind, crossover trial conducted in two populations, premenopausal breast cancer survivors and women at high risk for familial breast cancer. Supplementation with tomato lycopene for two months did not significantly alter serum total IGF-I and other IGF system components in the overall population. However, when the two populations were analyzed separately, a beneficial effect (a reduction in free IGF-I) was found in high-risk healthy women but not in breast cancer survivors. Partial effects on the IGF system were also evident in another study conducted by the same group in 40 men and 31 postmenopausal women, with a family history of colorectal cancer, a personal history of colorectal adenoma, or both (Vrieling et al. 2007). Tomato lycopene supplementation significantly increased serum IGFBP-1 and IGFBP-2 concentrations although total IGF-I, IGF-II, and IGFBP-3 concentrations were not significantly altered.

A possible beneficial role of lycopene has been suggested in a pilot study in patients diagnosed with benign prostate hyperplasia, at increased risk for developing prostate cancer (Schwarz et al. 2008). Fourty patients with benign prostate hyperplasia and free of prostate cancer were randomized to receive either synthetic lycopene or a placebo for 6 months. Plasma lycopene concentration increased in the group taking lycopene suggesting good compliance. This was not accompanied by a change in serum concentrations of IGF-I and IGFBP-3, however, prostate-specific antigen (PSA) level decreased in the lycopene but not in the placebo group. Moreover, prostate enlargement occurred in the placebo group but not in the lycopene group.

It may be concluded from the presented results of short intervention studies with healthy people or cancer patients that a small but significant reduction in IGF-I activity (either a decrease in IGF-I or an increase in IGFBP-3 or other binding proteins) could be obtained with tomato lycopene. Most of these studies were performed with tomato extract preparations (e.g. LycoMato® produced by LycoRed Ltd) which, in addition to the major tomato carotenoid lycopene, contain also other carotenoids such as phytoene, phytofleune and β-carotene. Combination of these carotenoids may produce additive or even synergistic effects on many end points including the inhibition of the IGF system. This may be at least a partial explanation for the failure of Schwarz et al. (2008), who used a synthetic lycopene and not the natural tomato lycopene, to show a beneficial effect on the IGF system in patients diagnosed with benign prostate hyperplasia.

An additional consideration in human studies with lycopene supplementations is the source of blood IGF-I and IGFBP-3, which may be different in healthy people and cancer patients (LeRoith and Roberts 2003). It is well established that tumors secrete many growth factors including IGF-I and IGF-II, which function as both endocrine and autocrine/paracrine agents (Daughaday and Deuel 1991). Consequently, in cancer patients, tumor tissue may be an important source of IGFs in the blood, and the effect of tomato carotenoids on IGF release from tumors may be different from their effect on IGF release from normal tissues. Thus, analysis of the effect of tomato carotenoids on IGF-I levels in healthy people appears to be more relevant for cancer prevention than such an analysis in individuals bearing tumors.

3.3.3 Hormone-Dependent Cancers

Evidence has been accumulated that lycopene may play a significant role in the prevention of sex hormone-dependent cancers. Among these are the major human malignancies, such as estrogen-dependent breast and endometrial cancers in women and androgen-dependent prostate cancer in men. This section will review the recent data on the inhibition of estrogenic and androgenic activities by lycopene.

3.3.3.1 Interference with Estrogenic Activity in Hormone-Dependent Cancers

Breast cancer is the second leading cause of cancer deaths in women today and the most common cancer among women in North America (Greenlee et al. 2001). There is substantial evidence to suggest that estrogens play an important role in both the development and progression of breast cancer, and that endogenous and exogenous estrogens increase the risk of developing this malignancy (Henderson et al. 1988).

The estrogen dependence of breast cancer represents a unique feature of the disease that can be manipulated to effectively control tumor development. This can be achieved by a family of drugs called Specific Estrogen Receptor Modulators (SERMs) such as tamoxifen (Early Breast Cancer Trialists' Collaborative Group 1998). The favorable outcome of such antiestrogen therapy led to the suggestion that it can be used for chemoprevention of breast cancer. However, the inability to precisely predict who will develop breast cancer, due to its complex etiologies, has required broad, population based strategies to prevent the disease. A successful chemopreventive strategy must therefore be effective and acceptable to the majority of women who are at risk to develop breast cancer. Fortunately, the recent success of clinical breast cancer prevention trials of tamoxifen (Fisher et al. 1998) and raloxifene (Cummings et al. 1999) in high-risk populations suggests that chemoprevention is not only rational and appealing but also practical. However, for long-term prevention in the general population, changes in diet rather than drug application has long been considered to be a more sensible approach.

As far as the importance of food ingredients in breast cancer prevention is concerned, the role of phytoestrogens in this malignancy appears to be one of the major issues. Phytoestrogens, constituting of isoflavones (abundant in soyfood), lignans and coumestans, are natural estrogen-like substances in plant foods that have been suggested to reduce breast cancer risk. In particular, much work was done on the role of soyfoods as a source of isoflavones and their potential to reduce risk of cancer, especially that of the breast. Isoflavones bind to estrogen receptors and exhibit weak estrogen-like effects under certain experimental conditions. This causes a controversy because of concerns that isoflavones may stimulate the growth of existing estrogen-sensitive breast tumors. This controversy carries considerable public health significance because of the increasing popularity of soy foods and the commercial availability of isoflavone supplements.

Whether fruit, vegetable, and antioxidant micronutrient consumption is associated with a reduction in breast cancer incidence was examined in several studies. A large population-based case-control study has shown that among postmenopausal women, reduced odds ratios were noted for the highest fifth, as compared with the lowest fifth, of intake of any vegetables and leafy vegetables (Gaudet et al. 2004). Similar results were found for postmenopausal breast cancer patients in relation to high intake of carotenoids and particularly lycopene. Inverse associations for fruits and vegetables were stronger for postmenopausal women with ER-positive tumors than ER-negative tumors. No similar inverse associations were observed among premenopausal women. Cui et al. (2008) also reported an inverse association of breast cancer risk with dietary intake of carotenoids (α-carotene, β-carotene and lycopene) for postmenopausal women with ER- and progesterone receptor-positive mammary tumors but not for other breast cancer groups. However, no evidence of association between breast cancer risk and dietary carotenoids was found in another recent study (Wang et al. 2009) in which extensive diet history questionnaire was used to assess dietary intake of carotenoids.

As estrogens are the most important risk factors for mammary and endometrial cancers, we aimed to determine whether carotenoids inhibit estrogen and phytoestrogen signaling in cancer cells, which could explain their cancer preventive activity (Hirsch et al. 2007). Genistein, the phytoestrogen mainly found in soy, shows significant estrogenic activity when tested at concentrations found in human blood. Similar to the known effect of 17β-estradiol, treatment of breast (T47D and MCF-7) and endometrial (ECC-1) cancer cells with genistein induced cell proliferation, cell-cycle progression and transactivation of the estrogen response element (ERE). However, each of the tested tomato carotenoids (lycopene, phytoene, phytofluene, and β-carotene) inhibited cell proliferation induced by either estradiol or genistein. The inhibition of cell growth by lycopene was accompanied by slow down of cell-cycle progression from G1 to S phase. Moreover, carotenoids inhibited estrogen-induced transactivation of ERE that was mediated by both ERα and ERβ (Hirsch et al. 2007) Preliminary studies suggest that the transcription factor Nrf2, known for its role in induction of detoxifying and antioxidant enzymes, is partially involved in the carotenoid inhibition of estrogenic activity in cancer cells. The results showing that dietary carotenoids inhibit estrogen signaling induced by both estradiol and genistein (Hirsch et al. 2007), imply that these nutrients can attenuate the deleterious estrogenic effect in estrogen-dependent malignancies. Other studies have shown that carotenoids and retinoids can also inhibit basal proliferation in the absence of added estrogen of ER-positive and ER-negative human breast cancer cells (Prakash et al. 2001; Wang and Zhang 2007).

BRCA1 and BRCA2 tumor suppressors interact with various proteins, including ERs to maintain genomic integrity and repress tumor formation (Deng and Brodie 2000). Mutations in BRCA1 and BRCA2 genes are associated with stimulation of estrogen-induced growth of mammary tumors. Interestingly, lycopene was found to increase BRCA1 mRNA levels in the ER-positive breast cancer cells (MCF-7 and HBL-100) (Chalabi et al. 2004). Moreover, treatment with lycopene increased the extent of BRCA1 and BRCA2 phosphorylation in MCF-7 cells but not in MDA-MB-231 (ER-negative breast cancer) or MCF-10a (fibrocystic, non-cancer) cell lines. The authors hypothesized that lycopene-induced BRCA1 phosphorylation may enhance its inhibition of ERα and, thus, of tumor progression (Chalabi et al. 2005).

The inhibition of estrogen signaling in mammary and endoemetrial tumor cells by lycopene and other carotenoids as shown in vitro, together with the results of epidemiological studies (Giovannucci 1999) may provide the basis for a preventive strategy for these malignancies. The accumulated evidence warrants further human studies of the long-term effects of tomato carotenoids and their combinations with other phyto-nutrients on reduction of risk for this disease.

3.3.3.2 Interference with Androgen Activity in Prostate Cancer

Prostate cancer is the most common solid cancer in males and is the second leading cause of cancer deaths in American men (Jemal et al. 2008). In addition, benign prostatic hyperplasia is the most common benign neoplasm, occurring in 50% of all men by the age of 60. Despite extensive research, the basis for these high rates of abnormal prostatic growth is not well understood. It is recognized, however, that steroid hormones, particularly androgens, play a role in the initiation and progression of prostate cancer (Kaarbo et al. 2007) and that this feature of androgens is the basis for hormonal treatment strategies for this malignancy. Castrated man does not develop prostatic carcinoma, and regression of the cancer can be initially achieved by castration and androgen blockade (Huggins and Hodges 1972).

Our understanding of the pivotal role of androgens in prostate disease led to the hypothesis that interventions to reduce the androgen activity in the prostate may have the potential to reduce the risk of disease development, to slow or even prevent disease progression, and to treat existing disease. However, androgen-ablative therapy is associated with significant adverse events such as sexual dysfunction, depression, osteoporosis, anemia and muscle weakness. While these events may be considered acceptable in the context of treatment of aggressive prostate cancer, they would appear too severe for the treatment of benign prostate hyperplasia, and certainly inappropriate for preventive approaches. Thus, an alternative approach is required to reduce androgen activity in the prostate, and the nutritional approach appears the most suitable for the wide population because of its complete absence of toxicity.

An increase in dietary consumption of lycopene was associated with declined prostate cancer development in multicenter case-control study conducted in Iran (Pourmand et al. 2007). The question if tomato consumption may affect androgen activity in the prostate was examined in elegant studies in rats (Boileau et al. 2003; Campbell et al. 2006). Male rats treated with carcinogen (N-methyl-N-nitrosourea) and testosterone to induce prostate cancer were fed diets containing whole tomato powder, synthetic lycopene beadlets, or control beadlets (Boileau et al. 2003). Risk of death from prostate cancer was lower for rats fed the tomato powder diet than for those fed control beadlets but pure lycopene beadlets were without effect. Thus consumption of tomato powder but not lycopene alone inhibited prostate carcinogenesis, suggesting that in addition to lycopene, tomato products contain compounds that modify prostate carcinogenesis. Indeed, the same group reported that short-term consumption of phytofluene, lycopene, or tomato powder reduces serum testosterone in rats (Campbell et al. 2006). These results suggest that short-term intake of tomato carotenoids alters androgen status, which may partially account for a mechanism by which tomato intake reduces prostate cancer risk. In an additional animal model of human prostate cancer cells in nude mice, synthetic lycopene alone failed to reduce prostate tumor volume. However, combined treatment with lycopene and vitamin E, suppressed the growth of PC-346C prostate tumors by 73% and increased median survival time by 40% (Limpens et al. 2006). These results strongly suggest that the concerted action of several tomato ingredients and not lycopene alone is pivotal for the reduction of prostate cancer risk.

The power of combinations of lycopene with other phytonutrients, as discussed above, is evident also from a study evaluating the combination of tomato and broccoli in the Dunning R3327-H prostate adenocarcinoma model (Canene-Adams et al. 2007). Male rats were fed diets containing tomato, broccoli, or the combination of tomato plus broccoli for 22 weeks starting 1 month prior to receiving s.c. tumor implants. Synthetic lycopene alone reduced tumor weight insignificantly, whereas a significant reduction was obtained with tomato or broccoli powder. The combination of the two powders caused the highest decrease in tumor weights. These results clearly show that the combination of tomato and broccoli was more effective at slowing tumor growth than either tomato or broccoli alone and support the public health recommendations to increase the intake of a variety of plant components.

The mechanism by which lycopene reduces prostate cancer risk was tested in the Dunning prostate cancer model to gain insight into the in vivo action of lycopene (Siler et al. 2004). Lycopene supplementation for 4 weeks, led to plasma levels comparable with those in humans. Macroscopic evaluation of the tumors by magnetic resonance imaging showed a significant increase in necrotic areas in the lycopene treatment group. Microarray analysis of tumor tissues revealed that lycopene interfered with local testosterone activation by down-regulating 5α-reductase and consequently reduced steroid target genes expression (Siler et al. 2004). This important enzyme, crucial for androgen activity in the prostate tissue, was inhibited also by astaxanthin and saw palmetto lipid extract in human prostate cancer cells in vitro (Anderson 2005). Drug inhibition of 5α-reductase has been reported to decrease the symptoms of benign prostate hyperplasia, help treat existing prostate cancer and reduce the risk of prostate cancer (Rittmaster 2008). Thus, The reduction of 5α-reductase by lycopene (Siler et al. 2004) suggests a non-drug alternative for the prevention of prostate cancer and alleviation of prostate diseases.

3.4 Safety of Lycopene

Carotenoid safety is of major concern. It has long been known that individuals who consume high-carotenoid diet may develop a condition known as carotenodermia – yellow discoloration of the skin caused by carotene accumulation. Carotenodermia is harmless, reversible and not considered as a safety concern. No other side effects were linked conclusively to high carotenoid consumption from food. However, in two clinical intervention studies, high dose supplemental β-carotene has been shown to increase the incidence of lung cancer in heavy smokers (Heinonen et al. 1994; Omenn et al. 1996).

From the safety aspect, supplementation with lycopene may differ from that of β-carotene. Reviewing intervention studies involving the two carotenoids shows an interesting difference in their maximal achievable plasma levels. In most studies, β-carotene serum levels were significantly higher than those found for lycopene (IARC 1998). Thus, serum levels reached for β-carotene were around 3 μM and may exceed 5 μM (Heinonen et al. 1994; Omenn et al. 1996). On the other hand, lycopene levels above 1.2 μM were rarely seen even after long-term supplementation. The reason for this difference is not known yet, but it may provide a safety gauge for the supplementation of lycopene. Moreover, the serum level achieved for lycopene was not directly correlated to the amount of the supplemented carotenoid. For example, even its 'mega doses' as high as 75 mg/d did not result in higher than 1 μM lycopene in serum (Paetau et al. 1998). Similarly, in a phase I-II prospective dose-escalating trial of lycopene in prostate cancer patients, the plasma levels for doses between 15 and 90 mg/d were similar, with additional elevation only at 120 mg/d to 1.4 μM (Clark et al. 2006).

The difference between lycopene and β-carotene in elevation of serum levels after supplementation is even more striking. Two-three fold increase was seen in most studies with lycopene (Aust et al. 2003; Olmedilla et al. 2002; Paetau et al. 1998; Richelle et al. 2002), whereas significantly higher increases were evident for β-carotene (IARC 1998; Aust et al. 2003; Olmedilla et al. 2002). Thus, in the most publicized trials, which yielded increased risk for lung cancer after β-carotene supplementation, the CARET (Omenn et al. 1996) and ATBC (Albanes et al. 1996) studies, the plasma carotenoid level increased more than 12- and 16-fold, respectively. In the Physicians' Health Study, designed to assess the balance of benefits and risks of supplementation with β-carotene, vitamin E, vitamin C, and multivitamins on cancer, cardiovascular, and eye diseases, only a 4-fold increase in the β-carotene serum level was achieved (Cook et al. 2000). However, no effect for β-carotene supplementation on total cancer risk was found in the latter study under that smaller increase in plasma level. Interestingly, the only study that demonstrated positive health results of β-carotene supplementation was conducted in Linxian County (China), where the population has very low carotenoid status. Although supplementation resulted in an 11-fold increase in β-carotene plasma levels, the final concentration reached for the carotenoid was relatively low, about 1.5 μM (Taylor et al. 1994) compared with e.g. 3–5 μM obtained in the CARET and ATBC studies trial.

Another support for lycopene safety was found in a recent questionnaire-based study that examined whether high-dose carotenoid supplementation is associated with increased lung cancer risk in the general population (not heavy smokers) (Satia et al. 2009). The results demonstrated that longer duration of use of β-carotene, retinol, and lutein supplements was associated with statistically significantly elevated risk of lung cancer. Interestingly, no such association was found for lycopene. Moreover, there was some beneficial effect of lycopene though it did not reach statistical significance. The authors concluded that long-term use of individual β-carotene, retinol, and lutein supplements should not be recommended for lung cancer prevention, particularly among smokers. These results reinforce the notion that lycopene supplementation is safe.

3.5 Concluding Remarks

Cancer prevention strategies based on nutritional changes have obvious advantages over drug-based intervention. The scientific research to date has demonstrated an array of health benefits clearly associated with tomato products in the diet. The biochemical processes involved in the chemoprotective effects of fruits and vegetables are not completely understood. In this review we addressed several mechanisms suggested for the cancer prevention activity of tomato lycopene, including induction of phase II enzymes, inhibition of growth factor and sex hormone activity. There is strong evidence that neither synthetic lycopene nor pure tomato lycopene alone will act as a magic bullet to prevent cancer by these mechanisms. We suggest that combinations of carotenoids themselves and with other micronutrients will produce significant health beneficial effects, most probably by synergistic interactions. Going back to the 'Mother nature' receipt, it is proposed that effectiveness and safety are married together in the whole tomato. Thus, health benefits can be achieved from the addition of tomato-based foods to the diet (particularly cooked tomato products containing oil) or from supplements of tomato extract suspended in oil. These tomato products are devoid of any significant toxicity and may be recommended for cancer prevention in the general healthy population.

References

Albanes D, Heinonen OP, Taylor PR et al (1996) Alpha-Tocopherol and beta-carotene supplements and lung cancer incidence in the alpha-tocopherol, beta-carotene cancer prevention study: effects of base-line characteristics and study compliance. J Natl Cancer Inst 88:1560–1570

Amir H, Karas M, Giat J et al (1999) Lycopene and 1,25-dihydroxyvitamin-D3 cooperate in the inhibition of cell cycle progression and induction of differentiation in HL-60 leukemic cells. Nutr Cancer 33:105–112

Anderson ML (2005) A preliminary investigation of the enzymatic inhibition of 5alpha-reduction and growth of prostatic carcinoma cell line LNCap-FGC by natural astaxanthin and Saw Palmetto lipid extract in vitro. J Herb Pharmacother 5:17–26

Astorg P, Berges R, Suschetet M (1994) Induction of gamma GT- and GST-P positive foci in the liver of rats treated with 2-nitropropane or propane 2-nitronate. Cancer Lett 79:101–106

Aust O, Ale-Agha N, Zhang L et al (2003) Lycopene oxidation product enhances gap junctional communication. Food Chem Toxicol 41:1399–1407

Balogun E, Hoque M, Gong P et al (2003) Curcumin activates the heme oxygenase-1 gene via regulation of Nrf2 and the antioxidant responsive element. Biochem J 371:887–895

Ben-Dor A, Steiner M, Gheber L et al (2005) Carotenoids activate the antioxidant response element transcription system. Mol Cancer Ther 4:177–186

Bohm V, Bitsch R (1999) Intestinal absorption of lycopene from different matrices and interactions to other carotenoids, the lipid status, and the antioxidant capacity of human plasma. Eur J Nutr 38:118–125

Boileau TW, Liao Z, Kim S et al (2003) Prostate carcinogenesis in N-methyl-N-nitrosourea (NMU)-testosterone-treated rats fed tomato powder, lycopene, or energy-restricted diets. J Natl Cancer Inst 95:1578–1586

Breinholt V, Lauridsen ST, Daneshvar B et al (2000) Dose-response effects of lycopene on selected drug-metabolizing and antioxidant enzymes in the rat. Cancer Lett 154:201–210

Buckley MF, Sweeney KJ, Hamilton JA et al (1993) Expression and amplification of cyclin genes in human breast cancer. Oncogene 8:2127–2133

Campbell JK, Stroud CK, Nakamura MT et al (2006) Serum testosterone is reduced following short-term phytofluene, lycopene, or tomato powder consumption in f344 rats. J Nutr 136:2813–2819

Canene-Adams K, Lindshield BL, Wang S et al (2007) Combinations of tomato and broccoli enhance antitumor activity in dunning r3327-h prostate adenocarcinomas. Cancer Res 67:836–843

Carroll JS, Prall OW, Musgrove EA et al (2000) A pure estrogen antagonist inhibits cyclin E-Cdk2 activity in MCF-7 breast cancer cells and induces accumulation of p130-E2F4 complexes characteristic of quiescence. J Biol Chem 275:38221–38229

Chalabi N, Le Corre L, Maurizis JC et al (2004) The effects of lycopene on the proliferation of human breast cells and BRCA1 and BRCA2 gene expression. Eur J Cancer 40:1768–1775

Chalabi N, Maurizis JC, Le Corre L et al (2005) Quantification by affinity perfusion chromatography of phosphorylated BRCAl and BRCA2 proteins from tumor cells after lycopene treatment. J Chromatogr B Analyt Technol Biomed Life Sci 821:188–193

Chan JM, Stampfer MJ, Giovannucci E et al (1998) Plasma insulin-like growth factor-I and prostate cancer risk: a prospective study. Science 279:563–566

Chiang HS, Wu WB, Fang JY et al (2007) Lycopene inhibits PDGF-BB-induced signaling and migration in human dermal fibroblasts through interaction with PDGF-BB. Life Sci 81: 1509–1517

Clark PE, Hall MC, Borden LS et al (2006) Phase I-II prospective dose-escalating trial of lycopene in patients with biochemical relapse of prostate cancer after definitive local therapy. Urology 67:1257–1261

Cook NR, Le IM, Manson JE et al (2000) Effects of beta-carotene supplementation on cancer incidence by baseline characteristics in the Physicians' Health Study (United States). Cancer Causes Control 11:617–626

Cui Y, Shikany JM, Liu S et al (2008) Selected antioxidants and risk of hormone receptor-defined invasive breast cancers among postmenopausal women in the Women's Health Initiative Observational Study. Am J Clin Nutr 87:1009–1018

Cummings SR, Eckert S, Krueger KA et al (1999) The effect of raloxifene on risk of breast cancer in postmenopausal women: results from the MORE randomized trial. Multiple Outcomes of Raloxifene Evaluation. JAMA 281:2189–2197

Daughaday WH, Deuel TF (1991) Tumor secretion of growth factors. Endocrinol Metab Clin North Am 20:539–563

Deng CX, Brodie SG (2000) Roles of BRCA1 and its interacting proteins. Bioessays 22:728–737

Dingley KH, Ubick EA, Chiarappa-Zucca ML et al (2003) Effect of dietary constituents with chemopreventive potential on adduct formation of a low dose of the heterocyclic amines PhIP and IQ and phase II hepatic enzymes. Nutr Cancer 46:212–221

Dinkova-Kostova AT, Holtzclaw WD, Cole RN et al (2002) Direct evidence that sulfhydryl groups of Keap1 are the sensors regulating induction of phase 2 enzymes that protect against carcinogens and oxidants. Proc Natl Acad Sci USA 99:11908–11913

Early Breast Cancer Trialists' Collaborative Group (1998) Tamoxifen for early breast cancer: an overview of the randomised trials. Lancet 351:1451–1467

Ferrucci L, Perry JR, Matteini A et al (2009) Common variation in the beta-carotene $15,15'$-monooxygenase 1 gene affects circulating levels of carotenoids: a genome-wide association study. Am J Hum Genet 84:123–133

Fisher B, Costantino JP, Wickerham DL et al (1998) Tamoxifen for prevention of breast cancer: report of the National Surgical Adjuvant Breast and Bowel Project P-1 Study. J Natl Cancer Inst 90:1371–1388

Gaudet MM, Britton JA, Kabat GC et al (2004) Fruits, vegetables, and micronutrients in relation to breast cancer modified by menopause and hormone receptor status. Cancer Epidemiol Biomarkers Prev 13:1485–1494

Giovannucci E (1999) Tomatoes, tomato-based products, lycopene, and cancer: review of the epidemiologic literature. J Natl Cancer Inst 91:317–331

Giovannucci E (2005) Tomato products, lycopene, and prostate cancer: A review of the epidemiological literature. J Nutr 135:2030S–2031S

Giovannucci E, Pollak M, Liu Y et al (2003) Nutritional predictors of insulin-like growth factor I and their relationships to cancer in men. Cancer Epidemiol Biomarkers Prev 12:84–89

Gradelet S, Astorg P, Leclerc J et al (1996) Effects of canthaxanthin, astaxanthin, lycopene and lutein on liver xenobiotic-metabolizing enzymes in the rat. Xenobiotica 26:49–63

Graydon R, Gilchrist SE, Young IS et al (2007) Effect of lycopene supplementation on insulin-like growth factor-1 and insulin-like growth factor binding protein-3: a double-blind, placebo-controlled trial. Eur J Clin Nutr 61:1196–1200

Greenlee RT, Hill-Harmon MB, Murray T et al (2001) Cancer statistics 2001. CA Cancer J Clin 51:15–36

Gunnell D, Oliver SE, Peters TJ et al (2003) Are diet-prostate cancer associations mediated by the IGF axis? A cross-sectional analysis of diet, IGF-I and IGFBP-3 in healthy middle-aged men. Br J Cancer 88:1682–1686

Heinonen OP, Huttunen JK, Albanes D et al (1994) Effect of vitamin E and beta carotene on the incidence of lung cancer and other cancers in male smokers. N Engl J Med 330:1029–1035

Henderson BE, Ross R, Bernstein L (1988) Estrogens as a cause of human cancer: the Richard and Hinda Rosenthal Foundation award lecture. Cancer Res 48:246–253

Herzog A, Siler U, Spitzer V et al (2005) Lycopene reduced gene expression of steroid targets and inflammatory markers in normal rat prostate. FASEB J 19:272–274

Hirsch K, Atzmon A, Danilenko M et al (2007) Lycopene and other carotenoids inhibit estrogenic activity of 17β-estradiol and genistein in cancer cells. Breast Cancer Res Treat 104:221–230

Holmes MD, Pollak MN, Willett WC et al (2002) Dietary correlates of plasma insulin-like growth factor I and insulin-like growth factor binding protein 3 concentrations. Cancer Epidemiol Biomarkers Prev 11:852–261

Hu KQ, Liu C, Ernst H et al (2006) The biochemical characterization of ferret carotene-9′, 10′-monooxygenase catalyzing cleavage of carotenoids in vitro and in vivo. J Biol Chem 281:19327–19338

Huang CS, Liao JW, Hu ML (2008) Lycopene inhibits experimental metastasis of human hepatoma SK-Hep-1 cells in athymic nude mice. J Nutr 138:538–543

Huggins C, Hodges CV (1972) Studies on prostatic cancer. I. The effect of castration, of estrogen and androgen injection on serum phosphatases in metastatic carcinoma of the prostate. CA Cancer J Clin 22:232–240

IARC Handbook of Cancer Prevention (1998) Carotenoids, WHO Press

Iqbal M, Sharma SD, Okazaki Y et al (2003) Dietary supplementation of curcumin enhances antioxidant and phase II metabolizing enzymes in ddY male mice: possible role in protection against chemical carcinogenesis and toxicity. Pharmacol Toxicol 92:33–38

Jemal A, Siegel R, Ward E et al (2008) Cancer statistics, 2008. CA Cancer J Clin 58:71–96

Kaarbo M, Klokk TI, Saatcioglu F (2007) Androgen signaling and its interactions with other signaling pathways in prostate cancer. Bioessays 29:1227–1238

Kanagaraj P, Vijayababu MR, Ravisankar B et al (2007) Effect of lycopene on insulin-like growth factor-I, IGF binding protein-3 and IGF type-I receptor in prostate cancer cells. J Cancer Res Clin Oncol 133:351–359

Karas M, Kleinman D, Danilenko M et al (1995) Components of the IGF system mediate the opposing effects of tamoxifen on endometrial and breast cancer cell growth. Prog Growth Factor Res 6:513–520

Karas M, Amir H, Fishman D et al (2000) Lycopene interferes with cell cycle progression and insulin-like growth factor I signaling in mammary cancer cells. Nutr Cancer 36:101–111

Khachik F, Carvalho L, Bernstein PS et al (2002) Chemistry, distribution, and metabolism of tomato carotenoids and their impact on human health. Exp Biol Med (Maywood) 227:845–851

Kong AN, Owuor E, Yu R et al (2001) Induction of xenobiotic enzymes by the map kinase pathway and the antioxidant or electrophile response element (ARE/EpRE). Drug Metab Rev 33: 255–271

Krinsky NI, Johnson EJ (2005) Carotenoid actions and their relation to health and disease. Mol Aspects Med 26:459–516

Kwak MK, Egner PA, Dolan PM et al (2001) Role of phase 2 enzyme induction in chemoprotection by dithiolethiones. Mutat Res 480–481:305–315

LeRoith D, Roberts CT Jr (2003) The insulin-like growth factor system and cancer. Cancer Lett 195:127–137

Levy J, Bosin E, Feldman B et al (1995) Lycopene is a more potent inhibitor of human cancer cell proliferation than either α-carotene or β-carotene. Nutr Cancer 24:257–267

Levy J, Walfisch S, Walfisch Y et al (2008) Tomato Carotenoids and the IGF System in Cancer. In: Preedy V, Watson R (ed) Tomatoes and tomato products: nutritional, medicinal and therapeutic properties. Science, Enfield, USA 397–412

Lian F, Smith DE, Ernst H et al (2007) Apo-10′-lycopenoic acid inhibits lung cancer cell growth in vitro, and suppresses lung tumorigenesis in the A/J mouse model in vivo. Carcinogenesis 28:1567–1574

Limpens J, Schroder FH, de Ridder CM et al (2006) Combined lycopene and vitamin E treatment suppresses the growth of PC-346C human prostate cancer cells in nude mice. J Nutr 136: 1287–1293

Linnewiel K, Hansgeorg E, Caris-Veyrat C et al (2009) Structure activity relationship of carotenoid derivatives in activation of the electrophile/antioxidant response element transcription system. Free Radic Biol Med. 47:659–667

Liu C, Lian F, Smith DE et al (2003) Lycopene supplementation inhibits lung squamous metaplasia and induces apoptosis via up-regulating insulin-like growth factor-binding protein 3 in cigarette smoke-exposed ferrets. Cancer Res 63:3138–3144

Liu X, Allen JD, Arnold JT et al (2008) Lycopene inhibits IGF-I signal transduction and growth in normal prostate epithelial cells by decreasing DHT-modulated IGF-I production in co-cultured reactive stromal cells. Carcinogenesis 29:816–823

Martin D, Rojo AI, Salinas M et al (2004) Regulation of Heme Oxygenase-1 Expression through the phosphatidylinositol 3-kinase/Akt pathway and the Nrf2 transcription factor in response to the antioxidant phytochemical carnosol. J Biol Chem 279:8919–8929

Mucci LA, Tamimi R, Lagiou P et al (2001) Are dietary influences on the risk of prostate cancer mediated through the insulin-like growth factor system? BJU Int 87:814–820

Murakoshi M, Takayasu J, Kimura O et al (1989) Inhibitory effects of α-Carotene on proliferation of the human neuroblastoma cell line GOTO. J Natl Cancer Inst 81:1649–1652

Musgrove EA, Swarbrick A, Lee CS et al (1998) Mechanisms of cyclin-dependent kinase inactivation by progestins. Mol Cell Biol 18:1812–1825

Nahum A, Hirsch K, Danilenko M et al (2001) Lycopene inhibition of cell cycle progression in breast and endometrial cancer cells is associated with reduction in cyclin D levels and retention of p27(Kip1) in the cyclin E-cdk2 complexes. Oncogene 20:3428–3436

Nahum A, Zeller L, Danilenko M et al (2006) Lycopene inhibition of IGF-induced cancer cell growth depends on the level of cyclin D1. Eur J Nutr 45:275–282

Okuzumi J, Nishino H, Murakoshi M et al (1990) Inhibitory effects of fucoxanthin, a natural carotenoid, on N-myc expression and cell cycle progression in human malignant tumor cells. Cancer Lett 55:75–81

Olmedilla B, Granado F, Southon S et al (2002) A European multicentre, placebo-controlled supplementation study with alpha-tocopherol, carotene-rich palm oil, lutein or lycopene: analysis of serum responses. Clin Sci 102:447–456

Omenn GS, Goodman GE, Thornquist MD et al (1996) Effects of a combination of beta carotene and vitamin A on lung cancer and cardiovascular disease. N Engl J Med 334: 1150–1155

Paetau I, Khachik F, Brown ED et al (1998) Chronic ingestion of lycopene-rich tomato juice or lycopene supplements significantly increases plasma concentrations of lycopene and related tomato carotenoids in humans. Am J Clin Nutr 68:1187–1195

Pastori M, Pfander H, Boscoboinik D et al (1998) Lycopene in association with alpha-tocopherol inhibits at physiological concentrations proliferation of prostate carcinoma cells. Biochem Biophys Res Commun 250:582–585

Planas Silva MD, Weinberg RA (1997) Estrogen-dependent cyclin E-cdk2 activation through p21 redistribution. Mol Cell Biol 17:4059–4069

Pourmand G, Salem S, Mehrsai A et al (2007) The risk factors of prostate cancer: a multicentric case-control study in Iran. Asian Pac J Cancer Prev 8:422–428

Prakash P, Russell RM, Krinsky NI (2001) In vitro inhibition of proliferation of estrogen-dependent and estrogen-independent human breast cancer cells treated with carotenoids or retinoids. J Nutr 131:1574–1580

Prochaska HJ, Talalay P (1988) Regulatory mechanisms of monofunctional and bifunctional anticarcinogenic enzyme inducers in murine liver. Cancer Res 48:4776–4782

Riboli E, Norat T (2003) Epidemiologic evidence of the protective effect of fruit and vegetables on cancer risk. Am J Clin Nutr 78:559S–569S

Richelle M, Bortlik K, Liardet S et al (2002) A food-based formulation provides lycopene with the same bioavailability to humans as that from tomato paste. J Nutr 132:404–408

Riso P, Brusamolino A, Martinetti A et al (2006) Effect of a tomato drink intervention on insulin-like growth factor (IGF)-1 serum levels in healthy subjects. Nutr Cancer 55: 157–1562

Rittmaster RS (2008) 5alpha-reductase inhibitors in benign prostatic hyperplasia and prostate cancer risk reduction. Best Pract Res Clin Endocrinol Metab 22:389–402

Satia JA, Littman A, Slatore CG et al (2009) Long-term use of β-carotene, retinol, lycopene, and lutein supplements and lung cancer risk: results from the VITamins and lifestyle (VITAL) study. Am J Epidemiol 169:815–828

Schwarz S, Obermuller-Jevic UC, Hellmis E et al (2008) Lycopene inhibits disease progression in patients with benign prostate hyperplasia. J Nutr 138:49–53

Sherr CJ (1995) D-type cyclins. Trends Biochem Sci 20:187–190

Signorello LB, Kuper H, Lagiou P et al (2000) Lifestyle factors and insulin-like growth factor 1 levels among elderly men. Eur J Cancer Prev 9:173–178

Siler U, Barella L, Spitzer V et al (2004) Lycopene and vitamin E interfere with autocrine/paracrine loops in the Dunning prostate cancer model. FASEB J 18:1019–1021

Stahl W, Sies H (1992) Uptake of lycopene and its geometrical isomers is greater from heat-processed than from unprocessed tomato juice in humans. J Nutr 122: 2161–2166

Talalay P (2000) Chemoprotection against cancer by induction of phase 2 enzymes. Biofactors 12:5–11

Talalay P, Fahey JW (2001) Phytochemicals from cruciferous plants protect against cancer by modulating carcinogen metabolism. J Nutr 131:3027S–3033S

Talegawkar SA, Johnson EJ, Carithers TC et al (2008) Carotenoid intakes, assessed by food-frequency questionnaires (FFQs), are associated with serum carotenoid concentrations in the Jackson Heart Study: validation of the Jackson Heart Study Delta NIRI Adult FFQs. Public Health Nutr 11:989–997

Taylor PR, Li B, Dawsey SM et al (1994) Prevention of esophageal cancer: the nutrition intervention trials in Linxian, China. Linxian Nutrition Intervention Trials Study Group. Cancer Res 54:2029S–2031S

Teixeira C, Pratt MAC (1997) CDK2 is a target for retinoic acid–mediated growth inhibition in MCF-7 human breast cancer cells. Mol Endocrinol 11:1191–1202

Temple NJ, Gladwin KK (2003) Fruit, vegetables, and the prevention of cancer: research challenges. Nutrition 19:467–470

Tran CD, Diorio C, Berube S et al (2006) Relation of insulin-like growth factor (IGF) I and IGF-binding protein 3 concentrations with intakes of fruit, vegetables, and antioxidants. Am J Clin Nutr 84:1518–1526

van Poppel G (1993) Carotenoids and cancer: An update with emphasis on human intervention studies. Eur J Cancer 29A:1335–1344

Voskuil DW, Vrieling A, Korse CM et al (2008) Effects of lycopene on the insulin-like growth factor (IGF) system in premenopausal breast cancer survivors and women at high familial breast cancer risk. Nutr Cancer 60:342–353

Vrieling A, Voskuil DW, Bueno de Mesquita HB et al (2004) Dietary determinants of circulating insulin-like growth factor (IGF)-I and IGF binding proteins 1, -2 and -3 in women in the Netherlands. Cancer Causes Control 15:787–796

Vrieling A, Voskuil DW, Bonfrer JM et al (2007) Lycopene supplementation elevates circulating insulin-like growth factor binding protein-1 and -2 concentrations in persons at greater risk of colorectal cancer. Am J Clin Nutr 86:1456–1462

Walfisch Y, Walfisch S, Agbaria R et al (2003) Lycopene in serum, skin and adipose tissues after tomato-oleoresin supplementation in patients undergoing haemorrhoidectomy or peri-anal fistulotomy. Br J Nutr 90:759–766.

Walfisch S, Walfisch Y, Kirilov E et al (2007) Tomato lycopene extract supplementation decreases insulin-like growth factor-I levels in colon cancer patients. Eur J Cancer Prev 16:298–303

Wang AH, Zhang LS (2007) Effect of lycopene on the proliferation of MCF-7 and MDA-MB-231 cells. Sichuan Da Xue Xue Bao Yi Xue Ban 38:958–960

Wang C, Baumgartner RN, Yang D et al (2009) No evidence of association between breast cancer risk and dietary carotenoids, retinols, vitamin C and tocopherols in Southwestern Hispanic and non-Hispanic White women. Breast Cancer Res Treat 114:137–145

Watts CK, Sweeney KJ, Warlters A et al (1994) Antiestrogen regulation of cell cycle progression and cyclin D1 gene expression in MCF-7 human breast cancer cells. Breast Cancer Res Treat 31:95–105

Wu WB, Chiang HS, Fang JY et al (2007) Inhibitory effect of lycopene on PDGF-BB-induced signalling and migration in human dermal fibroblasts: a possible target for cancer. Biochem Soc Trans 35:1377–1378

Zhou Q, Stetler Stevenson M, Steeg PS (1997) Inhibition of cyclin D expression in human breast carcinoma cells by retinoids in vitro. Oncogene 15:107–115

Ziouzenkova O, Orashanu G, Sukhova G et al (2007) Asymmetric cleavage of β-carotene yields a transcriptional repressor of RXR and PPAR responses. Mol Endocrinol 21:77–88

Chapter 4
β-Carotene and Other Carotenoids in Cancer Prevention

Yan Wang and Xiang-Dong Wang

Abstract Epidemiological evidence suggests associations between dietary and circulating carotenoids and reduced risk of cancer at multiple sites. However, clinical supplementation trials have returned null findings, or even evidence of harmful effects of beta-carotene supplementation in certain populations. Studies in animal models of lung cancer have provided possible mechanistic explanations for the discordance between the results of observational epidemiological studies and intervention trials using beta-carotene as a potential chemopreventive agent. As we await better scientific understanding of carotenoid metabolism and mechanisms of action, a prudent strategy to reduce the risk of cancer incidence and mortality would include increased consumption of vegetables and fruits as a part of a healthy, balanced diet.

Keywords Carotenoids · Chemoprevention

Contents

X.-D. Wang (✉)
Nutrition and Cancer Biology Laboratory, Jean Mayer United States Department of Agriculture
Human Nutrition Research Center on Aging at Tufts University, 711 Washington Street, Boston,
MA 02111, USA
e-mail: xiang-dong.wang@tufts.edu

M. Mutanen, A.-M. Pajari (eds.), *Vegetables, Whole Grains, and Their Derivatives*
in Cancer Prevention, Diet and Cancer 2, DOI 10.1007/978-90-481-9800-9_4,
© Springer Science+Business Media B.V. 2011

4.1 Introduction

Carotenoids are a family of pigmented compounds synthesized by plants including vegetables and are responsible for their yellow, orange and red colors. More than 600 carotenoids have been identified in nature whereas only about 40~50 of them are present in a typical human diet and can be absorbed, metabolized, or utilized by the human body (Rao and Rao 2007). Close to 90% of the carotenoids in the diet and human body is represented by: β-carotene, α-carotene, β-cryptoxanthin, lutein, zeaxanthin, and lycopene (Khachik et al. 1991) (Fig. 4.1). Some carotenoids such as β-carotene, α-carotene, and β-cryptoxanthin can be cleaved to generate vitamin A and therefore referred to as provitamin A carotenoids, whereas others like lutein, zeaxanthin and lycopene cannot be converted to vitamin A and are called non-provitamin A carotenoids. All carotenoids possess a polyisoprenoid structure, a long conjugated chain of double bond and a near bilateral symmetry around the central double bond, as common chemical features (Britton 1995). The presence of the conjugated double bonds makes carotenoids particularly susceptible to oxidative cleavage and geometric (*trans/cis*) conversion. Although the *trans* isomers are more common in foods and more stable, very little is known about the biological significance of carotenoid isomerization in human health. Epidemiological studies suggest that a higher dietary intake of carotenoids may offer protection against the development of certain cancers (e.g. lung, cervix, bladder, gastrointestinal tract, breast and prostate) (Ziegler 1989; van Poppel and Goldbohm 1995; Sesso and Gaziano 2004). However, two large double-blind clinical trials have shown that supplementation with β-carotene, alone or in combination with vitamin A, did not reduce the risk of lung cancer and even increased that risk in smokers (Albanes et al. 1996; Omenn et al. 1996). These observations have led to extensive research efforts over the last decade to better understand the mechanisms involved in the action of carotenoids on carcinogenic process. This chapter will focus on the roles of β-carotene in specific and other carotenoids in general, in cancer prevention and potential mechanisms involved (Fig. 4.2). The content related to lycopene has been discussed in another chapter in this book.

4.2 Dietary Sources, Bioavailability and Metabolism

4.2.1 Dietary Sources

Carotenoids are present in many common human foods whereas the deeply pigmented fruits and vegetables constitute the major dietary sources. β-Carotene is the most widely studied carotenoid and one of the major carotenoids in both diet and

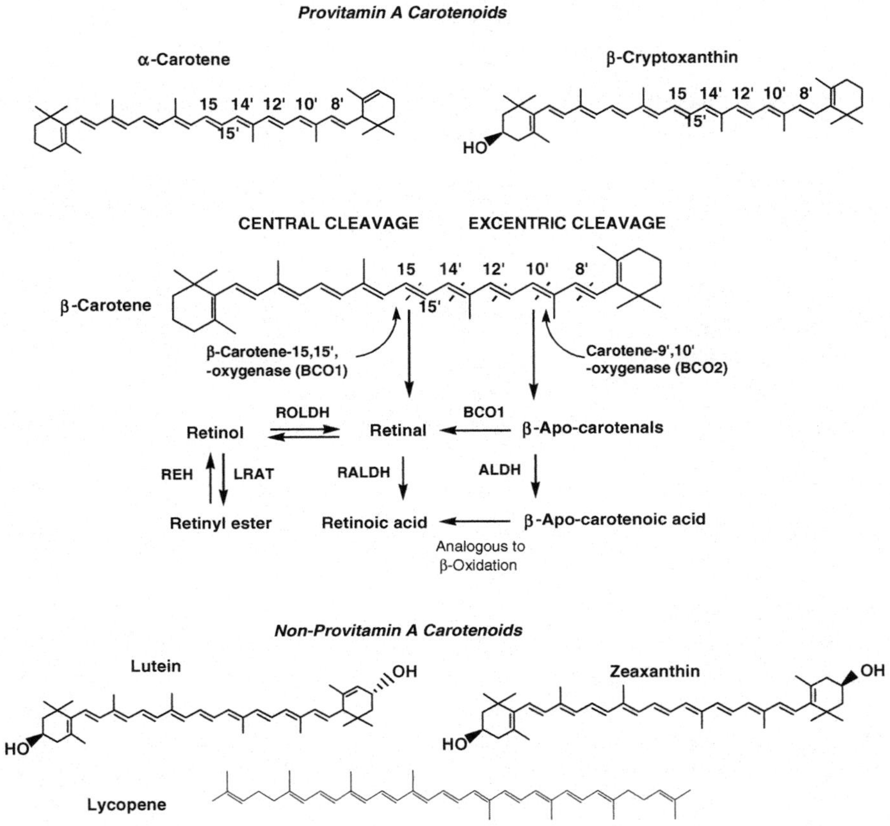

Provitamin A Carotenoids

α-Carotene

β-Cryptoxanthin

15 14' 12' 10' 8'
15'

15 14' 12' 10' 8'
15'

HO

CENTRAL CLEAVAGE   EXCENTRIC CLEAVAGE

β-Carotene

15 14' 12' 10' 8'
15'

β-Carotene-15,15',
-oxygenase (BCO1)

Carotene-9',10'
-oxygenase (BCO2)

ROLDH
Retinol ⇌ Retinal ← β-Apo-carotenals
                              BCO1

REH ↑↓ LRAT   RALDH ↓   ALDH ↓

Retinyl ester   Retinoic acid ← β-Apo-carotenoic acid

Analogous to
β-Oxidation

Non-Provitamin A Carotenoids

Lutein   OH   Zeaxanthin   OH

HO   HO

Lycopene

Fig. 4.1 Metabolic pathway of β-carotene and chemical structures of provitamin A carotenoids (α-carotene and β-cryptoxanthin) and non-provitamin A carotenoids (lutein, zeaxanthin and lycopene). Abbreviations used: BCO1, β-carotene-15,15'-oxygenase; BCO, β-carotene-9',10'-oxygenase; ROLDH, retinol dehydrogenase; REH, retinyl ester hydrolases; LRAT, lecithin:retinol acyltransferase; RALDH, retinal dehydrogenase; ALDH, aldehyde dehydrogenase. Figure adapted from Mernitz, Wang (2007)

human bodies (Schmitz et al. 1991; Enger et al. 1996). Beta-carotene ($C_{40}H_{56}$) has a chemical structure characterized by a large carbon chain with alternating double and single bonds, terminated at each end by a ring structure (Fig. 4.1). The richest dietary sources of β-carotene are yellow, orange, and leafy green fruits and vegetables, such as carrots, spinach, sweet potatoes, and cantaloupe. The National Health and Nutrition Examination Survey (1999–2000) reported dietary intakes of β-carotene to be 5.4 ± 0.3 mg/d among general American population (Ervin et al. 2004). Two major vegetables that are found to contain high amount of lutein and zeaxanthin are spinach and kale, respectively (During et al. 2002). In contrast, β-cryptoxanthin is mainly derived from orange fruits like tangerine and papaya.

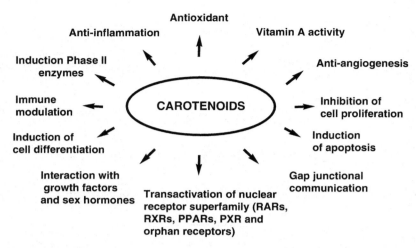

Fig. 4.2 Possible biologic functions of carotenoids. Figure adapted from Mein, Lian, Wang (2008)

4.2.2 Bioavailability

The bioavailability of β-carotene from vegetables is generally low (Castenmiller et al. 1999). Several factors are important for β-carotene absorption. For examples, food processing and cooking that cause mechanical breakdown of the food matrix and release of β-carotene can improve its intestinal absorption (Parker 1996, 1997; Gartner et al. 1997). The presence of dietary fat could be another factor to promote its absorption considering that β-carotene is lipophilic and absorbed by incorporation into the micelles at intestine (Wang 1994). Both the cellular uptake and secretion of β-carotene are saturable, concentration-dependent processes. The selective absorption of all-*trans* β-carotene versus its *cis* isomers, the differential absorption of individual carotenoids, and the specific interactions between carotenoids during their absorption has been discussed in detailed (During and Harrison 2004). After taken up by the mucosa of small intestine, β-carotene is packaged into chylomicrons and secreted into lymphatic system for transport to the liver and other peripheral tissues. Although factors influencing other carotenoid absorption are similar to those for β-carotene, more investigations are needed in terms of the varying absorption of individual carotenoids.

4.2.3 Metabolism

As a provitamin A carotenoid, β-carotene is the major source of vitamin A. Two metabolic pathways exist for its conversion to vitamin A, and they are known as the central cleavage pathway and the excentric cleavage pathway (Fig. 4.1). For provitamin A carotenoids, central cleavage is the main pathway leading to the formation of vitamin A (Goodman and Huang 1965; Olson and Hayaishi 1965). β-Carotene, α-carotene, and β-cryptoxanthin are cleaved symmetrically at their central double bond by β-carotene 15, 15′-monooxygenase (CMO1, formerly called β-carotene 15, 15′-dioxygenase). This enzyme has been cloned in several species and has been further characterized as a non-heme iron monooxygenase (von Lintig and Vogt 2000; Wyss et al. 2000). Besides central cleavage pathway, an alternative excentric cleavage pathway was reported by a serial of studies from our labs and others (Wang et al. 1991, 1992; Wang and Krinsky 1998). The existence of this pathway was further confirmed by molecular identification of an excentric cleavage enzyme, β-carotene 9′, 10′-monooxygenase (CMO2) in mice, humans, zebrafish and ferret (Kiefer et al. 2001; Hu et al. 2006). CMO2 has been demonstrated to have the ability to catalyze the asymmetric cleavage of β-carotene to produce β-apo-10′-carotenal and β-ionone (Kiefer et al. 2001). Apo-β-carotenals can be precursors of vitamin A in vitro and in vivo, by further cleavage enzyme, CMO1 (Lakshmanan et al. 1968; Liu et al. 1997). They can also be oxidized to their corresponding apo-β-carotenoic acids, which may then undergo a process similar to β-oxidation of fatty acids, to produce retinoic acid (Wang et al. 1996). The coexistence of these two cleavage pathways reveals a greater complexity of β-carotene metabolism in organisms and raises a potential link between effects from β-carotene (and its metabolites) and anti-carcinogenesis. An understanding of the impact of conversion of β-carotene into its bioactive metabolites is important in understanding the health effects of these compounds. Recent studies shown that common nonsynonymous single-nucleotide polymorphisms (SNPs) exist in the human *CMO1* gene that occur at high frequencies and that alter β-carotene metabolism (Ferrucci et al. 2009; Leung et al. 2009). These studies may provide an explanation for the various phenotypes in β-carotene metabolism, and indicate that genetic variability should be taken into account in future recommendations for vitamin A supplementation, particular in terms of cancer prevention.

4.3 Biological Activity of β-Carotene

4.3.1 Beneficial Effects

4.3.1.1 Growth Inhibition and Induction of Apoptosis

One of the actions of β-carotene on cells is its ability to alter growth patterns, and in particular, inhibit growth in tumor cell lines. The addition of 70 μM β-carotene inhibited the proliferation of cultured human squamous cells (SK-MES lung carcinoma or Scc-25 oral carcinoma) (Schwartz et al. 1990), further analysis found that this inhibitory effect was accompanied by a rapid appearance of a unique 70 kD protein, analogous to heat shock proteins. Another example of an effect on the molecular basis of growth inhibition is the observation that β-carotene inhibits cyclinD1-associated cdk4 kinase activity, along with a decrease in the levels of the hyperphosphorylated form of retinoblastoma protein in human fibroblast (Stivala et al. 2000).

It is well known that genetic loss or functional aberration of cellular control mechanism of apoptosis is considered to be a critical event in the initiation, promotion or progression of cancer (Thompson 1995). Apoptosis of pre-initiated and/or neoplastic processes represents a protective mechanism against neoplastic transformation and development of tumors by eliminating genetically damaged cells or cells that may have been inappropriately induced to divide by mitogenic and proliferative stimuli. There is a growing body of literatures showing a potential role of β-carotene in the induction of cell apoptosis in cancer cells. For example, in human cervical cancer cells 10 μM β-carotene caused chromatin condensation, a characteristic of apoptosis (Muto et al. 1995). Moreover, β-carotene was able to induce apoptosis in human colon adenocarcinoma (Palozza et al. 2001, 2002a) as well as in human leukemic cells (Palozza et al. 2002b). It is noteworthy that the concentration responsible for the pro-apoptotic effects of β-carotene in many of these in vitro studies are higher (2–20 μM) than those observed in the serum of normal human subjects, however, the concentration of carotenoids can be reached in the serum of humans supplemented with high doses of the carotenoids (Nierenberg et al. 1991; Prince and Frisoli 1993). Nierenberg and coworkers reported that supplementation with 50 mg/d of β-carotene in humans resulted in plasma carotenoids concentration of up to 16.1 μM. Prince and Frisoli demonstrated that human subject ingesting various dosage of β-carotene as supplements (51~102 mg/d) could have a steady serum concentrations of carotenoids ranging from 2 to 13.2 μM. The proapoptotic effect of β-carotene could be derived from its potential regulation on caspase cascade activation in tumor cells. A recent study also found a dose-dependent increase of cleaved form of Bid, which is known to induce the release of cytochrome c by a caspase-dependent mechanism, was observed in tumor cell line treated with β-carotene (Palozza et al. 2003a).

4.3.1.2 Antioxidant Function

Carotenoids are scavengers of singlet oxygen and other reactive oxygen species. Since cancer development has been linked to DNA damage, which can result from increased levels of oxidative stress, the antioxidant properties of carotenoids including β-carotene have been suggested as being one of the main mechanisms by which they afford their beneficial effects against carcinogenic process. Like the other members of the carotenoid family, β-carotene is indeed very effective in neutralizing singlet oxygen ($^1O_2$) and, to a lesser extent, in interrupting lipid peroxidation chain reactions. One of the well known beneficial effects of β-carotene is its ability to reduce the harmful effects of solar radiation on photosensitive individuals by contrasting the action of $^1O_2$ and other reactive species, such as free radicals deriving from the excitation of protoporphyrin (Krinsky 1991). β-Carotene can also result in a very significant decrease in lymphocyte DNA oxidative damage (Fabiani et al. 2001). In the work of Astley et al (Astley et al. 2004) examining the effects of carotenoids on DNA damage and susceptibility to oxidative damage in lymphocytes, it was reported that β-carotene was capable of exerting antioxidant protection by scavenging DNA-damaging free radicals and modulating DNA repair mechanism. Various animal species have been used for many years in attempts to evaluate the in vivo antioxidant effect of carotenoids. However, these studies are marred by the fact that most experimental animals are very poor absorbers of carotenoids. Some animals that can absorb dietary carotenoids, such as ferret, have been used to study carotenoids bioavailability but little has been done with respect to antioxidant effectiveness in these species (Lee et al. 1999a, b). In mice treated for 15 days with 4, 4′-diketo-β-carotene, a direct antioxidant effect was not observed but indirectly, a significant over-expression of the MnSOD gene was observed, suggesting that this carotenoid was capable of altering the antioxidant protection in this species (Palozza et al. 2000). Evidence from human subjects also found that in a group of Iranian men supplementation with 30 mg/d β-carotene for 10 weeks significantly reduced the plasma MDA level (Meraji et al. 1997). Another example is the ability of β-carotene to inhibit the invasion of rat mesentery derived hepatoma cells (Kozuki et al. 2000). This process is markedly increased by pre-treating cells with xanthine oxidase to generate ROS, and this enhanced effect is also inhibited by β-carotene, suggesting that antioxidation property of β-carotene is involved in its anti-invasive function.

4.3.1.3 Regulation of Transcriptional Receptors

Provitamin A carotenoids, such as β-carotene and its excentric cleavage metabolites, can serve as direct precursors for (all-*trans*)-retinoic acid and (9-*cis*)-retinoic acid which are ligands for retinoic acid receptors (RAR) and retinoid X receptors (RXR), respectively. Previously, we observed that β-carotene and its oxidative metabolite, apo-14′-carotenoic acid, reversed the down-regulation of RARβ by smoke-borne carcinogens in normal bronchial epithelial cells (Prakash et al. 2004). We further demonstrated that the transactivation of the RARβ2 promoter by β-apo-14′-carotenoic acid appears to occur, in large part, via its metabolism to all-*trans*-retinoic acid (Prakash et al. 2004). Therefore, the molecular mode of the action of β-carotene may be mediated by retinoic acid through transcriptional activation of a series of genes with distinct antiproliferative or proapoptotic activity, which allows for the elimination of cells with irreparable alterations in the genome and the killing of neoplastic cells. Interestingly, however, relatively more luciferase activity was observed from β-apo-14′-carotenoic acid than can be accounted for by the appearance of retinoic acid, when compared to the effect of retinoic acid alone (Prakash et al. 2004). Considering that retinoid X receptors (RXRs) may function not only as heterodimeric partners of other nuclear receptors, but also as active transducers of tumor suppressive signals (Altucci and Gronemeyer 2001), it will be interesting to investigate whether the biological activity of carotenoids or their metabolites are mediated through interaction with RXRs, thyroid hormone receptors, the vitamin D receptor (VDR), peroxisome proliferators-activated receptors (PPAR), or other orphan receptors.

4.3.1.4 Inhibition on Malignant Transformation

The profound effects of carotenoids on cell grown in culture have been reported with respect to the inhibition of malignant transformation. This phenomenon involves the process whereby normal cells are converted to cells that have the ability to induce tumors when injected into animals. For example, β-carotene can inhibit malignant transformation induced by 3-methylcholanthrene or X-ray treatment in the fibroblast cell line C3H/10T1/2 (Merriman and Bertram 1979). Interestingly, another study found that all-trans-β-carotene was consistently more active in suppressing neoplastic transformation in both murine 10T1/2 and human HaCaT keratinocytes as compared with 9-*cis*-β-carotene (Hieber et al. 2000).

4.3.1.5 β-Carotene and Antioxidant Combinations

Strong interactions among β-carotene, α-tocopherol, and ascorbic acid in vitro and the capability of these compounds to 'recycle' each other, regenerating efficient antioxidants from their radical cations, have led researchers to speculate about the potential utility of combined antioxidant therapy in vivo. It is possible that this additional protection against oxidative degradation of carotenoids may increase the utility of nutritional interventions targeting cancer, surpassing effects seen in single-agent intervention studies.

Previously, we have shown that vitamin E (α-tocopherol) enhances lymphatic transport of β-carotene and central cleavage of β-carotene to form vitamin A (rather than oxidative by-products) in vivo (Wang et al. 1995). We have further shown that α-tocopherol and ascorbic acid were able to decrease the production of undesirable oxidative metabolites and increase the formation of retinoids from β-carotene in the lung tissues of smoke-exposed ferrets in vitro (Liu et al. 2003b). The formation of excentric cleavage products in ferret lung post-nuclear fractions after incubation with β-carotene was greatly increased in animals that had been exposed to cigarette smoke, as compared with control ferrets. However, the enhanced formation of β-apo-carotenals after smoke exposure was much lower when 50 μM of α-tocopherol and 50 μM of ascorbic acid were added to the incubation mixture. Similarly, the formation of retinoic acid in ferret lung post-nuclear fractions after incubation with β-carotene was greatly decreased in animals that had been exposed to cigarette smoke, as compared with control ferrets, and this effect was reversed by the addition of α-tocopherol or ascorbic acid to the incubation mixture. Addition of both α-tocopherol and ascorbic acid led to a significant increase in both retinal and retinoic acid production after incubation with β-carotene, above the levels seen in non-smoke-exposed animals. These data indicate that α-tocopherol and ascorbic acid may act synergistically to prevent the enhanced oxidative excentric cleavage of β-carotene induced by exposure to cigarette smoke and to support the conversion of β-carotene in retinal and retinoic acid.

A recent study in our laboratory investigated the effectiveness of combined antioxidant therapy in vivo in a smoke-exposed, carcinogen-induced ferret model of lung cancer (Kim et al. 2006). Animals were supplemented with β-carotene in combination with α-tocopherol and ascorbic acid for six months. We observed that smoke exposure and carcinogen injections were associated with significant declines in lung levels of retinoic acid and ascorbic acid, but combined antioxidant supplementation restored lung levels of retinoic acid and also reversed changes in lung protein levels related to cellular proliferation and apoptosis. Further, while it has previously been shown that smoke exposure significantly reduces lung tissue levels of β-carotene in ferrets receiving supplemental β-carotene alone, there were no significant smoke-induced changes in lung levels of β-carotene in this combined antioxidant study. This suggests the α-tocopherol and ascorbic acid were able to protect β-carotene from smoke-enhanced degradation, preventing excessive formation of excentric cleavage products and the subsequent cascade of events that may result, including bioactivation of carcinogens, destruction of retinoic acid via induction of cytochrome P_{450} enzymes, and binding of benzo[a]pyrene metabolites to DNA. This was supported by a recent study that the combination of β-carotene with α-tocopherol and ascorbyl palmitate did not induce any pro-oxidant effects in the lung of ferrets (Fuster et al. 2008).

Combined antioxidant supplementation reversed the increased labeling of proliferating cellular nuclear antigen observed in the smoke-exposed, carcinogen-injected group, and also reversed smoke- and carcinogen-induced phosphorylation of mitogen-activated protein kinase (MAPK) proteins, c-jun N-terminal kinase (JNK), and extracellular signal-regulated kinase (ERK), previously associated with pathways leading to increased cellular proliferation. This inhibition of JNK activation by combined antioxidants may help maintain normal retinoid signaling, as it has recently been reported that activation of JNK contributes to RAR dysfunction by inducing the phosphorylation and proteasomal degradation of RARα. Further, phosphorylation of JNK and ERK mediate phosphorylation of p53 tumor suppressor protein. Following up on this, we found that total p53 protein and phosphorylated p53 were induced by smoke and carcinogen exposure, and this was prevented by supplementation with combined antioxidants, mirroring the changes in phospho-JNK and phospho-ERK. Further, a downstream target of p53, the Bax apoptotic protein, was similarly affected. This suggests that smoke and carcinogen exposure may lead to a loss of homeostasis between cellular proliferation and apoptosis that contributes to the process of carcinogenesis. In addition, we observed that combined antioxidants inhibited smoke-induced oxidative stress assessed by Comet analysis (Kim et al. 2006, 2007). These data may help to explain the conflicting results of the negative human β-carotene intervention trials (which used high doses of β-carotene) versus the positive observational epidemiological studies showing that diets high in fruits and vegetables containing β-carotene (but at much lower concentrations than in the intervention studies and with other antioxidants present) are associated with a decreased risk for lung cancer. Taken together, this data suggests that vitamin E and vitamin C can act together to inhibit the oxidation of β-carotene and facilitate the conversion of β-carotene into retinoic acid in smoke-exposed lung tissue in vivo. Combined antioxidant supplementation can maintain normal levels of lung retinoic acid and inhibit the phosphorylation of JNK, ERK, and p53, protecting against lung carcinogenesis instigated by smoke and carcinogen exposure. This offers in vivo evidence of the utility of combined nutrients as a chemopreventive strategy to reduce the risk of lung cancer in smokers. A very recent report from the Linxian Trial (Qiao et al. 2009) showed that the beneficial effects of combined beta-carotene, vitamin E, and selenium supplementation on mortality were still evident up to 10 years after the cessation of supplementation. In addition, the results of the Vitamins and Lifestyle (VITAL) Study (Satia et al. 2009) found that long-term use of individual beta-carotene and lutein supplements significantly increased lung cancer risk among smokers, but not in smokers using multivitamin supplementation.

4.3.2 Harmful Effects and Potential Mechanisms

It appears that while small quantities of carotenoids can offer protection against certain cancers related to free radical oxidation, larger amounts of carotenoids may actually be harmful especially when coupled with a highly oxidative environment, probably via their generated metabolites. Intervention trials using β-carotene as a potential chemopreventive agent have resulted in no evidence of an effect, or even increased risk of lung cancer in heavy smokers and asbestos workers (Albanes et al. 1996; Hennekens et al. 1996; Omenn et al. 1996; Lee et al. 1999a, b). Although the relevance of the outcome of the human study and the details of the study design are still being debated among the scientists, the recent experimental evidence also support the potential adverse effects mediated by high-dose of β-carotene during cancer development. For example, ferret receiving high-dose β-carotene had decreased levels of tumor suppressor protein RARβ, increased expression of the transcription factor AP-1 (a dimer of c-jun and c-fos proteins), increased levels of cyclinD1, and over-expression of proliferating cellular nuclear antigen (Wang et al. 1999). Effects were even more dramatic in animals when high-dose β-carotene was combined with exposure to cigarette smoke, where molecular alterations were associated with squamous metaplasia in ferret lung. We proposed that diminished retinoid signaling by the down regulation of RARβ expression could be a mechanism for enhancement of lung tumorigenesis after high-dose β-carotene supplementation and cigarette smoke exposure. More significantly, smoke exposure in the high dose β-carotene supplemented group resulted in an even greater decrease in lung retinoic acid levels, and accompanied an increase in oxidative metabolites of β-carotene. In contrast, ferrets receiving low-dose β-carotene, equivalent to the amount contained in 5~9 servings of fruits and vegetables, had no evidence of precancerous lesions and no changes in molecular biomarkers associated with carcinogenesis, and this level of supplementation was associated with protection against smoke-induced changes in lung retinoic acid levels (Liu et al. 2000). These evidence suggests a possible biphasic response of β-carotene that promotes health when taken at dietary levels, but may have adverse effects when taken in higher amounts. The dosages of β-carotene used in the ATBC and CARET trail studies were 20–30 mg/d for 2–8 years, and these doses are 10–15 fold higher than the average intake of β-carotene in a typical American diet (approximately 2 mg/d). Such a high dose of β-carotene in humans could result in an accumulation of a relatively high β-carotene level in lung tissue, especially after long periods of supplementation. This was supported by a recent study showing that β-carotene promoted the development of pulmonary adenocarcinoma in hamsters by subcutaneously injection of β-carotene for one and half years (Al-Wadei and Schuller 2009). Very recently, we evaluated whether β-carotene supplementation affects molecular markers of lung carcinogenesis in the Physicians'

Health Study (PHS) trial (Liu et al. 2009), which had much higher levels of blood β-carotene in the β-carotene placebo group compared with the levels for those groups in the CARET and ATBC studies (0.3 mg/l vs. 0.18 mg/l vs. 0.18 mg/l, respectively) but had much lower levels of blood β-carotene in the β-carotene group (1.2 mg/l vs. 2.1 mg/l vs. 3.0 mg/l, respectively). Our data suggest that 50-mg β-carotene supplementation on alternate days had no significant influence on the molecular markers of lung carcinogenesis that we evaluated in the PHS. This finding provides mechanistic support for the main PHS trial results of bcarotene, which indicated no benefit or harm on the risk of lung cancer.

The outcome of carotenoid supplementation depends on the carotenoid (or its metabolites), the dosage level, and the specific organs examined. This concept is supported by β-carotene human intervention studies, which indicate that β-carotene may prevent gastric carcinogenesis and esophagus precancerous lesions (Correa et al. 2000; Mayne et al. 2001). Unlike lung tissue, eliminating β-carotene through epithelial cells can prevent accumulation of excessive β-carotene in oral and gastric mucosa. Furthermore, animal studies reported that both dietary and topical β-carotene failed to act as a tumor promoter in the AJ mouse model of lung cancer (Obermueller-Jevic et al. 2002) and the two-stage model of skin tumorigenesis (Ponnamperuma et al. 2000). It is noteworthy that the extrapolation of the data from rodent models to human populations has to be paid more attention to the actual carotenoid levels in plasma and tissue and their relevance to those from humans.

4.3.2.1 Pro-oxidant Function

It is interesting to observe that β-carotene has also been reported to act as a pro-oxidant under certain situations. β-Carotene at a concentration of 0.2 μM augmented UVA-induced heme oxygenase-1 induction indicating a pro-oxidant effect (Obermuller-Jevic et al. 1999). Similarly, in another study β-carotene at a concentration of 10 μM increased the production of ROS and the levels of cellular oxidized glutathione in leukaemia and colon adenocarcinoma cell lines in vitro (Palozza et al. 2003a, b). The pro-oxidant effect of β-carotene was also demonstrated in rats that showed increased activity of phase I enzymes in liver, kidney and intestine as well as increased oxidative stress (Paolini et al. 2001). Lowe et al. further demonstrated that β-carotene protect against oxidative DNA damage (induced by xanthine/xanthine oxidase) in HT29 cells at relatively low concentrations (1–3 μM), but lose this capacity at higher concentrations (4–10 μM) (Lowe et al. 1999). Yeh and Hu demonstrated that β-carotene at a high concentration (20 μM) significantly enhanced levels of lipid peroxidation induced by a lipid-soluble radical generator, AMVN (2,2′-azobis[2,4-dimethylvaleronitrile]) (Yeh and Hu 2003).

Besides high concentration of β-carotene used in these experimental studies, there have been reports that high oxygen tensions, such as that observed in lung from heavy smokers, could be also responsible for the prooxidant effect of β-carotene even at its physiological concentration. Zhang and Omaye found that at the oxygen tensions up to 150 Torr, β-carotene inhibited the AAPH-induced production of protein carbonyls while at 760 Torr the addition of 1.6 μM β-carotene resulted in a

26% increase in carbonyl formation, suggesting a prooxidant action of β-carotene at high oxygen tension (Zhang and Omaye 2000). Zhang also demonstrated a specific prooxidant effect of β-carotene using human lung cells exposed to AAPH, at 143 Torr β-carotene protect cellular lipid, protein and DNA damage but at 722 Torr 1.5 μM promoted isoprostane formation and its protective effect against protein oxidation and DNA damage was decreased (Zhang and Omaye 2001a). Thus, it would appear that even at a physiological concentration, β-carotene could exhibit a prooxidant effect at high oxygen tensions. Similar effect was also observed using ex vivo system. For example, β-carotene added to rat liver microsomes was an effective antioxidant at 15 Torr, but a prooxidant at 150 Torr, when the lipid-soluble azo initiator 1,1′-azobis (cyclohexane-carbonitrile) was used to initiate lipid peroxidation, as evaluated by MDA formation (Zhang and Omaye 2001b).

Besides pro-oxidant effect from β-carotene itself, an alternative mechanism for the results observed in the human β-carotene trials is that the presentation of high doses of β-carotene *via* supplements to the highly oxidative environment of the lung in smokers results in increased levels of oxidative metabolites of β-carotene which may have detrimental effects (Wang and Russell 1999; Arora et al. 2001). One possible mechanism to explain the instability of the β-carotene molecule is that exposure of lung cells to smoke results in increased lung cell oxidative stress and thereby causes a decrease in other antioxidants, such as vitamin C and vitamin E, which normally have a stabilizing effect on the unoxidized form of β-carotene (Bohm et al. 1998). β-Carotene is capable of regenerating alpha-tocopherol from its radical. Conversely, vitamin E protect carotenoids from autoxidation; the combination of β-carotene and alpha-tocopherol results in inhibition of free radical induced lipid peroxidation which is significantly greater than the sum of the individual inhibitions (Palozza and Krinsky 1992). These data suggest that tocopherol may limit the prooxidant effects of carotenoids in biological systems. Moreover, we have shown that vitamin E enhances lymphatic transport of β-carotene and central cleavage of β-carotene to form vitamin A (rather than oxidative by-products) in vivo (Wang et al. 1995). It has also been reported that vitamin C is able to convert the β-carotene radical back to β-carotene and can help maintain β-carotene in its unoxidized form (Bohm et al. 1998). The combination of β-carotene (20 mg/d) and vitamin E (50 mg/d) were not found to be protective against smoke-related lung cancer in the ATBC study. However, vitamin C, which would facilitate both vitamin E recycling and β-carotene stability, was not used in the ATBC study. Epidemiologic studies have shown that smokers have significantly lower plasma levels of vitamin C compared with nonsmokers (Schectman et al. 1989). It is particularly important to have broad antioxidant protection when using high doses of β-carotene in order to prevent the production of carotene excentric cleavage products and the subsequent cascade of events that may result from them (i.e. bioactivating carcinogens and destroying retinoic acid via induction of CYP enzymes, or facilitating the binding of benzo[a]pyrene metabolites to DNA). Both vitamins E and C can also inhibit cytochrome P450 mediated lipid peroxidation and carcinogen activation. Possible protective effects of combined antioxidant supplementation in humans exposed to environmental tobacco smoke has been reported (Howard et al. 1998). Recent study using a ferret model has shown that β-carotene, used in combination with vitamins E and C, may have a possible chemopreventive effect against smoke-induced lung lesions (Kim et al. 2007). Results from these studies and the known biochemical interactions of β-carotene, vitamin E and vitamin C suggest that this combination of nutrients may be an effective chemopreventive strategy against lung cancer in smokers.

4.3.2.2 Induction of CYP450 Enzymes

In Sprague-Dawley rats, supplementation of 250 or 500 mg/kg body weight β-carotene at either single or repeated manner significantly induce a number of CYP isoforms in all tissues: CYP3A1/2, CYP2E1, CYP1A1/2 and CYP2B1/2 in the liver; CYP3A1/2, CYP2E1 and CYP1A1/2 in the kidney; CYP1A1/2 and CYP3A1/2 in the lung; and CYP3A1/2, CYP1A1/2 and CYP2E1 in the intestine (Paolini et al. 2001). It was also reported that β-apo-8'-carotenal, an excentric cleavage product of β-carotene, is a strong inducer of CYP1A1 in rats (Gradelet et al. 1996). This study is particularly interesting because the formation of β-apo-8'-carotenal from β-carotene was three fold higher in lung extracts of smoke-exposed ferrets than from non-smoke-exposed ferrets (Liu et al. 2004). The recorded CYP induction is consistent with the concept that β-carotene or its oxidative metabolites have co-carcinogenic potential. Indeed, if extrapolated to humans, similar increases in CYP levels could raise the risk of lung cancer in heavy smokers, due to the immense range of tobacco-smoke pro-carcinogens (a complex mixture of more than 4,000 substances, among which at least 40 have been identified as carcinogens, tumor initiators or promoters in laboratory animals. In addition, many tobacco-smoke pro-carcinogens are themselves CYP inducers, and they could act in a synergic way with β-carotene, thereby further contributing to the overall carcinogenic risk (Bartsch and Hietanen 1996). Increased bioactivation of pro-carcinogens to final carcinogens could facilitate lung tumorigenesis by saturating the DNA repair mechanisms and thus altering tumor suppressor genes. Besides bioactivation of carcinogen, induction of CYPs by β-carotene or its oxidative cleavage products may also destroy inherent retinoic acid level, thereby enhancing lung carcinogenesis (Fig. 4.1). We carried out a study to test whether the destruction of retinoic acid in the ferret lung after smoke alone or after high dose β-carotene (with or without smoke) treatment is due to CYP induction involving in the destruction of retinoic acid (Liu et al. 2003a, b). Using retinoic acid as the substrate, we found that the formation of the polar metabolites including 18-hydroxy-retinoic acid and 4-oxo-retinoic acid increased 6–10-fold after incubation with smoke-exposed, high dose β-carotene supplemented, or both treated ferret lung microsomes, as compared with the controls. Furthermore, this enhanced retinoic acid catabolism was substantially (~80%) inhibited by non-specific CYPs inhibitors (disulfiram and liarozole), but were partially (~50%) inhibited by resveratrol (CYP1A1 inhibitor), α-naphthoflavone (CYP1A2 inhibitor) and antibodies against CYP1A1 and CYP1A2. Cigarette smoke-exposure and/or pharmacological dose of β-carotene increased levels of CYP1A1 and 1A2 by 3–6 folds but not levels of 2E1 and 3A1 in ferret lung tissue. These findings suggest that low levels of RA in the lung of ferrets exposed to cigarette smoke and/or high dose of β-carotene may be caused by the enhanced retinoic acid catabolism *via* induction of CYPs (e.g. CYP1A1/1A2), which provides a possible explanation for enhanced lung carcinogenesis seen with pharmacological dose of β-carotene supplementation in cigarette smokers.

4.3.2.3 Enhancement of Carcinogen Binding to DNA

Several reports have appeared pertaining to the question of whether intact β-carotene or its metabolites can act as co-carcinogens. Carcinogenic metabolites of benzo[*a*]pyrene, can bind to DNA and form DNA adducts, thereby damaging DNA (Hecht et al. 1999). Salgo et al. reported that β-carotene decreases the binding of metabolites of benzo[*a*]pyrene (one of the most important smoke-borne carcinogens) to DNA, whereas the HPLC fractions containing β-carotene oxidative metabolites facilitate the binding of metabolites of benzo[*a*]pyrene to DNA (Salgo et al. 1999). Although the oxidative metabolites were not identified, this study provided a basis for the possible mechanism(s) for a harmful effect of the combination of smoking and β-carotene supplementation on initiation of carcinogenesis. Perocco et al., showed that induction of BALB/c 3T3 cell transformation by benzo[*a*]pyrene was markedly increased by the presence of β-carotene, although it is not clear whether the enhancement of cell transforming activity was due to β-carotene itself or to its metabolites (Perocco et al. 1999). Recently, it has been shown hat oxidative products/metabolites of β-carotene impair mitochondrial functions (Siems et al. 2005) and enhanced inflammation-induced oxidative DNA damage (Sommerburg et al. 2003; van Helden et al. 2009). In general, these studies indicate that β-carotene itself can act as an anticarcinogen, but its oxidized products may facilitate carcinogenesis (Fig. 4.1).

4.4 Other Carotenoids and Effects on Carcinogenesis

4.4.1 α-Carotene

Several studies showed that α-carotene possesses higher activity than β-carotene to suppress the tumorigenesis in skin, lung, liver and colon (Murakoshi et al. 1992; Narisawa et al. 1996). In skin tumorigenesis experiment (Murakoshi et al. 1992), the percentage of tumor-bearing mice in the control group was 69%, whereas the percentages of tumor-bearing mice in the groups treated with α- and β-carotene were 25 and 31%, respectively. The average number of tumors per mouse in the control group was 3.7, whereas the α-carotene-treated group had 0.3 tumors per mouse ($p < 0.01$, Student's *t*-test). β-Carotene treatment also decreased the average number of tumors per mouse (2.9 tumors per mouse), but the difference from the control group was not significant. The higher potency of α-carotene than β-carotene in the suppression of tumor promotion was further confirmed in this study. For example, in 4-nitroquinoline 1-oxide (4NQO)-initiated and glycerol-promoted mouse lung carcinogenesis model, the average number of tumors per mouse in the control group was 4.1, whereas the α-carotene treated group had 1.3 tumors per mouse ($p < 0.001$). β-Carotene treatment did not show any suppressive effect on the average number of tumors per mouse, but rather induced slight increase (4.9 tumors per mouse). In liver carcinogenesis experiment (Murakoshi et al. 1992), C3H/He mice, which have a high incidence of spontaneous liver tumor development, were treated for 40 weeks with α- and β-carotene (at the concentration of 0.05%, mixed as an emulsion into drinking water) or vehicle as a control. The mean number of hepatomas was significantly decreased by α-carotene treatment as compared with that in the control group; the control group developed 6.3 tumors per mouse, whereas the α-carotene-treated group had 3.0 tumors per mouse ($p < 0.001$). On the other hand, the β-carotene-treated group only showed a tendency toward a decrease of tumors, as compared with the control group (Murakoshi et al. 1992).

4.4.2 Lutein

The structures of lutein is characterized by the presence of a hydroxyl group attached to each of the 2 terminal β-ionone rings in the molecules (Fig. 4.1); these xanthophylls are more hydrophilic than other carotenoids and allow them to react with singlet oxygen generated in water phase more efficiently than nonpolar carotenoids (Ojima et al. 1993). Research involving animal models and human studies has been directed to the potential role of lutein in protecting against several chronic diseases particularly visual disease and cancer. In humans plasma lutein has been inversely associated with Cytochrome CYP1A2 activity, a hepatic enzyme responsible for the metabolic activation of a number of putative human carcinogens (Le Marchand et al. 1997). In contrast to β-carotene, data from ATBC trail reported that men in highest quintile of lutein plus zeaxanthin intake at baseline had a 17% lower risk of lung cancer (OR: 0.83; 95% CI: 0.71–0.99; P-trend = 0.006) (Holick et al. 2002) compared to men in the lowest quintile of lutein plus zeaxanthin intake. In a population based case-control study involving 332 lung cancer cases and 865 controls, Le Marchand et al. reported a significant dose-dependent inverse association for dietary lutein and risk of lung cancer (Le Marchand et al. 1993). Prospective cohort studies also reported that lung cancer risk was significantly increased in those with lowest quartile of lutein and zeaxanthin intake at study enrollment (Ziegler et al. 1996; Voorrips et al. 2000). In addition, the lower dietary lutein intake is also inversely related the risk for breast cancer, prostate cancer, colorectal cancer and gastric cancer (Albanes et al. 1996; Zhang et al. 1999; Cohen et al. 2000). In animal models of colon (Narisawa et al. 1996) and breast (Park et al. 1998) cancers lutein has been demonstrated to exhibit chemopreventive activity. The mechanisms for a potential protective role of lutein against carcinogenesis may include selective modulation of apoptosis (Muller et al. 2002), inhibition of angiogenesis (Chew et al. 2003), enhance of gap junctional intercellular communication (Zhang et al. 1991), induction of cell differentiation (Gross et al. 1997) and modulation of immune system (Jyonouchi et al. 1994).

4.4.3 Zeaxanthin

Zeaxanthin is dihydroxy-form of β-carotene (Fig. 4.1), and distributed in our daily foods, such as corn and various vegetables. Since awareness of zeaxanthin as a beneficial carotenoid is achieved recently, available data for zeaxanthin are little. Recently, some features of zeaxanthin were elucidated. For example, zeaxanthin suppressed TPA induced expression of early antigen of Epstein–Barr virus in Raji cells (Nishino et al. 2002). Anti-carcinogenic activity of zeaxanthin in vivo was also examined. For example, it was found that spontaneous liver carcinogenesis in C3H/He male mice was suppressed by the treatment with zeaxanthin (at the concentration of 0.005%, mixed as an emulsion with drinking water) (Nishino et al. 2002).

4.4.4 β-Cryptoxanthin

Recently, several epidemiological studies have brought attention to β-cryptoxanthin for its potential benefits against lung cancer (Yuan et al. 2001, 2003; Mannisto et al. 2004). In 2 cohort studies involving Chinese populations, among all carotenoids examined, only serum levels of β-cryptoxanthin or the dietary intake of β-cryptoxanthin were significantly associated with a reduced risk of lung cancer. Similarly, in a pooled analysis of data from 7 large cohorts in North America and Europe involving 3,155 incident cases of lung cancer, β-cryptoxanthin was the only dietary carotenoid found to be significantly associated with a reduction of lung cancer risk (RR 5 0.76, 0.67–0.86, the highest vs. the lowest quintile). Data from our lab (Lian et al. 2006) found that β-cryptoxanthin inhibited the growth of a premalignant human bronchial epithelial BEAS-2B cells, which was associated with a decrease of cells in S phase, lowered protein levels of cyclin D and cyclin E, and increased levels of the cell cycle inhibitor p21, without inducing apoptosis, indicating that the growth inhibitory effect of β-cryptoxanthin is predominantly through the inhibition of cell proliferation. Our observation further suggests that β-cryptoxanthin may function as a cancer preventive agent in the earlier promotion stage rather than in the later progression stage of carcinogenesis. In the present study, we show that the treatment with β-cryptoxanthin significantly increased the levels of RARβ mRNA in BEAS-2B cells. The effect of β-cryptoxanthin is, in part, due to the transactivation of RARs, supported by our further observation that β-cryptoxanthin dramatically increased RARE-dependent promoter activity in cells co-transfected with RAR expression vector.

Recent study demonstrate that cancer-preventive effects of β-cryptoxanthin may depend on the enhancement of DNA repair as well as antioxidant protection against damage (Lorenzo et al. 2009). At low concentrations, close to those found in plasma, β-cryptoxanthin protects transformed human cells (HeLa and Caco-2) from damage induced by H_2O_2 or by visible light in the presence of a photosensitizer. In addition, it has a striking effect on two kinds of DNA repair-SB rejoining and excision repair of oxidized bases (Lorenzo et al. 2009).

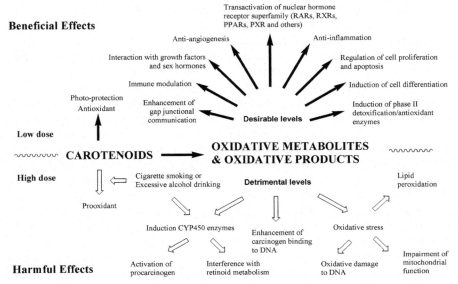

Fig. 4.3 Schematic illustration of beneficial and detrimental effects of carotenoids on human health, including possible mechanisms related to carotenoid dose and oxidative metabolite formation. The biological activities of carotenoids could be related to the function of intact carotenoids or their metabolic products, which can possess either more or less activity than their parent compounds, or have entirely different functions. It appears that while small quantities of carotenoids can offer protection against certain cancers and chronic diseases related to free radical oxidation, larger amounts of carotenoid metabolites may actually be harmful, especially when coupled with a highly oxidative environment, such as the lungs of a cigarette smoker or liver of an excessive alcohol drinker. Oxidative destruction of beta-carotene results in the formation of metabolites that may facilitate the carcinogenic process. Strong interactions among beta-carotene, vitamin E, and vitamin C, and the capability of these compounds to 'recycle' each other or antioxidant 'network', regenerating efficient antioxidants from their radical cations, have led researchers to speculate about the potential utility of combined antioxidant therapy in vivo. It is possible that this additional protection against oxidative degradation may increase the utility of nutritional interventions targeting lung cancer in smoke-exposed models, surpassing effects seen in single-agent intervention studies. The combination of carotenoids and other antioxidants, such as vitamins E and C, which provide complementary or synergistic protective effects, would be a valuable strategy against cancer risk. Figure adapted from Wang (2004)

4.5 Conclusions

Beneficial effects of carotenoid-rich vegetables and fruits on cancer risk have been found in many epidemiological studies; however, the metabolism and molecular biological properties of carotenoids remain to be determined through further research. In considering the efficacy and complex biological functions of carotenoids in human lung cancer prevention, it seems that provitamin A carotenoids (β-carotene, α-carotene, and β-cryptoxanthin) combined with other antioxidants (ascorbic acid, α-tocopherol, and lycopene), which limit oxidative cleavage products of carotenoids formed in large quantities in the highly oxidative conditions of the smoke-exposed lung and enhance retinoid signaling by blocking the activation of MAPK, would be a chemopreventive strategy against certain cancers.

However, there appear to be detrimental interactions between beta-carotene, cigarette smoke, and alcohol, and the molecular mechanisms that underlie these interactions need to be understood before β-carotene can be further pursued in the prevention of carcinogenesis in humans. As we await a better scientific understanding of carotenoid metabolism and mechanisms of action, a prudent strategy to reduce the risk of cancer incidence and mortality would include increased consumption of vegetables and fruits as a part of a healthy, balanced diet, such as eating between five to nine servings of fruits and vegetables every day. There is currently no evidence of any dangers associated with high levels of dietary beta-carotene from natural food sources, aside from the occasional appearance of carotenodermia, an accumulation of β-carotene in the skin that gives it a yellow or orange tint. At this time, supplemental doses of β-carotene beyond the recommended dietary intake to meet vitamin A needs are not advisable for the general population. Smokers and alcohol drinkers are especially encouraged to avoid high doses of supplemental β-carotene.

References

Al-Wadei HA, Schuller HM (2009) beta-Carotene promotes the development of NNK-induced small airway-derived lung adenocarcinoma. Eur J Cancer 45:1257–1264

Albanes D, Heinonen OP et al (1996) Alpha-Tocopherol and beta-carotene supplements and lung cancer incidence in the alpha-tocopherol, beta-carotene cancer prevention study: effects of base-line characteristics and study compliance. J Natl Cancer Inst 88: 1560–1570

Altucci L, Gronemeyer H (2001) The promise of retinoids to fight against cancer. Nat Rev Cancer 1:181–193

Arora A, Willhite CA et al (2001) Interactions of beta-carotene and cigarette smoke in human bronchial epithelial cells. Carcinogenesis 22:1173–1178

Astley SB, Elliott RM et al (2004) Evidence that dietary supplementation with carotenoids and carotenoid-rich foods modulates the DNA damage: repair balance in human lymphocytes. Br J Nutr 91:63–72

Bartsch H, Hietanen E (1996) The role of individual susceptibility in cancer burden related to environmental exposure. Environ Health Perspect 104(Suppl 3):569–577

Bohm F, Edge R et al (1998) Beta-carotene with vitamins E and C offers synergistic cell protection against NOx. FEBS Lett 436: 387–389

Britton G (1995) Structure and properties of carotenoids in relation to function. FASEB J 9: 1551–1558

Castenmiller JJ, Lauridsen ST et al (1999) beta-carotene does not change markers of enzymatic and nonenzymatic antioxidant activity in human blood. J Nutr 129:2162–2169

Chew BP, Brown CM et al (2003) Dietary lutein inhibits mouse mammary tumor growth by regulating angiogenesis and apoptosis. Anticancer Res 23:3333–3339

Cohen JH, Kristal AR et al (2000) Fruit and vegetable intakes and prostate cancer risk. J Natl Cancer Inst 92:61–68

Correa P, Fontham ET et al (2000) Chemoprevention of gastric dysplasia: randomized trial of antioxidant supplements and anti-helicobacter pylori therapy. J Natl Cancer Inst 92:1881–1888

During A, Harrison EH (2004) Intestinal absorption and metabolism of carotenoids: insights from cell culture. Arch Biochem Biophys 430:77–88

During A, Hussain MM et al (2002) Carotenoid uptake and secretion by CaCo-2 cells: beta-carotene isomer selectivity and carotenoid interactions. J Lipid Res 43:1086–1095

Enger SM, Longnecker MP et al (1996) Dietary intake of specific carotenoids and vitamins A, C, and E, and prevalence of colorectal adenomas. Cancer Epidemiol Biomarkers Prev 5: 147–153

Ervin RB, Wright JD, Wang CY, Kennedy-Stephenson J (2004) Dietary intake of selected vitamins for the United States population: 1999–2000. Advance data from vital and health statistics; no. 339. National Center for Health Statistics, Hyattsville, MD

Fabiani R, De Bartolomeo A et al (2001) Antioxidants prevent the lymphocyte DNA damage induced by PMA-stimulated monocytes. Nutr Cancer 39:284–291

Ferrucci L, Perry JR et al (2009) Common variation in the beta-carotene 15,15′-monooxygenase 1 gene affects circulating levels of carotenoids: a genome-wide association study. Am J Hum Genet 84:123–133

Fuster A, Pico C et al (2008) Effects of 6-month daily supplementation with oral beta-carotene in combination or not with benzo[a]pyrene on cell-cycle markers in the lung of ferrets. J Nutr Biochem 19:295–304

Gartner C, Stahl W et al (1997) Lycopene is more bioavailable from tomato paste than from fresh tomatoes. Am J Clin Nutr 66:116–122

Goodman DS, Huang HS (1965) Biosynthesis of vitamin a with rat intestinal enzymes. Science 149:879–880

Gradelet S, Leclerc J et al. (1996) beta-Apo-8′-carotenal, but not beta-carotene, is a strong inducer of liver cytochromes P4501A1 and 1A2 in rat. Xenobiotica 26:909–919

Gross MD, Bishop TD et al (1997) Induction of HL-60 cell differentiation by carotenoids. Nutr Cancer 27:169–173

Hecht SS, Kenney PM et al (1999) Evaluation of butylated hydroxyanisole, myo-inositol, curcumin, esculetin, resveratrol and lycopene as inhibitors of benzo[a]pyrene plus 4-(methylnitrosamino)-1-(3-pyridyl)-1-butanone-induced lung tumorigenesis in A/J mice. Cancer Lett 137:123–130

Hennekens CH, Buring JE et al (1996) Lack of effect of long-term supplementation with beta carotene on the incidence of malignant neoplasms and cardiovascular disease. N Engl J Med 334:1145–1149

Hieber AD, King TJ et al (2000) Comparative effects of all-trans beta-carotene vs. 9-cis beta-carotene on carcinogen-induced neoplastic transformation and connexin 43 expression in murine 10T1/2 cells and on the differentiation of human keratinocytes. Nutr Cancer 37:234–244

Holick CN, Michaud DS et al (2002) Dietary carotenoids, serum beta-carotene, and retinol and risk of lung cancer in the alpha-tocopherol, beta-carotene cohort study. Am J Epidemiol 156: 536–547

Howard DJ, Ota RB et al (1998) Oxidative stress induced by environmental tobacco smoke in the workplace is mitigated by antioxidant supplementation. Cancer Epidemiol Biomarkers Prev 7:981–988

Hu KQ, Liu C et al (2006) The biochemical characterization of ferret carotene-9′,10′-monooxygenase catalyzing cleavage of carotenoids in vitro and in vivo. J Biol Chem 281:19327–19338.

Jyonouchi H, Zhang L et al (1994) Immunomodulating actions of carotenoids: enhancement of in vivo and in vitro antibody production to T-dependent antigens. Nutr Cancer 21:47–58

Khachik F, Beecher GR et al (1991) Separation, identification, and quantification of carotenoids in fruits, vegetables and human plasma by high performance liquid chromatography. Pure Appl Chem 63:71–80

Kiefer C, Hessel S et al (2001) Identification and characterization of a mammalian enzyme catalyzing the asymmetric oxidative cleavage of provitamin A. J Biol Chem 276: 14110–14116

Kim Y, Chongviriyaphan N et al (2006) Combined antioxidant (beta-carotene, alpha-tocopherol and ascorbic acid) supplementation increases the levels of lung retinoic acid and inhibits the activation of mitogen-activated protein kinase in the ferret lung cancer model. Carcinogenesis 27:1410–1419

Kim Y, Lian F et al (2007) The effects of combined antioxidant (beta-carotene, alpha-tocopherol and ascorbic acid) supplementation on antioxidant capacity, DNA single-strand breaks and levels of insulin-like growth factor-1/IGF-binding protein 3 in the ferret model of lung cancer. Int J Cancer 120:1847–1854

Kozuki Y, Miura Y et al (2000) Inhibitory effects of carotenoids on the invasion of rat ascites hepatoma cells in culture. Cancer Lett 151:111–115

Krinsky NI (1991) Effects of carotenoids in cellular and animal systems. Am J Clin Nutr 53(1 Suppl):238S–246S

Lakshmanan MR, Pope JL et al (1968) The specificity of a partially purified carotenoid cleavage enzyme of rabbit intestine. Biochem Biophys Res Commun 33:347–352

Le Marchand L, Franke AA et al (1997) Lifestyle and nutritional correlates of cytochrome CYP1A2 activity: inverse associations with plasma lutein and alpha-tocopherol. Pharmacogenetics 7:11–19

Le Marchand L, Hankin JH et al (1993) Intake of specific carotenoids and lung cancer risk. Cancer Epidemiol Biomarkers Prev 2:183–187

Lee CM, Boileau AC et al (1999a) Review of animal models in carotenoid research. J Nutr 129:2271–2277

Lee IM, Cook NR et al (1999b) Beta-carotene supplementation and incidence of cancer and cardiovascular disease: the Women's Health Study. J Natl Cancer Inst 91: 2102–2106

Leung WC, Hessel S et al (2009) Two common single nucleotide polymorphisms in the gene encoding beta-carotene 15,15′-monoxygenase alter beta-carotene metabolism in female volunteers. FASEB J 23:1041–1053

Lian F, Hu KQ et al (2006) Beta-cryptoxanthin suppresses the growth of immortalized human bronchial epithelial cells and non-small-cell lung cancer cells and up-regulates retinoic acid receptor beta expression. Int J Cancer 119:2084–2089

Liu C, Lian F et al (2003a) Lycopene supplementation inhibits lung squamous metaplasia and induces apoptosis via up-regulating insulin-like growth factor-binding protein 3 in cigarette smoke-exposed ferrets. Cancer Res 63:3138–3144

Liu C, Russell RM et al (2003b) Exposing ferrets to cigarette smoke and a pharmacological dose of beta-carotene supplementation enhance in vitro retinoic acid catabolism in lungs via induction of cytochrome P450 enzymes. J Nutr 133:173–179

Liu C, Wang XD et al (1997) Biosynthesis of retinoic acid from β-apo-14′-carotenal in ferret in vivo. J Nutr Biochem 8:652–657

Liu C, Wang XD et al (2000) Effects of physiological versus pharmacological beta-carotene supplementation on cell proliferation and histopathological changes in the lungs of cigarette smoke-exposed ferrets. Carcinogenesis 21:2245–2253

Liu C, Wang XD et al (2009) Modulation of lung molecular biomarkers by beta-carotene in the Physicians' Health Study. Cancer 115:1049–1058

Lorenzo Y, Azqueta A et al (2009) The carotenoid beta-cryptoxanthin stimulates the repair of DNA oxidation damage in addition to acting as an antioxidant in human cells. Carcinogenesis 30:308–314

Lowe GM, Booth LA et al (1999) Lycopene and beta-carotene protect against oxidative damage in HT29 cells at low concentrations but rapidly lose this capacity at higher doses. Free Radic Res 30:141–151

Mannisto S, Smith-Warner SA et al (2004) Dietary carotenoids and risk of lung cancer in a pooled analysis of seven cohort studies. Cancer Epidemiol Biomarkers Prev 13:40–48

Mayne ST, Risch HA et al (2001) Nutrient intake and risk of subtypes of esophageal and gastric cancer. Cancer Epidemiol Biomarkers Prev 10:1055–1062

Mein J, Lian F, Wang XD (2008) Biological activity of lycopene metabolites: implications for cancer prevention. Nutr Rev 66:667–683

Meraji S, Ziouzenkova O et al (1997) Enhanced plasma level of lipid peroxidation in Iranians could be improved by antioxidants supplementation. Eur J Clin Nutr 51:318–325

Mernitz H, Wang XD (2007) The bioconversion of carotenoids into retinoids: implications for cancer prevention. In: Loessing IT (ed) Vitamin A: new research. Karger Press, New York, NY, pp 39–57

Merriman RL, Bertram JS (1979) Reversible inhibition by retinoids of 3-methylcholanthrene-induced neoplastic transformation in C3H/10T1/2 clone 8 cells. Cancer Res 39:1661–1666

Muller K, Carpenter KL et al (2002) Carotenoids induce apoptosis in the T-lymphoblast cell line Jurkat E6.1. Free Radic Res 36:791–802

Murakoshi M, Nishino H et al (1992) Potent preventive action of alpha-carotene against carcinogenesis: spontaneous liver carcinogenesis and promoting stage of lung and skin carcinogenesis in mice are suppressed more effectively by alpha-carotene than by beta-carotene. Cancer Res 52:6583–6587

Muto Y, Fujii J et al (1995) Growth retardation in human cervical dysplasia-derived cell lines by beta-carotene through down-regulation of epidermal growth factor receptor. Am J Clin Nutr 62(6 Suppl):1535S–1540S

Narisawa T, Fukaura Y et al (1996) Inhibitory effects of natural carotenoids, alpha-carotene, beta-carotene, lycopene and lutein, on colonic aberrant crypt foci formation in rats. Cancer Lett 107:137–142

Nierenberg DW, Stukel TA et al (1991) Determinants of increase in plasma concentration of beta-carotene after chronic oral supplementation. The skin cancer prevention study group. Am J Clin Nutr 53:1443–1449

Nishino H, Murakosh M et al (2002) Carotenoids in cancer chemoprevention. Cancer Metastasis Rev 21:257–264

Obermueller-Jevic UC, Espiritu I et al (2002) Lung tumor development in mice exposed to tobacco smoke and fed beta-carotene diets. Toxicol Sci 69:23–29

Obermuller-Jevic U, Francz PI et al (1999) Enhancement of the UVA induction of haem oxygenase-1 expression by beta-carotene in human skin fibroblasts. FEBS Lett 460:212–216

Ojima F, Sakamoto H et al (1993) Consumption of carotenoids in photosensitized oxidation of human plasma and plasma low-density lipoprotein. Free Radic Biol Med 15:377–384

Olson JA, Hayaishi O (1965) The enzymatic cleavage of beta-carotene into vitamin A by soluble enzymes of rat liver and intestine. Proc Natl Acad Sci USA 54:1364–1370

Omenn GS, Goodman GE et al (1996) Effects of a combination of beta carotene and vitamin A on lung cancer and cardiovascular disease. N Engl J Med 334:1150–1155

Palozza P, Calviello G et al (2000) Canthaxanthin supplementation alters antioxidant enzymes and iron concentration in liver of Balb/c mice. J Nutr 130:1303–1308

Palozza P, Calviello G et al (2001) beta-carotene at high concentrations induces apoptosis by enhancing oxy-radical production in human adenocarcinoma cells. Free Radic Biol Med 30:1000–1007

Palozza P, Krinsky NI (1992) beta-Carotene and alpha-tocopherol are synergistic antioxidants. Arch Biochem Biophys 297:184–187

Palozza P, Serini S et al (2002a) Induction of cell cycle arrest and apoptosis in human colon adenocarcinoma cell lines by beta-carotene through down-regulation of cyclin A and Bcl-2 family proteins. Carcinogenesis 23:11–18

Palozza P, Serini S et al (2002b) Regulation of cell cycle progression and apoptosis by beta-carotene in undifferentiated and differentiated HL-60 leukemia cells: possible involvement of a redox mechanism. Int J Cancer 97:593–600

Palozza P, Serini S et al (2003a) Mechanism of activation of caspase cascade during beta-carotene-induced apoptosis in human tumor cells. Nutr Cancer 47:76–87

Palozza P, Serini S et al (2003b) Beta-carotene regulates NF-kappaB DNA-binding activity by a redox mechanism in human leukemia and colon adenocarcinoma cells. J Nutr 133:381–388

Paolini M, Antelli A et al (2001) Induction of cytochrome P450 enzymes and over-generation of oxygen radicals in beta-carotene supplemented rats. Carcinogenesis 22:1483–1495

Park JS, Chew BP et al (1998) Dietary lutein from marigold extract inhibits mammary tumor development in BALB/c mice. J Nutr 128:1650–1656

Parker RS (1996) Absorption, metabolism, and transport of carotenoids. FASEB J 10:542–551

Parker RS (1997) Bioavailability of carotenoids. Eur J Clin Nutr 51(Suppl 1):S86–S90

Perocco P, Paolini M et al (1999) beta-carotene as enhancer of cell transforming activity of powerful carcinogens and cigarette-smoke condensate on BALB/c 3T3 cells in vitro. Mutat Res 440:83–90

Ponnamperuma RM, Shimizu Y et al (2000) beta-Carotene fails to act as a tumor promoter, induces RAR expression, and prevents carcinoma formation in a two-stage model of skin carcinogenesis in male Sencar mice. Nutr Cancer 37:82–88

Prakash P, Liu C et al (2004) Beta-carotene and beta-apo-14'-carotenoic acid prevent the reduction of retinoic acid receptor beta in benzo[a]pyrene-treated normal human bronchial epithelial cells. J Nutr 134:667–673

Prince MR, Frisoli JK (1993) Beta-carotene accumulation in serum and skin. Am J Clin Nutr 57:175–181

Qiao YL, Dawsey SM et al (2009) Total and cancer mortality after supplementation with vitamins and minerals: follow-up of the Linxian General Population Nutrition Intervention Trial. J Natl Cancer Inst 101:507–518

Rao AV, Rao LG (2007) Carotenoids and human health. Pharmacol Res 55:207–216

Salgo MG, Cueto R et al (1999) Beta carotene and its oxidation products have different effects on microsome mediated binding of benzo[a]pyrene to DNA. Free Radic Biol Med 26:162–173

Satia JA, Littman A et al (2009) Long-term use of beta-carotene, retinol, lycopene, and lutein supplements and lung cancer risk: results from the VITamins And Lifestyle (VITAL) study. Am J Epidemiol 169:815–828

Schectman G, Byrd JC et al. (1989) The influence of smoking on vitamin C status in adults. Am J Public Health 79:158–162

Schmitz HH, Poor CL et al (1991) Concentrations of selected carotenoids and vitamin A in human liver, kidney and lung tissue. J Nutr 121:1613–1621

Schwartz JL, Singh RP et al (1990) Induction of a 70 kD protein associated with the selective cytotoxicity of beta-carotene in human epidermal carcinoma. Biochem Biophys Res Commun 169:941–946

Sesso HD, Gaziano JM (2004) Heart and vascular diseases. Marcel Dekker, New York, NY

Siems W, Wiswedel I et al (2005) Beta-carotene breakdown products may impair mitochondrial functions – -potential side effects of high-dose beta-carotene supplementation. J Nutr Biochem 16:385–397

Sommerburg O, Langhans CD et al (2003) Beta-carotene cleavage products after oxidation mediated by hypochlorous acid – a model for neutrophil-derived degradation. Free Radic Biol Med 35:1480–1490

Stivala LA, Savio M et al (2000) The antiproliferative effect of beta-carotene requires p21waf1/cip1 in normal human fibroblasts. Eur J Biochem 267:2290–2296

Thompson CB (1995) Apoptosis in the pathogenesis and treatment of disease. Science 267:1456–1462

van Helden YG, Keijer J et al (2009) Beta-carotene metabolites enhance inflammation-induced oxidative DNA damage in lung epithelial cells. Free Radic Biol Med 46:299–304

van Poppel G, Goldbohm RA (1995) Epidemiologic evidence for beta-carotene and cancer prevention. Am J Clin Nutr 62(6 Suppl):1393S–1402S

von Lintig J, Vogt K (2000) Filling the gap in vitamin A research. Molecular identification of an enzyme cleaving beta-carotene to retinal. J Biol Chem 275:11915–11920

Voorrips LE, Goldbohm RA et al (2000) A prospective cohort study on antioxidant and folate intake and male lung cancer risk. Cancer Epidemiol Biomarkers Prev 9:357–365

Wang XD (1994) Review: absorption and metabolism of beta-carotene. J Am Coll Nutr 13: 314–325

Wang XD (2004) Carotenoid oxidative/decompositive products and their biological activities. In: Krinsky NI, Mayne ST, Sies H (eds) Carotenoids in health and disease. Marcel Dekker, New York, NY, pp 313–335

Wang XD, Krinsky NI (1998) The bioconversion of beta-carotene into retinoids. Subcell Biochem 30:159–180

Wang XD, Krinsky NI et al (1992) Retinoic acid can be produced from excentric cleavage of beta-carotene in human intestinal mucosa. Arch Biochem Biophys 293:298–304

Wang XD, Marini RP et al (1995) Vitamin E enhances the lymphatic transport of beta-carotene and its conversion to vitamin A in the ferret. Gastroenterology 108:719–726

Wang XD, Russell RM (1999) Procarcinogenic and anticarcinogenic effects of beta-carotene. Nutr Rev 57:263–272

Wang XD, Russell RM et al (1996) Beta-oxidation in rabbit liver in vitro and in the perfused ferret liver contributes to retinoic acid biosynthesis from beta-apocarotenoic acids. J Biol Chem 271:26490–26498

Wang XD, Tang GW et al (1991) Enzymatic conversion of beta-carotene into beta-apo-carotenals and retinoids by human, monkey, ferret, and rat tissues. Arch Biochem Biophys 285:8–16

Wyss A, Wirtz G et al (2000) Cloning and expression of beta,beta-carotene 15,15′-dioxygenase. Biochem Biophys Res Commun 271:334–336

Yeh SL, Hu ML (2003) Oxidized beta-carotene inhibits gap junction intercellular communication in the human lung adenocarcinoma cell line A549. Food Chem Toxicol 41:1677–1684

Yuan JM, Ross RK et al (2001) Prediagnostic levels of serum beta-cryptoxanthin and retinol predict smoking-related lung cancer risk in Shanghai, China. Cancer Epidemiol Biomarkers Prev 10:767–773

Yuan JM, Stram DO et al (2003) Dietary cryptoxanthin and reduced risk of lung cancer: the Singapore Chinese Health Study. Cancer Epidemiol Biomarkers Prev 12:890–898

Zhang LX, Cooney RV et al (1991) Carotenoids enhance gap junctional communication and inhibit lipid peroxidation in C3H/10T1/2 cells: relationship to their cancer chemopreventive action. Carcinogenesis 12:2109–2114

Zhang P, Omaye ST (2000) Beta-carotene and protein oxidation: effects of ascorbic acid and alpha-tocopherol. Toxicology 146:37–47

Zhang P, Omaye ST (2001a, b) Antioxidant and prooxidant roles for beta-carotene, alpha-tocopherol and ascorbic acid in human lung cells. Toxicol In Vitro 15:13–24

Zhang P, Omaye ST (2001a, b) beta-Carotene: interactions with alpha-tocopherol and ascorbic acid in microsomal lipid peroxidation. J Nutr Biochem 12:38–45

Zhang S, Hunter DJ et al (1999) Dietary carotenoids and vitamins A, C, and E and risk of breast cancer. J Natl Cancer Inst 91:547–556

Ziegler RG (1989) A review of epidemiologic evidence that carotenoids reduce the risk of cancer. J Nutr 119:116–122

Ziegler RG, Colavito EA et al (1996) Importance of alpha-carotene, beta-carotene, and other phytochemicals in the etiology of lung cancer. J Natl Cancer Inst 88:612–615

Chapter 5
The Role of Alliums and their Sulfur and Selenium Constituents in Cancer Prevention

Karam El-Bayoumy, Raghu Sinha, Arthur J.L. Cooper, and John T. Pinto

Abstract Garlic and its sulfur and selenium-containing components are widely known for their cancer preventive activities primarily in preclinical in vitro and in vivo model systems. Most of our common foods including garlic contain very low levels of selenium compounds relative to those of sulfur. Humans consume a substantial portion of their dietary sulfur and selenium in organic forms. Selenium-enriched foods such as garlic, broccoli and wheat are more effective chemopreventive agents than the corresponding regular dietary items. Naturally occurring and synthetic organoselenium compounds are superior cancer chemopreventive agents compared to their corresponding sulfur analogs. Mechanistic studies demonstrate that sulfur and selenium compounds are capable of cell growth inhibition, cell cycle arrest, induction of apoptosis, alterations of phase I and phase II enzyme activities, and histone deacetylase (HDAC) inhibition. The fact that organosulfur and organoselenium compounds can target multiple pathways suggests that these agents can be used directly as chemopreventive and/or therapeutic agents or in combination with other medicinal compounds. The effect of these agents on the aforementioned parameters varies depending on the dose and form (structure) and whether cells are normal or transformed. Whether the protective effects observed in animals and in cell cultures can be applicable to humans remain to be determined. Thus, studies using genomic, proteomic, and metabolomic techniques in well designed small-scale clinical trials are needed to unequivocally evaluate the potential of allium vegetable constituents on biomarkers of risk for specific cancers prior to entering into long-term expensive phase III clinical chemoprevention trials.

Keywords Allium vegetable · Organosulfur compounds · Organoselenium compounds · Chemoprevention

K. El-Bayoumy (✉)
Department of Biochemistry and Molecular Biology, Penn State College of Medicine, Penn State Hershey Cancer Institute, Hershey, PA, USA
e-mail: kee2@psu.edu

M. Mutanen, A.-M. Pajari (eds.), *Vegetables, Whole Grains, and Their Derivatives in Cancer Prevention*, Diet and Cancer 2, DOI 10.1007/978-90-481-9800-9_5,
© Springer Science+Business Media B.V. 2011

Contents

5.1 Introduction

Dietary factors are believed to account for about 40% of all human cancers (Doll and Peto 1981; Doll 1992; Hill 1997; Sinha and Potter 1997; Wynder and Gori 1977). The potential health benefits of certain plant based phytonutrients, in particular allium vegetables such as garlic (*Allium sativum*) and onion (*Allium cepa*) have been known since antiquity to affect human health. As early as 1,550 BC, Egyptians had recommended garlic as a remedy for a variety of diseases (Block 1985, 1992; Dausch and Nixon 1990; Nunn 1996). Garlic bulbs have been found in tombs of the Pharaohs, in Crete and in ancient cultures throughout the world. The Bible mentions garlic with regard to the Jews' flight from Egypt and indeed, Hippocrates considered garlic to be a vital part of his therapeutic armamentarium (Rivlin 2001).

Over 2,500 papers have been published on garlic and related allium vegetables; a book entitled 'Growth and Other Alliums-The Lore and the Science' has recently been published by The Royal Society of Chemistry, UK (Block 2009). Garlic contains a large number of potent bioactive organosulfur compounds (OSC) with anticancer properties such as allylsulfide derivatives; in addition it also contains amino acids, vitamins, and nutrients such as selenium containing compounds that will be discussed later in this chapter. Diallylsulfide (DAS), for example, is responsible in part for its strong odor and taste (Amagase 2006). Onion and garlic intakes could be simply considered markers of a healthier life-style, which includes complex aspects of quantity and quality of diet. At least 33 different types of OSC have been identified in garlic and their levels vary with different strains of garlic as well as environmental factors (e.g., climate and use of fertilizers). Structures of OSC discussed here are shown in Table 5.1. In addition to OSC, fresh garlic contains a

Table 5.1   Chemical structures for sulfur and selenium compounds

Alliin	$CH_2=CH-CH_2-S(O)-CH_2-CH(NH_2)-COOH$
Allicin	$CH_2=CH-CH_2-S(O)-S-CH_2-CH=CH_2$
Ajoene	$CH_2=CH-CH_2-S(O)-CH_2-CH=CH-S-S-CH_2-$ $CH=CH_2$
Diallylsulfide	$CH_2=CH-CH_2-S-CH_2-CH=CH_2$
Diallyldisulfide	$CH_2=CH-CH_2-S-S-CH_2-CH=CH_2$
Diallyltrisulfide	$CH_2=CH-CH_2-S-S-S-CH_2-CH=CH_2$
Allylmethyldisulfide	$CH_2=CH-CH_2-S-S-CH_3$
Allylmethyltrisulfide	$CH_2=CH-CH_2-S-S-S-CH_3$
S-Allylcysteine	$CH_2=CH-CH_2-S-CH_2-CH(NH_2)-COOH$
S-Allylmercaptocysteine	$CH_2=CH-CH_2-S-S-CH_2-CH(NH_2)-COOH$
Allylmercaptan	$CH_2=CH-CH_2-S-H$
Allylhydrodisulfide	$CH_2=CH-CH_2-S-S-H$
Se-Methylselenocysteine	$CH_3-Se-CH_2-CH(NH_2)-COOH$
Selenomethionine	$CH_3-Se-CH_2-CH_2CH(NH_2)-COOH$
Methylselenopyruvate	$CH_3-Se-CH_2-C\,(O)-COOH$
Ketomethylselenobutyrate	$CH_3-Se-CH_2-CH_2\,C(O)-COOH$
1,4-Phenylenebis-(methylene)selenocyanate	$N{\equiv}C-Se-CH_2-C_6H_4-CH_2-Se-C{\equiv}N$
Methylseleninic Acid	$CH_3-Se(O)-OH$

variety of organoselenium compounds whose presence and level (15–35 $\mu g/100$ g) depend on soil conditions and likewise contribute to garlic's odor and taste. When garlic is cut, chopped, or crushed, the clove's membrane disrupts and S-allylcysteine (SAC) sulfoxide (alliin) is transformed enzymatically into allicin by allinase (Block 1985). Allicin is responsible for the typical odor of garlic, but is unstable and converts readily into mono-, di-, and tri-sulfides and other compounds such as ajoene. The total allicin yield has been determined as 2.5 mg/g of fresh crushed garlic or about 5–20 mg per clove. Further transformation of OSC can occur after interaction with free sulfhydryl groups such as those present in cysteine, glutathione or proteins (Gilbert 1990; Weisberger and Pensky 1958). Incubation of cysteine with DAS produces allylmercaptan (Lawson and Wang 1993). Allylmethyl sulfide and DAS have been detected in breath of humans after ingestion of garlic (Laakso et al. 1989; Minami et al. 1989).

The potential anticarcinogenic action of onions may be related to their high content of organosulfur, organoselenium compounds as well as flavonoids. However, there are important differences in the composition, concentration, and beneficial activities of these bioactive compounds, which also are affected by cooking (Yang et al. 2004). The primary difference between the OSC in onion and garlic is the presence of a propyl ($CH_3CH_2CH_2-$) moiety attached to sulfur in onion rather than an allyl or 1-propenyl ($CH_2=CHCH_2-$) moiety in garlic.

Although, the known health benefits of allium vegetables constituents include cardiovascular effects, improvement of immune function, lowering blood glucose levels, radioprotection, protection against microbial infection and anticancer effects (Agarwal 1996; Milner 2001; Pelucchi et al. 2009; Rahman 2001; Rivlin 2001), this chapter however, focuses on the anticarcinogenicity. Nevertheless, there are excellent reviews available on the aforementioned health benefits of sulfur and selenium-containing foods (Powolny and Singh 2008; Shukla and Kalra 2007; El-Bayoumy and Sinha 2005).

5.2 Dietary Sources of Sulfur and Selenium Compounds

Both animals and humans consume a major portion of their dietary sulfur and selenium in organic forms. Plants synthesize the sulfur amino acids and their derivatives from sulfite and sulfate in soil. Similarly, plants are also capable of synthesizing selenoamino acids (e.g., selenomethionine (SM), selenocysteine, selenocystathionine and Se-methylselenocysteine (MSC)) from selenite and selenate. The metabolism of selenium compounds in plants has been described previously (Terry et al. 2000; Whanger 1989, 2003, 2004) and is not discussed in this chapter. Several selenium-containing compounds present in selenium-enriched foods have been identified (Whanger 2004). Briefly, SM, the most common organic form of selenium available commercially, is the major form of selenium in selenium-enriched wheat, maize, rice, and yeast. The major form of selenium in selenium-enriched garlic, onions, broccoli florets, broccoli sprouts and wild leeks is MSC (Whanger 2004).

Many foods (grain products, seafood, meat, and poultry) are major sources of selenium (Wolf and Schubert 1989). Seafood accounts for approximately 30% of the dietary selenium intake. Due to low levels of selenium in our common foods, the structural identities of the selenium compounds in food remain largely unknown but due to its properties as a chalcogen, selenium may mimic the chemical forms of organosulfur. As a naturally occurring element, selenium ranks 17th in abundance in the earth's crust. Its geographical distribution varies from high concentration in the soil in certain regions (e.g., certain regions of China, the former USSR, Venezuela, and the mid-western USA) to rather lower levels in New Zealand and Finland. Selenium intakes in most parts of Europe are considerably lower than those in the USA (Rayman 2000). With respect to recommended nutritional requirements and because of the wide distribution of food items grown on selenium rich soils, a sizeable percentage of the US population is not selenium-deficient.

As members of the chalcogen family of elements, sulfur and selenium share similar chemical and physical properties (Whanger 2004). Five common oxidation states of sulfur and selenium are known: -2, 0, $+2$, $+4$ and $+6$. Elemental sulfur (S) and perhaps selenium (Se) are not biologically inert and possess biological activity when formed in situ. For example, at neutral pH, L-thiocystine slowly breaks down to L-cystine and elemental or sulfane sulfur (S^0) which can then form persulfides with endogenous cysteine residues. As discussed later in this chapter, Toohey (1989), and in a recent review Iciek et al. (2009), suggest that several of the known molecular aspects of action of OSC may be mediated by sulfane sulfur-containing compounds or sulfane progenitors. With regard to the higher oxidation states, sulfite and selenite ($+4$) and sulfate and selenate ($+6$) are biologically active forms.

Two features that distinguish selenium from sulfur biological systems are as follows. (1) Sulfur compounds are metabolized to more oxidized states while selenium compounds are metabolized to more reduced states; (2) the hydride derived from selenium (H_2Se) is much more acidic than that derived from sulfur (H_2S); i.e., selenium is a good donor of hydrogen ions and H_2Se is completely ionized at normal blood pH levels. Thus, the lower pKa (5.3 vs. 8.3) of selenocysteine (Cys-SeH) versus cysteine (Cys-SH), respectively and the much greater nucleophilicity of Cys-SeH render selenocysteine catalytically much more reactive than Cys-SH.

Garlic and onion are seleniferous plants and thus have the ability to accumulate and transport selenium as selenite or selenate from the soil. MSC and γ-glutamyl-*Se*-methylselenocysteine are major selenium compounds identified in selenium-enriched garlic and onion; other selenium compounds in selenium-enriched garlic and onion remain to be identified (Arnault and Auger 2006). Future studies should focus on their identification and synthesis so that a larger panel of organoselenium compounds from allium foods could be investigated for their chemopreventive properties.

5.3 Uptake and Bioavailability

5.3.1 Uptake and Bioavailability of Organosulfur Compounds

Whether the biological effective dose of OSC can be achieved in plasma through dietary intake of allium vegetables or via pharmacological intervention with a single agent remains to be determined and thus further research in this area is urgently needed. It has been estimated that one gram of fresh garlic potentially can provide about 900–1,100 μg of diallyltrisulfide (DATS) and 530–610 μg of diallyldisulfide (DADS) (Shukla and Kalra 2007). One gram of freshly blended garlic can provide up to 2.5 mg of allicin and about 60 μg of DATS (Lawson and Gardner 2005). The bioavailability of SAC has been examined in rats, mice and dogs (Nagae et al. 1994). In this study it was documented that SAC was rapidly absorbed in the gastrointestinal tract and distributed in plasma, liver and kidney of these animals; its bioavailability in the rat, mouse and dog was 98.2, 103 and 87.2%, respectively. After a single oral administration of 200 mg/Kg of DADS to rats (Germain et al. 2002), the highest level was observed in the stomach within the first 24 h. An i.v. injection of ten mg DATS to rats resulted in peak blood concentration of about 31 μM (Sun et al. 2006). The metabolism of garlic constituents in the isolated perfused rat liver was examined and it was shown that allicin was very efficiently metabolized into DADS and allyl mercaptan, with DADS being the most likely precursor for allyl mercaptan (Egen-Schwind et al. 1992).

5.3.2 Uptake and Bioavailability of Organoselenium Compounds

Limited forms of selenium are available for use in chemoprevention trials. SM, which was used in the Selenium and Vitamin E Cancer Prevention Trial (SELECT)

(Taylor and Albanes 1998), is synthesized by plants and therefore has been considered to be the major form of selenium in the human diet. Selenium-enriched yeast (SeY), which was used in the study by Clark et al. (1996, 1998), is produced by growing yeast in medium enriched with selenium. The major organoselenium in SeY is SM (60–75%), with other selenium containing compounds making up the difference (Ip et al. 2000a). The effects of different chemical forms of selenium on plasma levels in high-dose supplementation trials in humans have been examined (Burk et al. 2006). Selenium supplements in three dose levels (200, 400, and 600 μg/d) in the forms of sodium selenite, SeY, and SM were administered to subjects (37.1 ± 10.6 year-old) randomized into groups for 16 weeks. No signs of any selenium toxicity (hair loss and nail changes) were observed in this study. While supplementation with SM and SeY were found to raise plasma selenium concentration in a dose-dependent manner, sodium selenite did not (Burk et al. 2006). Plasma selenium concentrations were responsive to the supplements in proportion to their SM contents. Therefore, the authors proposed that increment in plasma selenium concentration during supplementation can be used to assess compliance and to ensure safety of SM supplements during chemoprevention studies; urinary selenium levels were found to be useful for assessing bioavailability. Interestingly, endogenous selenium biomarkers, such as glutathione peroxidase and selenoprotein P, showed no tendency to increase during the study in any of the treatment groups, suggesting that the study subjects were selenium replete as far as nutritional requirements before supplementation was begun.

Typical dietary intakes of selenium in a variety of forms in North America are 80–140 μg/d (El-Bayoumy 2001). The current recommended daily allowance (RDA) for selenium in men is 55 μg/d, which reflects the selenium intake required to achieve maximal plasma glutathione peroxidase activity. But, there is growing consensus that nutritionally adequate selenium intake may be suboptimal with respect to reducing disease risk (Combs and Gray 1998; Waters et al. 2005). Indeed, it has been shown that selenium status sufficient to saturate the activity of plasma glutathione peroxidase did not necessarily minimize prostatic DNA damage in the canine model or prostate cancer risk in men (Waters et al. 2005). Although selenium is known to inhibit DNA damage in canine and rodent models, similar information in human subjects is limited (Karunasighe et al. 2004). In preliminary studies, we showed that SeY inhibited 8-hydroxy-2′-deoxyguanosine (8-OHdG) levels in men less than 40 years of age but the effect was not significant, due in part to limited sample size (El-Bayoumy et al. 2002). Clearly, there is a need to determine the effect of different forms and doses of organoselenium in preventing DNA damage in men older than 40 years of age since oxidative stress increases with age (Klein 2004; Morley and Baumgartner 2004; Ray et al. 2006). In a previous study, women who were enrolled in the Women's Health and Aging Studies I and II in Baltimore, MD ($n =$ 632; 70–79 year-old) who had serum selenium measured at baseline were followed for mortality for over 60 months (Ferrucci et al. 2005). Of the 14.1% of the women who died from five major causes, i.e., heart disease (32.6%), cancer (18.0%), stroke (9.0%), infection (6.7%), and chronic obstructive pulmonary disease (5.6%), women living in the community who maintained higher plasma selenium were at a lower risk of death from the five major causes.

The most frequently used dose (200 μg/d) (Clark et al. 1996; Lippman et al. 2009) of organoselenium in intervention trials has been in the form of SM or SeY. Accordingly, individuals taking such a supplement should not be expected to exceed the safe upper limit of 400 μg/d set by the Institute of Medicine (2000). Higher doses of selenium that might be toxic have also been used in trials (Reid et al. 2004) and regardless of the selenium dose, monitoring for selenium toxicity and compliance is often required.

5.4 Cancer Prevention and the Mechanisms of Action

5.4.1 Comparison of Sulfur and Selenium Analogs in Cancer Prevention

In view of the similarity between the two elements, it was our goal to develop novel synthetic organoselenium analogs of established sulfur-containing chemo-preventive agents to obtain compounds with optimal chemopreventive potency and low toxicity. The rationale for synthesizing these selenium compounds is based on the following concepts: (1) although the known inhibitors of carcinogen-induced neoplasia possess few common structural features, many have functional groups containing oxygen, sulfur, or selenium, all of which are elements of group VI of the periodic table; (2) replacement of oxygen and/or sulfur by selenium is known to modify the biological activity and therapeutic index of certain drugs, a phenomenon known as isosteric effect in drug design. Accordingly, we substituted selenium for oxygen and/or sulfur in known inhibitors of chemical carcinogenesis. The chemo-preventive agents were examined in several animal models and, in some instances, were compared with the historical inorganic selenite, oxygen, and sulfur analogs (El-Bayoumy 1985). To determine whether the substitution of sulfur with selenium in DAS would result in a more potent chemopreventive agent, we synthesized diallyl selenide after modification of the method described earlier (Amosova et al. 1991) and compared its efficacy with that of DAS in the 7,12-dimethylbenz[a]anthracene (DMBA)-induced mammary carcinogenesis model (El-Bayoumy et al. 1996). Rats were gavaged 3 times with diallyl selenide (6 or 12 mmol/ kg body wt) or DAS (300, 900, or 1,800 mmol/kg body wt) at 96, 48, and 24 h before DMBA treat-ment. Both doses of diallyl selenide showed significant tumor inhibition, but only the highest dose of DAS showed inhibition. Based on these results, diallyl selenide appeared to be at least 300 times more active than DAS. Volatile garlic sulfides, as exemplified by DAS, have reportedly modulated activities of cytochrome P450 isozymes, blocked carcinogen activation, and facilitated carcinogen detoxification through increased activities of glutathione S-transferases, epoxide hydrolase, and UDP-glucuronosyl transferase, as well as through induction of glutathione perox-idase. The last effect decreases the ratio of glutathione to glutathione disulfide.

Collectively, these results can account for cancer chemoprevention by DAS in various target organs, including the mammary gland (Wargovich 1987; Wargovich et al. 1988; El-Bayoumy 1994; El-Bayoumy et al. 1996; Dalvi 1992; Pan et al. 1993; Sumiyoshi and Wargovich 1990; Maurya and Singh 1991; Yang et al. 2001; Perchellet et al. 1986; Brady et al. 1991). In line with the effect of DAS on the above-mentioned biochemical parameters, Amagase et al. (1996) showed that garlic, as a whole, suppresses the formation of DMBA-DNA adducts in the mammary gland in vivo; certain dietary components can modulate this effect further. Based on these results, we conducted a biochemical investigation to determine whether diallyl selenide exerts effects similar to those of DAS. We examined the effect of diallyl selenide on the initiation phase of carcinogenesis, i.e., DMBA-DNA adduct formation in rat mammary glands. Analysis of total binding and individual DMBA-DNA adducts in the mammary gland and liver showed that diallyl selenide had no effect on these parameters, suggesting that it might influence critical events in carcinogenesis other than carcinogen activation and/or detoxification. Thus, further research is needed to evaluate whether diallyl selenide is more effective than DAS in eliciting responses such as the inhibition of cell proliferation, diminishing ornithine decarboxylase activity, and/or induction of apoptosis (Knowles and Milner 2001; Hu and Wargovich 1989; Baer and Wargovich 1989). To further support our concept that replacing sulfur with selenium in known chemopreventive agents will result in more effective analogs, we synthesized and compared benzyl selenocyanate (BSC) with benzyl thiocyanate (BTC) in several carcinogen-induced tumor animal models (El-Bayoumy 2001). Briefly, we demonstrated that BSC is superior to BTC as an inhibitor of benzo[a]pyrene-induced forestomach tumors in mice, as well as DMBA-induced mammary tumors and azoxymethane-induced colon tumors in rats (El-Bayoumy 1985; Nayini et al. 1989, 1991). The results of numerous studies conducted in our laboratory, as well as in other laboratories, clearly support the concept described above (El-Bayoumy et al. 2006). In short, selenium-enriched garlic, selenium-enriched yeast, and selenium-enriched broccoli are each more effective cancer chemopreventive agents in various animal models than regular garlic, yeast, and broccoli, respectively (Whanger 2004). In addition to diallyl selenide and BSC, comparative chemopreventive efficacy of selenocystamine, selenobetaine, and 1,4-phenylenebis(methylene)selenocyanate (p-XSC) with their sulfur-containing analogs in vivo has been reported (El-Bayoumy and Sinha 2004; El-Bayoumy et al. 2006). Collectively, the outcome of these studies led to the conclusion that selenium-enriched food items and selenium compounds are more effective than their corresponding sulfur analogs, respectively (Ip et al. 1992; Ip and Lisk 1995; Finley et al. 2001; Ip and Ganther 1992).

5.4.2 Preclinical Efficacy Studies

Numerous studies over the past 20 years have provided convincing evidence that administration of garlic as well as several of its naturally occurring OSC to laboratory animals provides protection against chemically induced carcinogens in various organs (lung, stomach, breast, cervix, oral cavity, colon, liver, esophagus and skin) (Belman 1983; Cohen et al. 1999; Hayes et al. 1987; Hong et al. 1982; Ip et al. 1992; Knowles and Milner 2001; Sadhana et al. 1988; Schaffer et al. 1996; Sparnins et al. 1988; Suzui et al. 1997; Wargovich et al. 1988; Wattenberg et al. 1989; Weisberger and Pensky 1958). Several of these studies indicated that the oil-soluble organosulfur compounds, such as DAS, DATS, and ajoene, were more effective than the water-soluble SAC in reducing the incidence and delaying the onset of N-methyl-N-nitrosourea-induced mammary tumors (Ip et al. 1992; El-Bayoumy et al. 2006). Collectively, preclinical investigations consistently demonstrate that cancer chemoprevention by garlic and several of its OSC is clearly evident and appears to be independent of the organ site or the type of carcinogen employed; several reviews are available on this topic (de Boer et al. 2004; Dwivedi et al. 1992; Hadjiolov et al. 1993; Hussain et al. 1990; Herman-Antosiewicz and Singh 2004; Mori et al. 1999; Morris and Levander 1970; Nishikawa et al. 2002; Reddy et al. 1993; Schaffer et al. 1996; Shukla and Kalra 2007; Singh and Shukla 1998a, b; Singh et al. 2004; Takahashi et al. 1992; Wargovich et al. 1996; Wilpart et al. 1986).

By contrast to organosulfur constituents, most commercially available foods contain lower levels of organoselenium; for example garlic grown in typical soils within the USA contain 0.05–0.35 μg selenium/g of fresh garlic (Medina et al. 2001). The protective role of selenium is supported by numerous epidemiological studies as well as most of the preclinical studies and some but not all clinical chemoprevention intervention trials; this area of research has been reviewed extensively and in general it is evident that the dose and the form (structure) are important factors that determine the chemopreventive efficacy of selenium. We were the first to show that synthetic organoselenium compounds are superior chemopreventive agents to their sulfur analogs (El-Bayoumy 2001; El-Bayoumy and Sinha 2004; Herman-Antosiewicz et al. 2007a; Ip et al. 2002; Sinha and El-Bayoumy 2004; El-Bayoumy et al. 2006).

5.4.3 Mechanisms of Cancer Prevention by Organosulfur Compounds

The underlying mechanisms of the inhibitory effects of allium-derived compounds may involve both the initiation and promotion phases of carcinogenesis. Prevention by OSC can be due in part to its effects on phase I and phase II enzymes that are involved in the metabolism of a variety of chemical carcinogens (Brady et al. 1991; Knowles and Milner 2000; Shukla and Kalra 2007; Wattenberg et al. 1989).

It has also been reported that OSC can halt cell cycle progression in neoplastic cells. For example treatment of human colon cancer cells with DADS resulted in G2/M phase cell cycle arrest (Arunkumar et al. 2006). Sriram et al. (2008) showed that DAS could increase reactive oxygen species (ROS) thus leading to DNA damage and apoptosis with concomitant decrease in cell proliferation in human colon cancer cell (Colo320DM). The apoptotic induction capacity of DAS may be attributed to its ability to activate caspases through the NFκB pathway by increasing the production of ROS. The inhibition of ERK-2 expression by DAS may account for its antiproliferative activity. The effect of two water-soluble constituents of garlic (SAC and S-allylmercaptocysteine [SAMC]) was investigated on proliferation and cell cycle progression in two human colon cancer cell lines (SW480, HT29) (Shirin et al. 2001). In this study, sulindac sulfone (SS), an established colon cancer chemo-preventive agent, was used for comparison. Inhibition of cell growth by SAMC was observed in both cell lines at doses similar to that of SS while SAC had no effect. The induction of apoptosis by SAMC was associated with an increased caspase-3-like activity, induction of jun kinase activity, and a marked increase in endogenous levels of GSH. SAMC inhibited progression at G2/M. Co-administration of SAMC with SS enhanced the growth inhibitory and apoptotic effects of SS. These results suggest that a combination approach of using drugs and dietary constituents may be a highly effective strategy for colon cancer chemoprevention. DATS suppressed the growth and caused G2/M arrest of human colon cancer cells HCT-15 and DLD-1, while DAS and DADS had little or no effect at similar doses (Seki et al. 2008). These studies strongly suggest that the chemical forms of OSC exhibit different chemo-preventive efficacies depending on their sulfur content and reactivity of the sulfur moiety, i.e., thioethers, such as DAS, differ from that of disulfides, such as DADS, which differ from trisulfides such as DATS. Each organosulfur constituent may pos-sess its own intrinsic protective quality when used either singly or in combination such as those found in allium vegetables.

In preclinical model systems, both water- and lipid-soluble allyl sulfur com-pounds arising from processed garlic inhibited formation of aberrant crypt foci (ACF) which are considered precursors to colorectal tumors. However, the response to these allyl sulfur compounds appears to depend on several factors including the speciation, quantity and duration of exposure to these agents (Ross et al. 2006). Clearly there is a need for clinical pilot studies to determine the inhibitory effect of these OSC on ACF in humans. Studies aimed at comparing the relative efficacy of water- and lipid-soluble allyl sulfur compounds suggest little difference in response, whereas tumor proliferation/apoptosis is highly dependent on the species provided (Milner 2006).

Similarly, DADS caused G2/M phase cell cycle arrest in a prostate cancer cell line (PC-3) (Arunkumar et al. 2006), human gastric cancer cell line (MGC803) (Yuan et al. 2004) and lung cancer cell line (A549) (Wu et al. 2005). Using other OSC, Singh and associates elucidated mechanisms of DATS-induced cell cycle arrest in human prostate cancer cells (PC-3, DU145) (Antosiewicz et al. 2006; Herman-Antosiewicz and Singh 2005; Herman-Antosiewicz et al. 2007b; Xiao et al. 2005). This team demonstrated that G2/M arrest mediated by DATS was associated with the generation of ROS-dependent hyperphosphorylation and destruction of the cell division cyclin 25C (cdc25) phosphatase. The effect of DATS on cell cycle arrest appeared to be selective for prostate cancer cells since normal prostatic epithe-lial cells were resistant to cell cycle arrest (Xiao et al. 2005). Singh et al. (2008a) were the first to report that DATS administered by oral gavage inhibits progression to poorly differentiated prostate carcinoma and pulmonary metastasis multiplicity in transgenic adenocarcinoma of mouse prostate (TRAMP) mice. The dorsolateral prostate from DATS-treated TRAMP mice exhibited decreased cellular proliferation in association with induction of cyclin B1 and securin protein levels and suppression of the expression of neuroendocrine marker synaptophysin. DATS, however, had no appreciable effect on apoptosis induction, angiogenesis or natural killer and dendritic cell function. Stan and Singh (2009) showed that DATS treatment also suppresses androgen receptor (AR) function in prostate cancer cells (LNCaP, C4-2, and TRAMP-C1) by decreasing the concentration of AR protein levels, which was accompanied by suppression of intracellular and secreted levels of prostate specific antigen (PSA).

Previous reports have also demonstrated that cell cycle arrest can be achieved by other organosulfur compounds (SAMC, ajoene, allicin) in a variety of cancer cell lines (Xiao et al. 2003; Li et al. 2002a; Hirsch et al. 2000). In addition to G2/M phase cell cycle arrest using DATS or DADS, treatment of human mammary cancer cells with allicin resulted in cell cycle arrest at both G2/M and G0/G1 phases (Druesne et al. 2004a). Aboyade-Cole et al. (2008) showed that DAS inhibits DNA strand breaks induced by the heterocyclic aromatic amine, 2-amino-1-methyl-6-phenylimidazo-[4,5-*b*]pyridine – found in grilled foods and attenuates cell viability in MCF10A human breast epithelial cells. Lei et al. (2008) showed that DADS inhibits cell proliferation and induces apoptosis in MCF-7 and that inhibition of ERK and the activation of the SAPK/JNK and p38 pathways may in part account for its chemopreventive properties.

DATS suppressed viability of cultured human lung cancer cell lines (H358, H460) by causing G2/M phase cell cycle arrest and apoptotic cell death; however, compared to lung cancer cells a normal human bronchial epithelial cell line BEAS-2B was significantly more resistant to growth inhibition and apoptosis induction by DATS. The DATS-induced apoptosis correlated with the induction of proapoptotic proteins Bax, Bak and BID, coupled with a concomitant decrease in the antiapoptotic proteins Bcl2 and Bcl-xL in lung cancer, but not in BEAS-2B (Xiao et al. 2009). Wu et al. (2009) showed that oil-soluble allyl sulfides such as DADS and DATS induced significant apoptosis in human lung adenocarcinoma A549 cells whereas DAS did not. The mechanisms of apoptotic induction by DADS and DATS appear to include activation of JNK, up-regulation of p53 and down-regulation of Bcl-2 expression. DADS, DATS and DAS had no effect on the expression of MAPK, p38, Bax and bcl-xL in these studies. The use of *N*-acetylcysteine, a precursor to glutathione synthesis, blocked DADS and DATS-induced apoptosis, whereas ERK inhibitors did not. In addition, Wu et al. (2009) and Xiao et al. (2009) provide the first evidence that Fas-mediated cell death pathway is partly involved in DADS, but not DATS-mediated cell death.

Ibrahim and Nassar (2008) provided evidence that DAS exerts a protective role on liver functions and tissue integrity against *N*-nitrosodiethylamine-induced liver tumorigenesis, as well as improving cancer-sensitivity to chemotherapy. The protective role of DAS can be mediated by inhibiting oxidative stress, improving the metabolic state of the cell and enhancing the activity of glutathione-*S*-transferases, glucose-6-phosphatase and aldose reductase; the last parameter was measured as an index for cancer cell resistance to chemotherapy. A study by Bergès et al. (2004)

demonstrated that consumption of garlic is efficient in protecting against aflatoxin B1-induced liver carcinogenesis in the rat. This study also showed that by controlling some cropping factors for garlic, in particular increasing the sulfur supply in the soil, it was possible to enhance the chemopreventive efficacy of garlic in a preclinical investigation. Whether the protective effects observed in animals can be applicable in humans remains to be determined. Taken together, structurally diverse OSCs are capable of causing cell cycle arrest in cancer cells and this mechanism may account, in part, for their cancer preventive properties.

In general, modification of histones by various compounds including OSC has been documented (Druesne et al. 2004b; Lea et al. 1999, 2002; Myzak and Dashwood 2006). Treatment of Caco-2 and HT-29 colon cancer cells with DADS resulted in accumulation of these cells in G2/M phase of the cell cycle, which correlated with inhibition of histone deactylase leading to hyperacetylation of H3 and H4 histones as well as upregulation of p21 mRNA and protein levels (Druesne et al. 2004a; Lea et al. 1999).

In vitro studies that employed garlic powder, garlic extracts as well as their constituents such as DAS, DADS, DATS, SAMC and ajoene showed that these agents are capable of suppressing several pathways associated with proliferation and inducing apoptosis in a variety of cancer cells in culture (reviewed by Shukla and Kalra 2007). Apoptosis is a cellular event, which is critical to decreasing tumor mass and limiting the growth of cancer cells. Several investigators have reported on the efficacy of OSC to induce apoptosis in cancer cell lines (colon, lung, and neuroblastoma) and the mechanisms that are responsible for this effect (Hong et al. 2000; Karmakar et al. 2007; Sundaram and Milner 1996). For example, treatment of MDA-MB-231 breast cancer cell lines with DADS has been shown to increase the level of the pro-apoptotic protein, Bax, and concomitantly to decrease the anti-apoptotic protein, Bcl-2 (Nakagawa et al. 2001). Other studies have demonstrated that the sensitivity of cancerous cells to apoptosis for example in human prostate cancer cell lines (PC-3, DU145) depends on the molecular structure of OSC and the type of cell line used (Xiao et al. 2004).

Ajoene and DADS are known to induce apoptosis in the HL60 cells; the induction of apoptosis by the former compound correlates with caspase-mediated cleavage of Bcl-2 (Li et al. 2002b), which correlates with levels of ROS generated (Kwon et al. 2002). Studies by Kim et al. (2007) have also implicated ROS generation in apoptotic induction by DATS in a prostate cancer cell line (LNCaP). Ajoene-induced apoptosis in human promyeloleukemic cells was accompanied by generation of ROS and accompanied by activation of NFκB (Dirsch et al. 1998). It is important to emphasize here that OSC induce apoptosis in numerous cancer cells and that normal cells exhibit either weak or have refractory responses to these agents (Dirsch et al. 1998; Karmakar et al. 2007; Kim et al. 2007).

The anti-angiogenic effects of organosulfur compounds have been reported in several systems including human endothelial cells, ex vivo neovascularization models and in vivo metastasis models (Meyer et al. 2004; Mousa and Mousa 2005;

Taylor et al. 2006; Xiao et al. 2006). Briefly, molecular targets (VEGF, AKT, MMP-2, MMP-9, nitric oxide, p53 protein expression) which are critical to the angiogenic process have been shown to be altered by OSC.

5.4.4 Mechanisms of Cancer Prevention by Organoselenium Compounds

The mechanisms by which selenium compounds inhibit tumor formation during the initiation phase of carcinogenesis have been explored in vitro and in well-defined animal models (reviewed in El-Bayoumy 2001). Oxidative damage has been implicated in the development of cancer during the initiation phase but more so during the promotion phase of carcinogenesis. The effects of various forms of selenium on molecular and cellular targets critical in the multistep carcinogenesis process have been reviewed (El-Bayoumy 2001). Inorganic selenium compounds appear to cause distinctly different cellular effects from those elicited by organic forms of selenium compounds. Inorganic selenium at levels of 5–10 μM can induce single strand breaks in DNA and cell death by necrosis in cell culture systems (Ip 1998). However, certain organoselenium compounds, even at higher levels (10–50 μM), can cause cell death by apoptosis without the evidence of DNA single strand breaks. It has also been shown that the chemopreventive effects of selenium are due, in part, to its inhibitory effects on cell growth, DNA, RNA, and protein synthesis in transformed cells. Because protein kinases play a role in regulation of cell growth, tumor promotion, and differentiation, several reports described the inhibition of kinase activities by selenium (Rao et al. 2000; Sinha et al. 1999, 2008b). However, recent results suggest that the cancer preventive actions of selenium may be negated both by an over-expression of PKCε, which is a redox-sensitive target of methylseleninic acid, and by the selenoprotein thioredoxin reductase, which reverses PKC sulfhydryl redox modification (Gundimeda et al. 2009). Cell cycle cdk2 or cell signaling protein kinases and/or a number of redox-regulated proteins-including the critical transcriptional factors (AP1 and NFκB)-have been proposed as targets for cancer prevention by selenium. In a recent report, Sinha et al. (2008) hypothesized that the inhibition of cell growth is due, in part, to selenium interaction with redox-sensitive proteins. Using androgen responsive and androgen-independent human prostate cancer cells and two-dimensional gel electrophoresis, these investigators showed that SM and the synthetic organoselenium compound p-XSC altered the expression, to a varied extent, of several previously unrecognized selenium-responsive proteins. Using MALDI-TOF-TOF, they identified several proteins, including redox-sensitive proteins such as the pro-apoptotic cofilin-2, which may be critical in prostate cancer prevention. Chen et al. (2007) showed that the synthetic chemopreventive organoselenocyanates (e.g., p-XSC) may exert their chemopreventive activity by inhibiting transcription factor, NFκB through covalent modification of Cys62 of the p50 subunit. Activation of NFκB, can lead to activation of numerous inflammatory genes such as COX-2 that can be inhibited by bio-active food components (Kim et al. 2009) among which organoselenium has been shown to be efficacious (Kawamori et al. 1998; El-Bayoumy et al. 2006). Studies with cell cultures suggest that organoselenium may exert its chemopreventive effect via the induction of apoptosis and inhibition of cell growth (reviewed in Sinha and El-Bayoumy 2004). The induction of the p53 gene by organoselenium compounds was demonstrated. However, the induction of apoptosis may not be entirely due to the response of p53 to organoselenium (Lanfear et al. 1994). Following the development of an improved assay to assess methyltransferase activity, Fiala et al. (1998) suggested that the inhibition of methyltransferase activity may be an important mechanism of chemoprevention by organoselenium compounds at the post-initiation phase of carcinogenesis. Clearly the effect of organoselenium compounds on cell proliferation, cell cycle regulation, and apoptosis is dependent on the form and dose of the organoselenium compound and whether cells are normal or transformed (Ip et al. 2000b).

Histone deacetylase (HDAC) inhibitors reactivate epigenetically-silenced genes in cancer cells, triggering cell cycle arrest and apoptosis. As described above OSC present in garlic can act as HDAC inhibitors; an excellent recent review on this topic is available (Nian et al. 2009b). The effects of organoselenium compounds on HDAC inhibition (Lee et al. 2009; Nian et al. 2009a) are discussed below. Collectively, the results reported in this review provide new insights into the relationships among reversible histone modifications, dietary sources including garlic, and cancer chemoprevention. Detailed studies are required to rank the importance of HDAC inhibition with other cellular targets that are critical factors in chemoprevention.   .

5.4.5 Aminotransferases, L-Amino Acid Oxidase and β-Lyases Metabolize Allium-Derived Organosulfur and Organoselenium L-Cysteine Conjugates

As described above several OSC isolated from extracts of fresh and aged garlic have been shown to possess antiproliferative and chemopreventive properties. Although freshly prepared garlic extracts contain a variety of pro-oxidant polyallylsulfides (Table 5.1) (e.g., DAS, DATS, allylmethyl disulfide, allylmethyl trisulfide, and diallyl tetrasulfide), upon consumption these derivatives immediately cross-react in situ with endogenous cysteine and produce cysteinyl S-conjugates, in particular, S-allylmercapto-L-cysteine (see reactions 5.1 and 5.2). Reaction 5.2 also depicts the formation of sulfane sulfur ($S°$). The importance of this reaction product to cancer prevention and control will be discussed below. Polyallylsulfides can also conjugate with glutathione within the enterocyte and be metabolized via the mercapturic acid pathway. This involves sequential removal of the glutamyl and glycine moieties via γ-glutamyltranspeptidase and cysteinylglycinase, respectively, forming the cysteinyl S-conjugate. The ability of allylpolysulfides to be transformed in situ to cysteinyl S-conjugates may be a prerequisite for their potential anticancer effects. In addition to reacting with sulfhydryl groups of cysteine and GSH, allylpolysulfides can react with sulfhydryl moieties in proteins, causing formation of either a disulfide bond between vicinal cysteinyl moieties within the same (reaction 5.3) or neighboring protein (reaction 5.4) or an allyl- or allylmercaptoprotein S-conjugate (reaction 5.5). These reactions demonstrate the possible interactions among endogenous OSC and those acquired through consumption of allium vegetables. Formation of cysteinyl disulfides or S-cysteinyl conjugates have the potential of causing either loss or initiation of enzymatic activity as well as modifying function of redox responsive signal proteins, which may ultimately affect cell cycle components (Burhans and Heintz 2009). Thus, the objective evaluation of allylsulfides and cysteinyl S-conjugates as chemopreventive agents must be viewed in the light of their interactions with endogenous organosulfur components and other cellular metabolites as well as their capacity to affect the redox environment of cells.

$$(CH_2=CH-CH_2-S)_2 + HSCH_2CH(NH_3^+)CO_2^-$$

Diallyldisulfide   Cysteine

$$\rightarrow CH_2=CH-CH_2-S-S-CH_2CH(NH_3^+)CO_2^- + CH_2=CH-CH_2-SH$$

   S-Allylmerapto-L-cysteine (SAMC)   Allylmercaptan

(5.1)

$$(CH_2=CH-CH_2-S)_2S + HSCH_2CH(NH_3^+)CO_2^-$$

Allyltrisulfide   Cysteine

$$\rightarrow CH_2=CH-CH_2-S-S-CH_2CH(NH_3^+)CO_2^- + S° + CH_2=CH-CH_2-SH$$

   SAMC   Sulfane sulfur   Allylmercaptan

(5.2)

$$(CH_2=CH-CH_2-S)_2 + Protein-(SH2)$$

Diallyldisulfide

$$\rightarrow Protein-(S_2) + 2CH_2=CH-CH_2-SH$$

       Allylmercaptan

(5.3)

$$(CH_2=CH-CH_2-S)_2 + 2\ Protein-SH$$

Diallyldisulfide

$$\rightarrow (Protein-S)_2 + 2CH_2=CH-CH_2-SH$$

        Allylmercaptan

(5.4)

$$(CH_2=CH-CH_2-S)_2 + protein-S-S-protein$$

Diallyldisulfide

$$\rightarrow 2\,Protein-S-S-CH_2CH=CH_2 \tag{5.5}$$

Protein-S-S-allyl

Studies using S-cysteinyl conjugates have focused primarily on S-allyl-L-cysteine (SAC), S-allylmercapto-L-cysteine, S-propylmercapto-L-cysteine, and S-methylmercapto-L-cysteine (Cooper and Pinto 2005). In a similar fashion, naturally-occurring organoselenium, e.g., MSC and SM, present in selenized-enriched garlic or yeast as well as Brazil nuts also play a critical role in chemoprevention and exhibit anticancer effects through their ability to alter cell signaling pathways and induce cellular apoptosis (Cooper and Pinto 2006). Research studies using these S-cysteinyl or Se-cysteinyl derivatives should identify relevant mechanisms that help direct human intervention trials with garlic-enriched or organoselenium supplements for not only cancer prevention but also metastatic control (Rooseboom et al. 2001).

Allylmercapto-S-cysteinyl and Se-cysteinyl conjugates may undergo transformations by aminotransferases, L-amino acid oxidase and/or β- and γ-lyase reactions (Cooper and Pinto 2005). SAC, SAMC, S-propylmercapto-L-cysteine, S-penta-1,3-dienylmercapto-L-cysteine are substrates of rat kidney and human glutamine transaminase K (GTK), L-amino acid oxidase, and cysteine S-conjugate β-lyases present in rat liver cytosol. S-Methylmercapto-L-cysteine is a substrate of GTK and L-amino acid oxidase, but not of cysteine S-conjugate β-lyase. Liver contains cystathionine γ-lyase (γ-cystathionase), which is responsible for the cysteine S-conjugate β-lyase reactions. The possible role of cystathionine γ-lyase in generating sulfane sulfur from the disulfide-containing cysteine S-conjugates present in allium extracts, and the possible role of sulfane sulfur in enzyme regulations, targeting of cancer cells and detoxification reactions has been considered by Toohey (1989).

Anti-proliferative and pro-apoptotic effects of garlic-derived cysteinyl S-conjugates against a number of hormone-sensitive and -refractory human tumor cell lines may be mediated by sulfane sulfur-containing compounds or sulfane progenitors. A paucity of sulfane sulfur in these cells may be related to proliferation of malignant cells, which would normally be inactivated by sulfane sulfur (Toohey 1989). In this manner, the anti-cancer effects of allyl-S-cysteine conjugates may be due at least in part to their ability to act as progenitors of sulfane sulfur via interactions involving cystathionine γ-lyase (Toohey 2001). Because of the interaction of garlic-derived S-allylsulfides with cystathionine γ-lyase and GTK to produce reactive sulfhydryl and/and or sulfane sulfur intermediates, the chemopreventive activity of these dietary factors may be due in part to their ability to modify intracellular redox potentials, to generate sulfane sulfur and/or to interact with thiols associated with cysteine moieties in regulatory or catalytic signal proteins (Toohey 2001).

Several pyridoxal $5'$ phosphate (PLP)-containing enzymes catalyze either β-lyase reactions with cysteinyl S- and cysteinyl Se-conjugates or γ-lyase reactions with methionine (methionine cleavage is not present in mammals) and SM resulting in generation of a keto acid, ammonium and a methylthiol or methylselenol fragment (reactions 5.6 and 5.7). Since chalcogens have excellent electron withdrawing properties, their presence in cysteinyl conjugates combined with the nature of the R constituent group can facilitate β-elimination reactions (Commandeur et al. 2000; Rooseboom et al. 2002). If the initial catalytic reaction results in formation of pyruvate and ammonia as well as regeneration of the PLP coenzyme, the chalcogen would be β-eliminated as RSH (Eq. 5.6) or RSeH (Eq. 5.7).

$$RSCH_2CH(NH_3^+)CO_2^- + H_2O \rightarrow CH_3C(O)CO_2^- + NH_4^+ + RSH \qquad (5.6)$$

$$RSeCH_2CH(NH_3^+)CO_2^- + H_2O \rightarrow CH_3C(O)CO_2^- + NH_4^+ + RSeH \qquad (5.7)$$

For example, serine dehydratase catalyzes β-elimination reactions (Ogawa et al. 2006). In addition, cystathionine γ-lyase can catalyze a β-elimination reaction with certain cysteine S- and cysteinyl Se-conjugates (Rooseboom et al. 2002; Cooper and Pinto 2005, 2006) Thus, chemopreventive activity of the β-eliminated product of MSC, e.g., methylselenol, is purported to be manifested through the oxidation of thiol moieties on redox responsive signal proteins and transcription factors thereby maintaining a non-proliferative intracellular environment (Suzuki et al. 2008; Wang et al. 2002). By contrast, if a half-transamination reaction occurs leaving the PLP coenzyme as pyridoxamine 5′-phosphate, the α-keto acid analogue of the cysteine S- or Se-conjugate will be formed. In such reactions, a competing transamination reaction may result. Thus, aminotransferases with syncatalytic properties as a β-lyase may exhibit a competing transamination (aminotransferase) reaction (reactions 5.8 and 5.9).

$$RSCH_2CH(CO_2^-)NH_3^+ + R'C(O)CO_2^- \leftrightarrow RSCH_2C(O)CO_2^- + R'C(NH_3^+)CO_2^-$$
$$(5.8)$$

$$RSeCH_2CH(CO_2^-)NH_3^+ + R'C(O)CO_2^- \leftrightarrow RSeCH_2C(O)CO_2^- + R'CH(NH_3^+)CO_2^-$$
$$(5.9)$$

Mammalian cysteinyl S- and Se-conjugate β-lyases with this feature include several aminotransferases (Cooper et al. 2008). Aminotransferases that conduct syncatalytic reactions as β-lyases include glutamine transaminase K (Stevens 1985) and mitochondrial aspartate aminotransferase (Cooper et al. 2002).

Recent studies using the keto acid product of MSC showed that after transamination of MSC, the resultant methylselenopyruvate (MSP) increases levels of histone-H3 acetylation in human prostate and colon cancer cells (Lee et al. 2009; Nian et al. 2009a). MSP and the α-keto acid product of SM, α-keto-γ-methylselenobutyrate (KMSB) resemble butyrate, an inhibitor of HDAC. In addition, formation of MSP and KMSB by reaction of MSC and SM, respectively, with L-amino acid oxidase, inhibits HDAC 3 and 8 activities in a dose dependent manner (Nian et al. 2009a). Thus, the α-keto acid metabolites of MSC and SM, along with methylselenol derived from β- and γ-lyase reactions, may be potential direct acting metabolites of organoselenium that lead to de-repression of silenced tumor suppressor proteins and/or responses to signal factors in prostate and colon cancers.

5.5 Epidemiology, Clinical Intervention Studies and Safety Aspects

Epidemiologic investigations have shown that risk of several types of cancer is inversely related to intake of garlic (Buiatti et al. 1989; Kelloff et al. 1992; Pelucchi et al. 2009; You et al. 1988, 1989). In a published case-control study (Key et al. 1997), risk of prostate cancer was significantly less (relative risk 0.56) in individuals who regularly consumed garlic food items 2 or more times per week compared to other food items. There was a significant trend of decreasing risk with an increase in garlic consumption of less than once per month, increasing to 1–4 times per month and then to 2 or more times per week ($p = 0.038$). These findings provide incentive for further mechanistic evaluation of the potential effects of garlic constituents to control growth of prostate cancer. The uniquely large data set from southern European populations shows an inverse association between the frequency of use of allium vegetables and the risk of several common cancers. Allium vegetables are a favorable correlate of cancer risk in Europe (Galeone et al. 2006). Devrim and Durak (2007) have reviewed the role that garlic may play in benign hyperplasia and prostate cancer. Hsing et al. (2002) administered in-person interviews and collected information on 122 food items from 238 case subjects with incident, histologically confirmed prostate cancer and from 471 male population control subjects. The reduced risk of prostate cancer associated with allium vegetables was independent of body size, intake of other foods, and total calorie intake and was more pronounced for men with localized than with advanced prostate cancer.

Despite the large base of preclinical studies showing potent anticancer effects of multiple water- and organic soluble constituents of garlic, the evidence that garlic reduces cancer risk in humans is at best modest (Kim and Kulon 2009). For example, there is insufficient evidence to show any relation between garlic and cancer of the stomach, breast, lung or endometrium and there is only limited evidence of an effect of garlic on cancers oral cavity, larynx, esophagus, colon, prostate, ovary and kidney; an excellent review in epidemiological studies is available (Shukla and Kalra 2007). Using data from an Italian case-control study, Galeone et al. (2009) found a moderately protective role of allium vegetables on the risk of endometrial cancer. Clinical trials that are scientifically sound are limited and the number of subjects involved in these trials is generally small. Thus, well-designed clinical trials are needed to unequivocally evaluate the chemopreventive potential of allium vegetable constituents in humans.

The effects of DATS, 200 mg/d and selenium (100 μg every other day) in 2,526 subjects for duration of one month were examined; the control group (2,507 subjects) was given placebo. After 5-years follow-up the results revealed that the intervention group had 22% lower incidence of all cancers and about 47% lower incidence of gastric cancer (Li et al. 2004). In this trial, DATS had no noticeable side effects. In a later study by You et al. (2006), 3,365 eligible subjects were randomly assigned to three intervention arms or placebo control, amoxicillin and omeprazole for two weeks (*Helicobacter pylori* treatment), vitamins C and E, and selenium for

7.3 years, and a blend of aged garlic extract (AGE) and steam-distilled garlic oil (that may contain DADS and DATS) for 7.3 years. The results showed that subjects received *H. pylori* treatment had significantly lower severe chronic atrophic gastritis, intestinal metaplasia, dysplasia and gastric cancer. On the other hand, subjects who received garlic or vitamins had no significant favorable effects. Another study examined the effects of two doses of AGE (high: 2–4 ml/d, low 0.16 ml/d) in patients with colorectal polyps over 12-months period (Tanaka et al. 2006). The high dose significantly reduced the number and size of colon adenomas after 12 months of treatment. In a therapeutic trial, Tilli et al. (2003) topically applied ajoene onto tumors of 21 patients with nodular or superficial basal carcinoma for 6 months; a significant reduction in tumor size in 17 cases and a reduction in the expression of anti-apoptotic protein Bcl-2 in these tumors was reported as evaluated by immunohistochemical analysis.

Epidemiological studies have suggested that an increased risk for certain human diseases, including cancer, is related to insufficient intake of selenium; however, there remains some inconsistency (Combs and Gray 1998; Shamberger and Frost 1969; Yoshizawa et al. 1998). Selenium has been used in several human clinical chemoprevention trials which have been conducted in China, India, Italy and the USA with selenium, in the form of selenized-yeast, selenite, selenate and SM. Populations having different risk factors were enrolled in these trials. Some of the studies performed in China suffered from methodological problems such as lack of quality controls (Yu et al. 1991, 1997). The Linxian (China) cancer prevention trials have shown that giving a combination of selenium (in the form of selenate), β-carotene, and α-tocopherol resulted in significantly fewer cases and a lower mortality from stomach cancer than were observed in the placebo groups (Blot et al. 1993). When selenium was given in combination with another 25 vitamins and minerals, it had no effect on the development of esophageal cancer (Li et al. 1993). In a study conducted in India, selenium was given in combination with vitamin A, C, and E, as well as zinc (Prasad et al. 1995); the results showed a protective effect of this cocktail against the development of oral lesions in subjects who practice reverse smoking. In a double-blind-randomized trial in Italy, inhibition of adenoma in the large bowel by selenium has been demonstrated (Bonelli 1998).

The results of the Nutritional Prevention of Cancer trial have had a profound effect on the field of cancer chemoprevention (Clark et al. 1996). The trial, designed to determine the effect of selenium on the incidence of recurrent nonmelanoma skin cancer in high-risk individuals, showed an increase in incidence of basal or squamous cell carcinoma of the skin, but a 63% decrease in prostate cancer incidence, a secondary end point, in the selenium-supplemented arm of the study. This sparked the initiation of multiple trials worldwide to elucidate the role of selenium (in various forms and doses) in the prevention of prostate cancer. Two large-scale double-blind, placebo-controlled clinical intervention trials are following the incidence of prostate cancer in healthy men supplemented with selenium: the SELECT study in the United States and the Prevention of Cancer by Intervention with Selenium Trial (PRECISE) in Europe. The SELECT study used 200 μg daily SM, the major form of selenium in SeY, alone or in combination with vitamin E, to track prostate cancer in healthy men above the age of 50 years with no history of cancer (Lippman et al. 2009). Data analysis showed a non-significant increase in prostate cancer in men taking only vitamin E, but SM had no effect; the use of SM alone, however, caused a non-significant increase in diabetes (Lippman et al. 2009). Although the potential association of selenium with increased diabetes remains controversial, the mechanisms by which SM increased diabetes in the SELECT population deserve further exploration. The SELECT trial was halted in October 2008, but subjects will be monitored for the next 3 years. These results do not prove there is a risk from the supplement and may be 'due to chance' as stressed by Dr. Scott Lippman, co-chair of the SELECT scientific steering committee [National Cancer Institute (NCI) Cancer Bulletin, November 4, 2008] and the Principal author on the respective publication (Lippman et al. 2009). Considering the potential limitations that the dose and form of selenium used in SELECT were wrong, it may be difficult to predict whether SeY would have been more effective than SM without credible information comparing the effects of both forms of organoselenium on intermediate biomarkers of prostate cancer risk. Nevertheless, based on extensive preclinical data, we believe that the protective effect of SeY in the Nutritional Prevention of Cancer trial could be due to the presence of several forms of organoselenium, some of which (e.g., MSC) show differential responses to both β-lyases and aminotransferases than does SM, the compound chosen in the SELECT study (Lippman et al. 2009). Furthermore, there is ample opportunity to develop even more effective and less toxic synthetic organoselenium compounds than known naturally occurring selenium compounds such as SM (El-Bayoumy and Sinha 2004). It is intriguing that the PRECISE trial, which includes cohorts in three European countries (United Kingdom, Denmark, and Sweden) supplemented participants with a range of doses (100–300 μg) of SeY, the form shown to be effective in the Nutritional Prevention of Cancer trial (Clark et al. 1998; Rayman 2000). A third large-scale trial, the Australian Prostate Cancer Prevention Trial Using Selenium (APPOSE), is being conducted in high-risk individuals. The APPOSE trial will survey the incidence of prostate cancer in healthy males with a family history of the disease supplemented with 200 μg SeY daily (Costello 2001). Although the results of these studies will not be known for several years, we conducted a pilot study in healthy adult males supplemented with 240 μg/d SeY for 9 months to provide some insights on the role of selenium in cancer prevention. Our study showed increases in serum glutathione levels, an endogenous antioxidant, accompanied by decreases in protein-bound serum glutathione and PSA in individuals supplemented with SeY, suggesting that selenium may protect against oxidative stress, a risk factor for prostate cancer (El-Bayoumy et al. 2002). It was intriguing to learn that in contrast to SeY, SM seems to lack an inhibitory effect on prostate-specific antigen levels (Lippman et al. 2009). Furthermore, the effects of SM on levels of antioxidants in men in the SELECT trial need to be determined. In fact, a clinical pilot study is currently being conducted in our laboratory aimed at comparing the effect of SM and SeY on biomarkers of prostate cancer risk.

5.6 Summary and Future Recommendations

Garlic and its organosulfur and organoselenium containing components are widely known for their cancer preventive activities primarily in preclinical in vitro and in vivo model systems. The protective effects of garlic are not limited to specific tissues or species and appear to be independent of the carcinogen-employed. In general plants synthesize sulfur-amino acids from sulfide and sulfate; similarly, they also synthesize seleno-amino acids from selenite and selenate and selenium can easily substitute for sulfur in plant metabolism. The sulfur and selenium contents of garlic are dependent upon the level of the respective elements in the soil. Most of our common foods including garlic contain very low levels of selenium compared to sulfur constituents. At least 33 different types of OSC have been identified in garlic. About ten selenium compounds have been identified in garlic and onion and more than 20 selenium compounds have been reported in selenium-enriched yeast; SM is the major form of selenium in the selenium-enriched yeast. The major form of selenium in selenium-enriched garlic and onion is MSC at low concentration and γ-glutamyl-*Se*-methylselenocysteine at high concentration (Arnault and Auger 2006). The analysis of selenium compounds in our common foods (non-enriched plants) remains an obstacle primarily because of the extremely low levels of selenium. Synthesis of selenium analogs of sulfur compounds found in garlic can serve as standards in the identification of such compounds in these plants. Furthermore, synthetic selenium analogs can also aid in the identification of such compounds in human biological fluids.

Humans consume a substantial portion of their dietary sulfur and selenium in organic forms. Selenium-enriched foods such as garlic, broccoli and wheat are more effective chemopreventive agents that the corresponding regular dietary items. Naturally-occurring and synthetic organoselenium compounds are superior cancer chemopreventive agents compared to their corresponding sulfur analogs.

Mechanistic studies demonstrate that sulfur and selenium compounds are capable of cell growth inhibition, cell cycle arrest, induction of apoptosis, alterations in phase I and phase II enzyme activities and HDAC inhibition (Fig. 5.1). Detailed studies are required to rank the importance of HDAC inhibition with other cellular targets that are critical in chemoprevention. Furthermore, careful evaluation of sulfur and selenium compounds as cancer chemopreventive agents must be viewed in light of their interactions with endogenous organosulfur components and other cellular metabolites as well as their capacity to affect the redox environment of the cells. The fact that OSC and organoselenium compounds can target multiple pathways, it is possible that these agents can be used as chemopreventive and/or therapeutic agents alone or in combination with other medicinal compounds. The effect of these agents on the aforementioned parameters varies depending on the dose and form (structure) and whether cells are normal or transformed.

Whether the protective effects of OSC and organoselenium compounds observed in animals and in cell cultures can be applicable in humans remain to be determined. Many epidemiological studies, but not all, provide some support to the

Fig. 5.1 Mechanisms that can account for cancer prevention and therapy by sulfur and selenium containing compounds described in the chapter

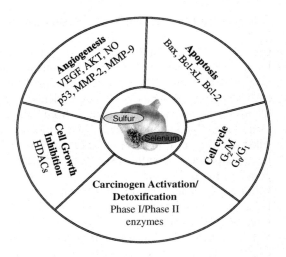

protective effects of garlic, and clinical chemoprevention trials are either scarce or poorly designed and in general the outcomes of these trials remain inconsistent. Clearly the disconnect between nutritional epidemiology and preclinical studies on the one hand and the phase III clinical chemoprevention trials is a testimony to the complex interactive biochemistry of organosulfur and selenium compounds with proteins and genes and to our limited understanding on how such agents work in humans. Thus, using technological advances in genomics, proteomics, metabolomics (El-Bayoumy and Sinha 2005), in well designed small-scale clinical trials are needed to unequivocally evaluate the potential of allium vegetable constituents on biomarkers of risk of specific cancer prior to entering into long-term expensive phase III clinical chemoprevention trials (El-Bayoumy 2009). In fact we are currently comparing the effect of SeY and SM on biomarkers of prostate cancer risk in men. These types of studies are necessary toward better understanding whether the results obtained in preclinical systems are applicable to humans.

Acknowledgments Studies performed in the authors' laboratories are supported by CA 70972, CA100924, CA127729, CA111842.

References

Aboyade-Cole A, Darling-Reed S, Oriaku E et al (2008) Diallyl sulfide inhibits PhIP-induced cell death via the inhibition of DNA strand breaks in normal human breast epithelial cells. Oncol Rep 20:319–323

Agarwal KC (1996) Therapeutic actions of garlic constituents. Med Res Rev 16:111–124

Amagase H, Schaffer EM, Milner JA (1996) Dietary components modify the ability of garlic to suppress 7,12 dimethylbenz[*a*]anthracene-induced mammary DNA adducts. J Nutr 126: 817–824

Amagase H (2006) Clarifying the real bioactive constituents of garlic. J Nutr 136:716S–725S

Amosova SV, Potapur VA, Nosyreva VV (1991) Synthesis of diallyl selenide. Org Prep Proced Int 23:207–208

Antosiewicz J, Herman-Antosiewicz A, Marynowski AW et al (2006) c-Jun NH(2)-terminal kinase signaling axis regulates diallyl trisulfide-induced generation of reactive oxygen species and cell cycle arrest in human prostate cancer cells. Cancer Res 66:5379–5386

Arnault I, Auger J (2006) Seleno-compounds in garlic and onion. J Chromatogr A 1112:23–30

Arunkumar A, Vijayababu MR, Srinivasan N et al (2006) Garlic compound, diallyl disulfide induces cell cycle arrest in prostate cancer cell line PC-3. Mol Cell Biochem 288:107–113

Baer AR, Wargovich MJ (1989) Role of ornithine decarboxylase in diallyl sulfide inhibition of colonic radiation injury in the house. Cancer Res 49:5073–5076

Belman S (1983) Onion and garlic oils inhibit tumor promotion. Carcinogenesis 4:1063–1065

Bergès R, Siess MH, Arnault I et al (2004) Comparison of the chemopreventive efficacies of garlic powders with different alliin contents against aflatoxin B1 carcinogenicity in rats. Carcinogenesis 25:1953–1959

Block E (1985) The chemistry of garlic and onions. Sci Am 252:114–119

Block E (1992) The organosulfur chemistry of the genus Allium-implications for the organic chemistry of sulfur. Angew Chem Int Ed (Eng) 31:1135–1178

Block E (2009) Growth and other alliums-the lore and the science. The Royal Society of Chemistry, UK

Blot WJ, Li JY, Taylor PR et al (1993) Nutrition intervention trials in Linxian, China: supplementation with specific vitamin/mineral combinations, cancer incidence, and disease-specific mortality in the general population. J Natl Cancer Inst 85:1483–1492

Bonelli L (1998) Chemoprevention of metachronous adenomas of the large bowel by means of antioxidants: a double-blindrandomized trial. In: Proceedings of the Presentation at the International Selenium Tellurium Development Association Meeting, Scottsdale, AZ

Brady JF, Ishizaki, H, Fukuto, JM et al (1991) Inhibition of cytochrome P-450 2E1 by diallyl sulfide and its metabolites. Chem Res Toxicol 4:642–647

Buiatti E, Palli D, Decarli A et al (1989) A case-control study of gastric cancer and diet in Italy. Int J Cancer 44:611–616

Burhans WC, Heintz NH (2009) The cell cycle is a redox cycle; linking phase-specific targets to cell fate. Free Radic Biol Med 47:1282–1293

Burk RF, Norssworthy BK, Hill KE (2006) Effects of chemical form of selenium on plasma biomarkers in a high-dose human supplementation trial. Cancer Epidemiol Biomarkers Prev 15:804–810

Chen KM, Spratt TE, Stanley BA et al (2007) Inhibition of nuclear factor-kappaB DNA binding by organoselenocyanates through covalent modification of the p50 subunit. Cancer Res 67: 10475–10483

Clark LC, Combs GF Jr, Turnbull, BW et al (1996) Effects of selenium supplementation for cancer prevention in patients with carcinoma of the skin. A randomized controlled trial. Nutritional Prevention of Cancer Study Group. J Am Med Assoc 276:1957–1963

Clark LC, Dalkin B, Krongrad A et al (1998) Decreased incidence of prostate cancer with selenium supplementation: results of a double-blind cancer prevention trial. Br J Urol 81:730–734

Cohen LA, Zhao Z, Pittman B et al (1999) S-Allylcysteine, a garlic constituent, fails to inhibit N-methylnitrosourea-induced rat mammary tumorigenesis. Nutr Cancer 35:58–63

Combs GF Jr, Gray WP (1998) Chemopreventive agents: selenium. Pharmacol Ther 79:179–192

Commandeur JNM, Andreadou I, Rooseboom M et al (2000) Bioactivation of selenocysteine Se-conjugates by a highly purified rat renal cysteine conjugate β-lyase/glutamine transaminase K. J Pharmacol Exp Ther 294:753–761

Costello AJ (2001) A randomized, controlled chemoprevention trial of selenium in familial prostate cancer: rationale, recruitment, and design issues. Urology 57:182–184

Cooper AJL, Bruschi SA, Iriarte A et al (2002) Mitochondrial aspartate aminotransferase catalyses cysteine S-conjugate β-lyase reactions. Biochem J 368:253–261

Cooper AJL, Pinto JT (2005) Aminotransferase, L-amino acid oxidase and β-lyase reactions involving L-cysteine S-conjugates found in allium extracts. Relevance to biological activity? Biochem Pharmacol 69:209–220

Cooper AJL, Pinto JT (2006) Cysteine S-conjugate β-lyases. Amino Acids 30:1–15

Cooper AJL, Pinto JT, Krasnikov BF et al (2008) Substrate specificity of human glutamine transaminase K as an aminotransferase and as a cysteine S-conjugate β-lyase. Arch Biochem Biophys 474:72–81

Dalvi RR (1992) Alterations in hepatic phase I and phase II biotransformation enzymes by garlic oil in rats. Toxicol Lett 60:299–305

Dausch JG, Nixon DW (1990) Garlic: a review of its relationship to malignant disease. Prev Med 19:346–361

de Boer GH, Yang J, Holcroft K et al (2004) Chemoprotection against N-nitrosomethylbenzylamine-induced mutation in the rat esophagus. Nutr Cancer 50: 168–173

Devrim E, Durak I (2007) Is garlic a promising food for benign prostatic hyperplasia and prostate cancer? Mol Nutr Food Res 51:1319–1323

Dirsch VM, Gerbes AL, Vollmar AM (1998) Ajoene, a compound of garlic, induces apoptosis in human promyeloleukemic cells, accompanied by generation of reactive oxygen species and activation of nuclear factor kappa B. Mol Pharmacol 53:402–407

Doll R (1992) The lessons of life: keynote address to the nutrition and cancer conference. Cancer Res 52:2024s–2029s

Doll R, Peto R (1981) The causes of cancer: quantitative estimates of avoidable risks of cancer in the United States today. J Natl Cancer Inst 66:1191–1308

Druesne N, Pagniez A, Mayeur C et al (2004a) Diallyl disulfide (DADS) increases histone acetylation and p21(waf1/cip1) expression in human colon tumor cell lines. Carcinogenesis 25:1227–1236

Druesne N, Pagniez A, Mayeur C et al (2004b) Repetitive treatments of colon HT-29 cells with diallyl disulfide induce a prolonged hyperacetylation of histone H3 K14. Ann N Y Acad Sci 1030:612–621

Dwivedi C, Rohlfs S, Jarvis D et al (1992) Chemoprevention of chemically induced skin tumor development by diallyl sulfide and diallyl disulfide. Pharm Res 9:1668–1670

Egen-Schwind C, Eckard R, Kemper FH (1992) Metabolism of garlic constituents in the isolated perfused rat liver. Planta Med 58:301–305

El-Bayoumy K (1985) Effects of organoselenium compounds on induction of mouse fore stomach tumors by benzo[a]pyrene. Cancer Res 45:3631–3615

El-Bayoumy K (1994) Evaluation of chemopreventive agents against breast cancer and proposed strategies for future clinical intervention trials. Carcinogenesis 15:2395–2420

El-Bayoumy K (2001) The protective role of selenium on genetic damage and on cancer. Mutat Res 475:123–139

El-Bayoumy K (2009) The negative results of the SELECT study do not necessarily discredit the selenium-cancer prevention hypothesis. Nutr Cancer 61:285–286

El-Bayoumy K, Sinha R (2004) Mechanisms of mammary cancer chemoprevention by organoselenium compounds. Mutation Res 551:181–197

El-Bayoumy K, Sinha R (2005) Molecular chemoprevention by selenium: a genomic approach. Mutat Res 591:224–236

El-Bayoumy K, Chae Y, Upadhyaya P et al (1996) Chemoprevention of mammary cancer by diallyl selenide, a novel organoselenium compound. Anticancer Res 16:2911–2915

El-Bayoumy K, Richie JP Jr, Boyiri T et al (2002) Influence of selenium-enriched yeast supplementation on biomarkers of oxidative damage and hormone status in healthy adult males: a clinical pilot study. Cancer Epidemiol Biomarkers Prev 11:1459–1465

El-Bayoumy K, Sinha R, Pinto JT et al (2006) Cancer chemoprevention by garlic and garlic-containing sulfur and selenium compounds. J Nutr 136:864S–869S

Ferrucci L, Corsi A, Lauretani F et al (2005) The origin of age-related proinflammatory state. Blood 105:2294–2299

Fiala ES, Staretz ME, Pandya GA et al (1998) Inhibition of DNA cytosine methyltransferase by chemopreventive selenium compounds, determined by an improved assay for DNA cytosine methyltransferase and DNA cytosine methylation. Carcinogenesis 19:597–604

Finley JW, Ip C, Lisk DJ et al (2001) Cancerprotective properties of high-selenium broccoli. J Agric Food Chem 49:2679–2683

Galeone C, Pelucchi C, Dal Maso L et al (2009) Allium vegetables intake and endometrial cancer risk. Public Health Nutr 12:1576–1579

Galeone C, Pelucchi C, Levi F, Negri E, Franceschi S, Talamini R, Giacosa A, La Vecchia C (2006) Onion and garlic use and human cancer. Am J Clin Nutr 84:1027–1032

Germain E, Auger J, Ginies C (2002) In vivo metabolism of diallyl disulphide in the rat: identification of two new metabolites. Xenobiotica 32:1127–1138

Gilbert HF (1990) Molecular and cellular aspects of thioldisulfide exchange. Adv Enzymol Relat Areas Mol Biol 63:69–172

Gundimeda U, Schiffman JE, Gottlieb SN et al (2009) Negation of the cancer-preventive actions of selenium by over-expression of protein kinase Cepsilon and selenoprotein thioredoxin reductase. Carcinogenesis 30:1553–1561

Hadjiolov D, Fernando RC, Schmeiser HH et al (1993) Effect of diallyl sulfide on aristolochic acid-induced forestomach carcinogenesis in rats. Carcinogenesis 14:407–410

Hayes MA, Rushmore TH, Goldberg MT (1987) Inhibition of hepatocarcinogenic responses to 1,2-dimethylhydrazine by diallyl sulfide, a component of garlic oil. Carcinogenesis 8: 1155–1157

Herman-Antosiewicz A, Singh SV (2004) Signal transduction pathways leading to cell cycle arrest and apoptosis induction in cancer cells by Allium vegetable-derived organosulfur compounds: a review. Mutat Res 555:121–131

Herman-Antosiewicz A, Singh SV (2005) Checkpoint kinase 1 regulates diallyl trisulfide-induced mitotic arrest in human prostate cancer cells. J Biol Chem 280:28519–28528

Herman-Antosiewicz A, Powolny AA, Singh SV (2007a) Molecular targets of cancer chemoprevention by garlic-derived organosulfides. Acta Pharmacol Sin 28:1355–1364

Herman-Antosiewicz A, Stan SD, Hahm ER et al (2007b) Activation of a novel ataxia-telangiectasia mutated and Rad3 related/checkpoint kinase 1-dependent prometaphase checkpoint in cancer cells by diallyl trisulfide, a promising cancer chemopreventive constituent of processed garlic. Mol Cancer Ther 6:1249–1261

Hill MJ (1997) Nutrition and human cancer. Acad Sci 833:68–78

Hirsch K, Danilenko M, Giat J et al (2000) Effect of purified allicin, the major ingredient of freshly crushed garlic, on cancer cell proliferation. Nutr Cancer 38:245–254

Hong JY, Wang ZY, Smith TJ et al (1982) Inhibitory effects of diallyl sulfide on the metabolism and tumorigenicity of the tobacco-specific carcinogen 4-(methylnitrosamino)-1-(3-pyridyl)-1-butanone (NNK) in A/J mouse lung. Carcinogenesis 13:901–904

Hong YS, Ham YA, Choi JH et al (2000) Effects of allyl sulfur compounds and garlic extract on the expression of Bcl-2, Bax, and p53 in non small cell lung cancer cell lines. Exp Mol Med 32:127–134

Hsing AW, Chokkalingam AP, Gao YT et al (2002) Allium vegetables and risk of prostate cancer: a population-based study. J Natl Cancer Inst 94:1648–1651

Hu PJ, Wargovich MJ (1989) Effect of diallyl sulfide on MNNG-induced nuclear aberrations and ornithine decarboxylase activity in the glandular stomach mucosa of the wistar rat. Cancer Lett 47:153–158

Hussain SP, Jannu LN, Rao, AR (1990) Chemopreventive action of garlic on methylcholanthrene-induced carcinogenesis in the uterine cervix of mice. Cancer Lett 49:175–180

Institute of Medicine (2000) Selenium. In: Dietary reference intakes for vitamin C, vitamin E, selenium and carotenoids. National Academy Press, Washington, DC

Ibrahim SS, Nassar NN (2008) Diallyl sulfide protects against N-nitrosodiethylamine-induced liver tumorigenesis: role of aldose reductase. World J Gastroenterol 14:6145–6153

Iciek M, Kwiecien I, Wlodek L (2009) Biological properties of garlic and garlic-derived organosulfur compounds. Environ Mol Mutagen 50:247–265

Ip C (1998) Lessons from basic research in selenium and cancer prevention. J Nutr 128:1845–1854

Ip C, Ganther HE (1992) Comparison of selenium and sulfur analogs in cancer prevention. Carcinogenesis 13:1167–1170

Ip C, Lisk DJ (1995) Efficacy of cancer prevention by high-selenium garlic is primarily dependent on the action of selenium. Carcinogenesis 16:2649–2652

Ip C, Birringer M, Block E (2000a) Chemical speciation influences comparative activity of selenium-enriched garlic and yeast in mammary cancer prevention. J Agric Food Chem 48:2062–2070

Ip C, Dong Y, Ganther HE (2002) New concepts in selenium chemoprevention. Cancer Metastasis Rev 21:281–289

Ip C, Lisk DJ, Stoewsand GS (1992) Mammary cancer prevention by regular garlic and selenium-enriched garlic. Nutr Cancer 17:279–286

Ip C, Thompson HJ, Ganther HE (2000b) Selenium modulation of cell proliferation and cell cycle biomarkers in normal and premalignant cells of the rat mammary gland. Cancer Epidemiol Biomarkers Prev 9:49–54

Karmakar S, Banik NL, Patel SJ et al (2007) Garlic compounds induced calpain and intrinsic caspase cascade for apoptosis in human malignant neuroblastoma SH-SY5Y cells. Apoptosis 12:671–684

Karunasighe N, Ryan J, Tuckey J (2004) DNA stability and serum selenium levels in a high-risk group for prostate cancer. Cancer Epidemiol Biomarkers Prev 13:391–397

Kawamori T, El-Bayoumy K, Ji BY et al (1998) Evaluation of benzyl selenocyanate glutathione conjugate for potential chemopreventive properties in colon carcinogenesis. Int J Oncol 13:29–34

Kelloff GJ, Boone CW, Malone WF et al (1992) Introductory remarks: development of chemopreventive agents for prostate cancer. J Cell Biochem 16:1–8

Key TJ, Silcocks PB, Davey GK et al (1997) A case-control study of diet and prostate cancer. Br J Cancer 76:678–687

Kim Jr, Kulon O (2009) Garlic intake and cancer risk: an analysis using the food and drug administration: evidence-based review system for the scientific evaluation of health claims. Am J Clin Nutr 89:257–264

Kim YA, Xiao D, Xiao H et al (2007) Mitochondria mediated apoptosis by diallyl trisulfide in human prostate cancer cells is associated with generation of reactive oxygen species and regulated by Bax/Bak. Mol Cancer Ther 6:1599–1609

Kim YS, Young MR, Bobe G et al (2009) Bioactive food components, inflammatory targets, and cancer prevention. Cancer Prev Res (Phila Pa) 2:200–208

Klein EA (2004) Selenium: epidemiology and basic science. J Urol 171:S50–S53

Knowles LM, Milner JA (2000) Diallyl disulfide inhibits p34(cdc2) kinase activity through changes in complex formation and phosphorylation. Carcinogenesis 21:1129–1134

Knowles LM, Milner JA (2001) Possible mechanism by which allyl sulfides suppress neoplastic cell proliferation. J Nutr 131:1061s–1066s

Kwon KB, Yoo SJ, Ryu DG et al (2002) Induction of apoptosis by diallyl disulfide through activation of caspase-3 in human leukemia HL-60 cells. Biochem Pharmacol 63:41–47

Laakso I, Seppanen-Laaskso T, Hiltunen R et al (1989) Volatile garlic odor components: gas phase and adsorbed exhaled air analysed by head space gas chromatography–mass spectrometry. Planta Med 55:257–261

Lanfear J, Fleming J, Wu L et al (1994) The selenium metabolite selenodiglutathione induces p53 and apoptosis: relevance to the chemopreventive effects of selenium? Carcinogenesis 15:1387–1392

Lawson LD, Gardner CD (2005) Composition, stability, and bioavailability of garlic products used in a clinical trial. J Agric Food Chem 53:6254–6261

Lawson LD, Wang ZJ (1993) Pre-hepatic fate of the organosulfur compounds derived from garlic (Allium sativum). Planta Med 59:688–689

Lea MA, Randolph VM, Patel M (1999) Increased acetylation of histones induced by diallyl disulfide and structurally related molecules. Int J Oncol 15:347–352

Lea MA, Rasheed M, Randolph VM et al (2002) Induction of histone acetylation and inhibition of growth of mouse erythroleukemia cells by Sallylmercaptocysteine. Nutr Cancer 43:90–102

Lee J-I, Nian H, Cooper AJL, et al (2009) α-Keto acid metabolites of naturally-occurring organoselenium compounds as inhibitors of histone deacetylase in human prostate cancer cells. Cancer Prev Res (Phila Pa) 2:683–693

Lei XY, Yao SQ, Zu XY et al (2008) Apoptosis induced by diallyl disulfide in human breast cancer cell line MCF-7. Acta Pharmacol Sin 29:1233–1239

Li M, Ciu JR, Ye Y et al (2002a) Antitumor activity of Z-ajoene, a natural compound purified from garlic: antimitotic and microtubule-interaction properties. Carcinogenesis 23:573–579

Li H, Li HQ, Wang Y et al (2004) An intervention study to prevent gastric cancer by microselenium and large dose of allitridum. Chin Med J (Engl) 117:1155–1160

Li M, Min JM, Cui JR et al (2002b) Z-ajoene induces apoptosis of HL-60 cells: involvement of Bcl-2 cleavage. Nutr Cancer 42:241–247

Li JY, Taylor PR, Li B et al (1993) Nutrition intervention trials in Linxian, China: multiple vitamin/mineral supplementation, cancer incidence, and disease-specific mortality among adults with esophageal dysplasia. J Natl Cancer Inst 85:1492–1498

Lippman SM, Klein EA, Goodman PJ et al (2009) Effect of selenium and vitamin E on risk of prostate cancer and other cancers: the Selenium and Vitamin E Cancer Prevention Trial (SELECT). J Am Med Assoc 301:39–51

Maurya AK, Singh SV (1991) Differential induction of glutathione transferase isoenzymes of mice stomach by diallyl sulfide, a naturally occurring anticarcinogen. Cancer Lett 57:121–129

Medina D, Thompson H, Ganther H et al (2001) Se-methylselenocysteine: a new compound for chemoprevention of breast cancer. Nutr Cancer 40:12–17

Meyer K, Ueberham E, Gebhardt R (2004) Influence of organosulphur compounds from garlic on the secretion of matrix metalloproteinases and their inhibitor TIMP-1 by cultured HUVEC cells. Cell Biol Toxicol 20:253–260

Milner JA (2001) Mechanisms by which garlic and allyl sulfur compounds suppress carcinogen bioactivation. Garlic and carcinogenesis. Adv Exp Med Biol 492:69–81

Milner JA (2006) Preclinical perspectives on garlic and cancer. J Nutr 136:827S–831S

Minami T, Boku T, Inada K et al (1989) Odor components of human breath after the ingestion of grated raw garlic. J Food Sci 54:763–765

Mori H, Sugie S, Rahman W et al (1999) Chemoprevention of 2-amino-1-methyl-6-phenylimidazo[4,5 b]pyridineinduced mammary carcinogenesis in rats. Cancer Lett 143:195–198

Morley JE, Baumgartner RN (2004) Cytokine-related aging process. J Gerontol A Biol Sci Med Sci 59:924–929

Morris VC, Levander OA (1970) Selenium content of foods. J Nutr 100:1383–1388

Mousa AS, Mousa SA (2005) Anti-angiogenesis efficacy of the garlic ingredient alliin and antioxidants: role of nitric oxide and p53. Nutr Cancer 53:104–110

Myzak MC, Dashwood RH (2006) Histone deacetylases as targets for dietary cancer preventive agents: lessons learned with butyrate, diallyl disulfide, and sulforaphane. Curr Drug Targets 7:443–452

Nagae S, Ushijima M, Hatono S et al (1994) Pharmacokinetics of the garlic compound S-allylcysteine. Planta Med 60:214–217

Nakagawa H, Tsuta K, Kiuchi K et al (2001) Growth inhibitory effects of diallyl disulfide on human breast cancer cell lines. Carcinogenesis 22:891–897

Nayini JR, El-Bayoumy K, Sugie S et al (1989) Chemoprevention of experimental mammary carcinogenesis by the synthetic organoselenium compound, benzylselenocyanate, in rats. Carcinogenesis 10:509–512

Nayini JR, Sugie S, El-Bayoumy K et al (1991) Effect of dietary benzylselenocyanate on azoxymethane-induced colon carcinogenesis in male F344 rats. Nutr Cancer 15:129–139

Nian H, Bisson WH, Dashwood W, et al (2009a) Alpha-keto acid metabolites of organoselenium compounds inhibit histone deacetylase activity in human colon cancer cells. Carcinogenesis 30:1416–1423

Nian H, Delage B, Ho E et al (2009b) Modulation of histone deacetylase activity by dietary isothiocyanates and allyl sulfides: studies with sulforaphane and garlic organosulfur compounds. Environ Mol Mutagen 50:213–221

Nishikawa T, Yamada N, Hattori A et al (2002) Inhibition by ajoene of skin-tumor promotion in mice. Biosci Biotechnol Biochem 66:2221–2223

Nunn J (1996) Ancient Egyptian Medicine. University of Oklahoma Press, Oklahoma

Ogawa H, Gomi T, Nishizawa M et al (2006) Enzymatic and biochemical properties of a novel human serine dehydratase isoform. Biochim Biophys Acta 1764:961–971

Pan J, Hong JY, Ma BL et al (1993) Transcriptional activation of cytochrome P450 2B1/2 genes in rat liver by diallyl sulfide, a compound derived from garlic. Arch Biochem Biophys 302: 337–342

Pelucchi C, Bosetti C, Rossi M et al (2009) Selected aspects of Mediterranean diet and cancer risk. Nutr Cancer 61:756–766

Perchellet JP, Perchellet EM, Abney NL et al (1986) Effects of garlic and onion oils on glutathione peroxidase activity, the ratio of reduced/ oxidized glutathione and ornithine decarboxylase induction in isolated mouse epidermal cells treated with tumor promoters. Cancer Biochem Biophys 8:299–312

Powolny AA, Singh SV (2008) Multitargeted prevention and therapy of cancer by diallyl trisulfide and related Allium vegetable-derived organosulfur compounds. Cancer Lett 269: 305–314

Prasad MP, Mukundan MA, Krishnaswamy K (1995) Micronuclei and carcinogen DNA adducts as intermediate end points in nutrient intervention trial of precancerous lesions in the oral cavity. Eur J Cancer B Oral Oncol 31B:155–159

Rahman K (2001) Historical perspective on garlic and cardiovascular disease. J Nutr 131: 977S–979S

Rao CV, Simi B, Hirose Y et al (2000) Mechanisms in the chemoprevention of colon cancer: modulation of protein kinase C, tyrosine protein kinase and diacylglycerol kinase activities by 1,4-phenylenebis(methylene) and impact of low-fat diet. Int J Oncol 16:519–527

Ray AL, Semba RD, Walstron J et al (2006) Low serum selenium and total carotenoids predict mortality among older women living in the community: The women's health and aging studies. J Nutr 136:172–176

Rayman MP (2000) The importance of selenium to human health. Lancet 356:233–241

Reddy BS, Rao CV, Rivenson A et al (1993) Chemoprevention of colon carcinogenesis by organosulfur compounds. Cancer Res 53:3493–3496

Reid ME, Stratton MS, Lillico AJ et al (2004) A report of high-dse selenium supplementation: response and toxicities. J Trace Elem Med Biol 18:69–74

Rivlin RS (2001) Historical perspective on the use of garlic. J Nutr 131:951S–954S

Rooseboom M, Vermeulen NP, van Hemert E et al (2001) Bioactivation of chemopreventive selenocysteine Se-conjugates and related compounds by amino acid oxidases. Novel route of metabolism of selenoaminoacids. Chem Res Toxicol 14:996–1005

Rooseboom M, Vermeulen NPE, Durgut F et al (2002) Comparative study on the bioactivation mechanisms and toxicity of Te-phenyl-L-tellurocysteine, Se-phenyl-L-selenocysteine, and S-phenyl-L-cysteine. Chem Res Toxicol 15:1610–1618

Ross SA, Finley JW, Milner JA (2006) Allyl sulfur compounds from garlic modulate aberrant crypt formation. J Nutr 136:852S–854S

Sadhana AS, Rao AR, Kucheria K et al (1988) Inhibitory action of garlic oil on the initiation of benzo[a]pyrene-induced skin carcinogenesis in mice. Cancer Lett 40:193–197

Schaffer EM, Liu JZ, Green J (1996) Garlic and associated allyl sulfur components inhibit N-methyl-N-nitrosourea induced rat mammary carcinogenesis. Cancer Lett 102:199–204

Seki T, Hosono T, Hosono-Fukao T et al (2008) Anticancer effects of diallyl trisulfide derived from garlic. Asia Pac J Clin Nutr 17:249–252

Shamberger RJ, Frost DV (1969) Possible protective effect of selenium against human cancer. Can Med Assoc J 100:682

Shirin H, Pinto JT, Kawabata Y et al (2001) Antiproliferative effects of S-allylmercaptocysteine on colon cancer cells when tested alone or in combination with sulindac sulfide. Cancer Res 61:725–731

Shukla Y, Kalra N (2007) Cancer chemoprevention with garlic and its constituents. Cancer Lett 247:167–181

Singh A, Shukla Y (1998a) Antitumour activity of diallyl sulfide on polycyclic aromatic hydrocarbon induced mouse skin carcinogenesis. Cancer Lett 131:209–214

Singh A, Shukla Y (1998b) Antitumor activity of diallyl sulfide in two-stage mouse skin model of carcinogenesis. Biomed Environ Sci 11:258–263

Singh A, Arora A, Shukla Y (2004) Modulation of altered hepatic foci induction by diallyl sulphide in Wistar rats. Eur J Cancer Prev 13:263–269

Singh SV, Powolny AA, Stan SD et al (2008a) Garlic constituent diallyl trisulfide prevents development of poorly differentiated prostate cancer and pulmonary metastasis multiplicity in TRAMP mice. Cancer Res 68:9503–9511

Singh U, Null K, Sinha R (2008b) In vitro growth inhibition of mouse mammary epithelial tumor cells by methylseleninic acid: involvement of protein kinases. Mol Nutr Food Res 52: 1281–1288

Sinha R, Potter JD (1997) Diet, nutrition, and genetic susceptibility. Cancer Epidemiol Biomarkers Prev 6:647–649

Sinha R, Kiley SC, Lu JX et al (1999) Effects of methylselenocysteine on PKC activity, cdk2 phosphorylation and gadd gene expression in synchronized mouse mammary epithelial tumor cells. Cancer Lett 146:135–145

Sinha R, El-Bayoumy K (2004) Apoptosis is a critical cellular event in cancer chemoprevention and chemotherapy by selenium compounds. Curr Cancer Drug Targets 4:13–428

Sinha R, Pinto JT, Facompre N et al (2008) Effects of naturally occurring and synthetic organoselenium compounds on protein profiling in androgen responsive and androgen independent human prostate cancer cells. Nutr Cancer 60:267–275

Sparnins VL, Barany G, Wattenberg, LW (1988) Effects of organosulfur compounds from garlic and onions on benzo[a]pyrene-induced neoplasia and glutathione S-transferase activity in the mouse. Carcinogenesis 9:131–134

Sriram N, Kalayarasan S, Ashokkumar P et al (2008) Diallyl sulfide induces apoptosis in Colo 320 DM human colon cancer cells: involvement of caspase-3, NF-kappaB, and ERK-2. Mol Cell Biochem 311:157–165

Stan SD, Singh SV (2009) Transcriptional repression and inhibition of nuclear translocation of androgen receptor by diallyl trisulfide in human prostate cancer cells. Clin Cancer Res 15:4895–4903

Stevens JL (1985) Isolation and characterization of a rat liver enzyme with both cysteine conjugate β lyase and kynureninase activity. J Biol Chem 260:7945–7950

Sumiyoshi H, Wargovich MJ (1990) Chemoprevention of 1,2-dimethylhydrazineinduced colon cancer in mice by naturally occurring organosulfur compounds. Cancer Res 50:5084–5087

Sun X, Guo, T, He J (2006) Determination of the concentration of diallyl trisulfide in rat whole blood using gas chromatography with electroncapture detection and identification of its major metabolite with gas chromatography mass spectrometry. Yakuga Zasshi 126:521–527

Sundaram SG, Milner JA (1996) Diallyl disulfide induces apoptosis of human colon tumor cells. Carcinogenesis 17:669–673

Suzui N, Sugie S, Rahman KM et al (1997) Inhibitory effects of diallyl disulfide or aspirin in 2-amino-1-methyl-6-phenylimidazo[4,5-b]pyridine-induced mammary carcinogenesis on rats. Jpn J Cancer Res 88:705–711

Suzuki KT, Tsuji Y, Ohta Y et al (2008) Preferential organ distribution of methylselenol source Se-methylselenocysteine relative to methylseleninic acid. Toxicol Appl Pharmacol 227:76–83

Takahashi S, Hakoi K, Yada H et al (1992) Enhancing effects of diallyl sulfide on hepatocarcinogenesis and inhibitory actions of the related diallyl disulfide on colon and renal carcinogenesis in rats. Carcinogenesis 13:1513–1518

Tanaka S, Haruma K, Yoshihara M et al (2006) Aged garlic extract has potential suppressive effect on colorectal adenomas in humans. J Nutr 136:821S–826S

Taylor P, Albanes D (1998) Selenium, vitamin E, and prostate cancer- ready for prime time? J Natl Cancer Inst 90:440–446

Taylor P, Noriega R, Farah C et al (2006) Ajoene inhibits both primary tumor growth and metastasis of B16/BL6 melanoma cells in C57BL/6 mice. Cancer Lett 239:298–304

Terry N, Zayed AM, De Souza MP et al (2000) Selenium in higher plants. Annu Rev Plant Physiol Plant Mol Biol 51:401–432

Tilli CM, Stavast-Kooy AJ, Vuerstaek JD et al (2003) The garlic-derived organosulfur component ajoene decreases basal cell carcinoma tumor size by inducing apoptosis. Arch Dermatol Res 295:117–123

Toohey JI (1989) Sulphane sulfur in biological systems: a possible regulatory role. Biochem J 264:625–632

Toohey JI (2001) Possible involvement of sulfane sulfur in homocysteine-induced atherosclerosis. Med Hypotheses 56:259–261

Wang Z, Jiang C, Lu J (2002) Induction of caspase-mediated apoptosis and cell-cycle G1 arrest by selenium metabolite methylselenol. Mol Carcinog 34:113–120

Wargovich MJ (1987) Diallyl sulfide, a flavor component of garlic (*Allium sativum*), inhibits dimethylhydrazine-induced colon cancer. Carcinogenesis 8:487–489

Wargovich MJ, Chen CD, Jimenez A et al (1996) Aberrant crypts as a biomarker for colon cancer: evaluation of potential chemopreventive agents in the rat. Cancer Epidemiol Biomarkers Prev 5:355–360

Wargovich MJ, Woods C, Eng VW et al (1988) Chemoprevention of N-nitrosomethylbenzylamine-induced esophageal cancer in rats by the naturally occurring thioether, diallyl sulfide. Cancer Res 48:6872–6875

Waters DJ, Shen S, Glickman LT (2005) Prostate cancer risk and DNA damage: translational significance of selenium supplementation in a canine model. Carcinogenesis 26:1256–1262

Wattenberg LW, Sparnins VL, Barany G (1989) Inhibition of *N*-Nitrosodiethylamine carcinogenesis in mice by naturally occurring organosulfur compounds and monoterpenes. Cancer Res 49:2689–2692

Weisberger AS, Pensky J (1958) Tumor inhibition by a sulfhydryl-blocking agent related to an active principle of garlic (*Allium sativum*). Cancer Res 18:1301–1308

Whanger PD (1989) Seleno compounds in plants and their effects on animals. In: Cheeke PR (ed) Toxicants of plant origins. CRC Press, Boca Raton, FL pp 141–167

Whanger PD (2003) Metabolic pathways of selenium in plants and animals and their nutritional significance. In: Lyone TP, Jacques KA (ed) Nutritional biotechnology in the feed and food industries. Nottingham University Press, UK pp 51–58

Whanger PD (2004) Selenium and its relationship to cancer: an update dagger. Br J Nutr 91:11–28

Wilpart M, Speder A, Roberfroid M (1986) Anti-initiation activity of N-acetylcysteine in experimental colonic carcinogenesis. Cancer Lett 31:319–324

Wolf WR, Schubert A (1989) Foods. In: Inhant M (ed) Occurrence and distribution of selenium. CRC Press, Boca Raton, FL

Wu XJ, Kassie F, Mersch-Sundermann V (2005) The role of reactive oxygen species (ROS) production on diallyl disulfide (DADS) induced apoptosis and cell cycle arrest in human A549 lung carcinoma cells. Mutat Res 579:115–124

Wu XJ, Hu Y, Lamy E et al (2009) Apoptosis induction in human lung adenocarcinoma cells by oil-soluble allyl sulfides: triggers, pathways, and modulators. Environ Mol Mutagen 50:266–275

Wynder EL, Gori GB (1977) Contribution of the environment to cancer incidence: an epidemiology exercise. J Natl Cancer Inst 58:825–832

Xiao D, Pinto JT, Soh JW et al (2003) Induction of apoptosis by the garlic-derived compound S-allylmercaptocysteine (SAMC) is associated with microtubule depolymerization and c-Jun NH(2)-terminal kinase 1 activation. Cancer Res 63:6825–6837

Xiao D, Choi S, Johnson DE et al (2004) Diallyl trisulfide-induced apoptosis in human prostate cancer cells involves c-Jun Nterminal kinase and extracellular-signal regulated kinasemediated phosphorylation of Bcl-2. Oncogene 23:5594–5606

Xiao D, Herman-Antosiewicz A, Antosiewicz J et al (2005) Diallyl trisulfide-induced G(2)-M phase cell cycle arrest in human prostate cancer cells is caused by reactive oxygen species-dependent destruction and hyperphosphorylation of Cdc 25 C. Oncogene 24: 6256–6268

Xiao D, Li M, Herman-Antosiewicz A et al (2006) Diallyl trisulfide inhibits angiogenic features of human umbilical vein endothelial cells by causing Akt inactivation and down-regulation of VEGF and VEGF-R2. Nutr Cancer 55:94–107

Xiao D, Zeng Y, Hahm ER et al (2009) Diallyl trisulfide selectively causes Bax- and Bak-mediated apoptosis in human lung cancer cells. Environ Mol Mutagen 50:201–212

Yang CS, Chhabra SK, Hong JY et al (2001) Mechanisms of inhibition of chemical toxicity and carcinogenesis by diallyl sulfide (DAS) and related compounds from garlic. J Nutr 131: 1041s–1045s

Yang J, Meyers KJ, van der Heide J et al (2004) Varietal differences in phenolic content and antioxidant and antiproliferative activities of onions. J Agric Food Chem 52:6787–6793

Yoshizawa K, Willett WC, Morris SJ et al (1998) Study of prediagnostic selenium level in toenails and the risk of advanced prostate cancer. J Natl Cancer Inst 90:1219–1224

You WC, Blot WJ, Chang YS et al (1988) Diet and high risk of stomach cancer in Shandong, China. Cancer Res 48:3518–3523

You WC, Blot WJ, Chang YS et al (1989) Allium vegetables and reduced risk of stomach cancer. J Natl Cancer Inst 81:162–164

You WC, Brown LM, Zhang L et al (2006) Gail, Randomized double-blind factorial trial of three treatments to reduce the prevalence of precancerous gastric lesions. J Natl Cancer Inst 98: 974–983

Yu SY, Zhu YJ, Li WG et al (1991) A preliminary report on the intervention trials of primary liver cancer in high-risk populations with nutritional supplementation of selenium in China. Biol Trace Elem Res 29:289–294

Yu SY, Zhu YJ, Li WG (1997) Protective role of selenium against hepatitis B virus and primary liver cancer in Qidong. Biol Trace Elem Res 56:117–124

Yuan JP, Ling H, Zhang MX et al (2004) Diallyl disulfide-induced G2/M arrest of human gastric cancer MGC803 cells involves activation of p38 MAP kinase pathways. Ai Zheng 23:169–172

Chapter 6
Molecular Mechanisms of Chemoprevention with Capsaicinoids from Chili Peppers

Young-Joon Surh and Joydeb Kumar Kundu

Abstract Chemoprevention is one of the most practical strategies to prevent cancer. Numerous dietary phytochemicals present in fruits, vegetables and spices have been reported to possess cancer preventive properties. Chili peppers are widely consumed spices throughout the world. The non-nutritive pungent phytochemicals present in chili peppers are capsaicinoids. While the principal capsaicinoid from hot chili pepper is a pungent alkaloid capsaicin [(*E*)-*N*-(4-hydroxy-3-methoxybenzyl)-8-methyl-6-nonenamide], the major nonpungent vanilloid from sweet red pepper is capsiate [4-hydroxy-3-methoxybenzyl (*E*)-8-methyl-6-nonenoate]. Both capsaicinoids and capsiates have been shown to possess antioxidant, anti-inflammatory and chemopreventive properties. Biochemical mechanisms underlying chemopreventive effects of capsaicinoids include inhibition of carcinogen activation, stimulation of carcinogen detoxification, attenuation of oxidative and inflammatory responses, inhibition of proliferation, induction of apoptosis in cancer cells, and the blockade of tumor angiogenesis and metastasis. This chapter will focus on the mechanistic aspect of cancer chemoprevention with vanilloids.

Keywords Capsaicinoids · Chili peppers · Chemoprevention · Cell signaling

Contents

Y.-J. Surh (✉)
National Research Laboratory of Molecular Carcinogenesis and Chemoprevention, College of Pharmacy, Seoul National University, Seoul, 151 742, South Korea
e-mail: surh@plaza.snu.ac.kr

M. Mutanen, A.-M. Pajari (eds.), *Vegetables, Whole Grains, and Their Derivatives in Cancer Prevention*, Diet and Cancer 2, DOI 10.1007/978-90-481-9800-9_6,
© Springer Science+Business Media B.V. 2011

6.1 Chili Peppers: A Potential Source of Chemopreventive Phytochemicals

'Chemoprevention', the term coined by Micheal B. Sporn, refers to the use of non-toxic chemical substances derived from either natural or synthetic sources to inhibit, retard or even reverse the multistage carcinogenic processes (Sporn 1976). Parallel to the population-based studies, numerous laboratory studies have highlighted the chemopreventive potential of substances derived from plant-based diets, collectively termed 'phytochemicals'. Interestingly, a wide variety of chemopreventive phytochemicals are present in fruits, vegetables and spices (Surh 2003). Chili peppers that belong to genus *Capsicum*. (family-Solanaceae) are widely consumed as spices throughout the world.

Chemical analysis of chili peppers revealed the presence of high content of antioxidant vitamins, and several non-nutritive phytochemicals including pungent (e.g., capsaicin, dihydrocapsaicin, nordihydrocapsaicin, homocapsaicin, homodihydrocapsaicin, and nonivamide) (Reilly et al. 2001a, b) and nonpungent (e.g., capsiate and dihydrocapsiate) (Macho et al. 2003a) vanilloids (Fig. 6.1). While capsaicin is the principal pungent ingredient of hot chili pepper (*Capsicum frutescence*) or hot red pepper (*Capsicum annum*), capsiate is a major nonpungent analog of capsaicin

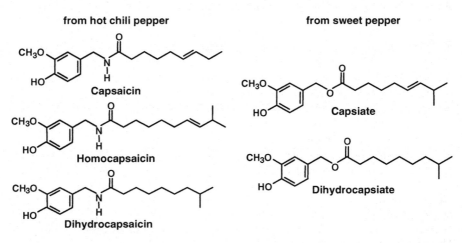

Fig. 6.1 Chemical structures of major pungent and nonpungent capsaicinoids from chili peppers

isolated from sweet peppers (*Capsicum annum.* var. CH-19 Sweet L.). The only structural difference between capsaicin and capsiate is the arrangement of vanillyl and the acyl moieties, respectively. The vanillyl moiety in capsaicin is linked through an amide bond, whereas the acyl moiety in capsiate is joined by an ester linkage. Although capsaicin has long been studied for its chemopreventive activities (Park and Surh 1997; Surh 2002; Surh et al. 1995), nonpungent capsaicinoids, such as capsiate and related vanilloids have received lesser attention (Macho et al. 2003a; Pyun et al. 2008). The scope of this chapter is limited to focus on the molecular mechanisms of chemoprevention with capsaicinoids derived from chili peppers.

6.2 Chemoprevention with Capsaicinoids: In Vivo Studies

Although the effects of chili pepper consumption on human carcinogenesis have long been under debate, some studies addressed the cancer preventive potential of capsaicinoids. Several studies suggested that capsaicin may act as a carcinogen or a co-carcinogen in laboratory animals (Kim et al. 1985; Toth and Gannett 1992) as well as in humans (Lopez-Carrillo et al. 2003). Other studies have demonstrated that capsaicin is not carcinogenic but rather inhibits experimentally induced tumorigenesis (Jang et al. 1989; Park and Surh 1997; Tanaka et al. 2002). This disparity may be attributed to the impurity profile of isolated capsaicin used in several studies as compared to the use of synthesized pure capsaicin in other studies. The evidence supporting the lack of carcinogenic potential of capsaicin was reported by several investigators. For example, repeated topical application of capsaicin failed to induce papillomagenesis in 7,12-dimethylbenz[α]anthracene (DMBA)-treated mouse skin (Park et al. 1998). Topical application of a proto-type tumor promoter 12-O-tetradecanoylphorbol-13-acetate (TPA), but not *trans*-capsaicin, induced skin papillomas in a *v*-Ha-*Ras*-transgenic (Tg.Ac) mouse model (Chanda et al. 2007). Moreover, prolonged dietary administration of capsaicinoids (a mixture of 64.5% capsaicin and 32.5% dihydrocapsaicin) was devoid of tumorigenic effects in B6C3F1 mice (Akagi et al. 1998).

Capsaicin inhibits experimentally induced tumorigenesis by interfering with initiation and promotion stages. Pretreatment of female ICR mice with capsaicin lowered the multiplicity of vinyl carbamate (VC)-induced skin tumors partly by inhibiting the activity of cytochrome P450 (CYP) 2E1, an enzyme responsible for the metabolic activation of VC (Surh et al. 1995). When capsaicin was topically applied to DMBA-initiated mouse skin prior to each topical application of TPA, there was a significant reduction in the skin tumor formation (Park and Surh 1997). Likewise, topical application of nor-dihydrocapsiate, a synthetic analog of capsiate, to DMBA-treated mouse skin before each TPA administration reduced the multiplicity and the volume of skin tumors (Macho et al. 2003a). Capsaicin and related pungent capsaicinoids act as agonists of vanilloid receptor-1 (VR1), alternatively known as transient receptor potential of vanilloids type-1 (TRPV1). TRPV1 has recently been reported to protect against mouse skin carcinogenesis through blockade of epidermal growth factor receptor-mediated signaling (Bode et al. 2009). Thus, it is worthwhile to investigate whether the chemopreventive activity of capsaicin is linked to its activation of TRPV1 in mouse skin.

Treatment of NIH(GP) mice with chemical carcinogens, such as benzo[α] pyrene (BP) or DMBA within 24 h of birth, and dietary administration of capsaicin (0.01%) to these animals at the post-weanling age for 6 weeks resulted in a significant decrease in the incidence of BP-induced pulmonary adenomas and the multiplicity of DMBA-induced lung tumors (Jang et al. 1989). Dietary administration of capsaicin (0.01%) also significantly inhibited the formation of glutathione-S-transferase-π-positive (GST-P+) hepatic foci and pulmonary adenomas in rats treated with diethylnitrosoamine, N-methylnitrosourea or N,N-dibutylnitrosoamine (Jang et al. 1991). In contrast, intragastric administration of capsaicin failed to inhibit tobacco-specific carcinogen 4-(methylnitrosamino)-1-(3-pyridyl)-1-butanone (NNK)-induced lung tumorigenesis in female A/J mice (Teel and Huynh 1999).

Dietary administration of capsaicin (500 ppm), either at the initiation or the promotion phase, reduced the incidence of azoxymethane (AOM)-induced formation of aberrant crypt foci and colonic adenocarcinomas (Yoshitani et al. 2001), and 4-nitro-quinoline-1-oxide (4-NQO)-induced tongue carcinoma formation as well as dysplasia in male F344 rats (Tanaka et al. 2002).

6.3 Molecular Mechanisms of Chemoprevention with Capsaicinoids

Abnormal amplification of intracellular signaling network comprising a wide spectrum of protein kinases and transcription factors is implicated in the premalignant and malignant transformation of cells. The mechanistic basis of chemoprevention involves the normalization of dysregulated signaling pathways associated with carcinogen activation and detoxification, cellular redox regulation, inflammation, cell proliferation, programmed cell death, metastasis and angiogenesis (Kundu et al. 2008). The following sections will provide molecular insights into the mechanisms of chemoprevention with capsaicinoids (also summarized in Table 6.1).

6.3.1 Effects on Carcinogen Metabolism

Many carcinogens acquire the DNA damaging potential through activation by phase I metabolizing enzymes. These metabolically activated carcinogens are usually eliminated by phase II detoxifying enzymes. Thus, inhibition of phase I metabolizing enzymes to block carcinogen activation, and the induction of phase II enzymes to facilitate carcinogen detoxification are generally considered to block carcinogen-induced DNA damage and subsequent mutation. Capsaicin has been reported to inhibit the metabolic activation of certain chemical carcinogens. For instance, the tobacco-specific carcinogen NNK is metabolically activated through

Table 6.1 Molecular mechanisms of chemoprevention with capsaicinoids

Capsaicinoids	Mechanisms/Targets	References
Capsaicin	*Inhibition of carcinogen activation*	
	↓BP metabolism and [^{3}H]-BP DNA binding; ↓arylhydrocarbon hydrolase activity	Modly et al. (1986)
	↓VC-induced mouse skin carcinogenesis; ↓NDMA-N-demethylation; ↓CYP 2E1 activity	Surh et al. (1995)
	↓Metabolic activation of NNK; ↓CYP2A2, 3A1, 2C11, 2B1, 2B2, and 2C6	Zhang et al. (1993)
	↓Methylation of NNK, ↓α-carbon hydroxylation of NNK	Zhang et al. (1997)
	Antioxidant effects	
	↓Ethanol-induced lipid peroxidation and myeloperoxidase activity in rat gastric mucosa	Park et al. (2000)
	↓BP-induced lipid peroxidation; restored BP-depleted activities of SOD	Anandakumar et al. (2008b, c)
	↑GST and quinone reductase activity in F344 rat liver	Yoshitani et al. (2001)
	↑Activation of Nrf2, ↑expression and activity of HO-1 in HepG2 cells	Joung et al. (2007)
	Inhibition of cell proliferation	
	Arrests the growth of CE 81T/VGH cells at G0-G1 phase; ↓expression of cyclin E, Cdk4 and Cdk6; ↓E2F level and ↑p16 expression	Wu et al. (2006)
	Arrests the growth of human leukemia cells at G0-G1 phase; ↓expression of retinoblastoma (Rb) and cyclin D1	Ito et al. (2004)
	G1 arrest in human multiple myeloma cells; ↓phosphorylation and the DNA binding of STAT3; ↓expression of survivin, cyclin D1, cSrc; ↓phosphorylation of JAK1; inhibits myeloma cell xenograft in nude mice	Bhutani et al. (2007)
	Induction of apoptosis	
	↑Intracellular ROS and Ca^{+2}; ↓mitochondrial membrane potential; ↑expression of p53, p21, Bax; ↓Bcl-2; ↑cytochrome c release; ↑caspase-3 activity in CE 81T/VGH cells	Wu et al. (2006)
	↑ROS and Ca^{2+}; ↓mitochondric membrane potential; ↑caspase-3 activity;	Sanchez et al. (2006, 2007, 2008)
	↑iNOS expression and peroxynitrite formation; ↑nitrotyrosine containing proteins in C6 glioma cells	Qiao et al. (2005)
	↑Phosphorylation of p38 MAP kinase and JNK in H-ras-transformed MCF-10A cells	Kang et al. (2003)
	↑Phosphorylation of AMPK and acetyl CoA carboxylase in HT-29 cells	Kim et al. (2007)
	↑Expression of p53, p21 and Bax in LnCaP, DU-145, and PC3 cells	Mori et al. (2006)

Table 6.1 (continued)

Capsaicinoids	Mechanisms/Targets	References
	Activation of PPAR-γ in HT-29 cells	Kim et al. (2004)
	$\downarrow$Mitochondrial membrane potential; $\uparrow$caspase-3 cleavage; $\uparrow$intracellular Ca^{2+}; $\uparrow$p38 MAP kinase phosphorylation; TRPV1-dependent apoptosis in Glioma cells	Amantini et al. (2007)
	Anti-inflammatory effects	
	$\downarrow$Expression of COX-2 and iNOS; $\downarrow$production of PGE_2 and NO; $\downarrow$phosphorylation of MAP kinases; $\downarrow$IKK activity; $\downarrow$NF-κB and AP-1 DNA binding in LPS-stimulated Raw 264.7 cells	Chen et al. (2003)
	$\downarrow$NF-κB activation and IL-8 production in IL-1β-stimulated melanoma cells	Patel et al. (2002a)
	$\downarrow$DNA binding of NF-κB and AP-1 and $\downarrow$PGE$_2$ production in LPS-stimulated macrophages	Kim et al. (2003)
	$\downarrow$DNA binding of NF-κB and AP-1 in TPA-treated mouse skin and HL-60 cells	Han et al. (2001)
	Inhibition of angiogenesis	
	$\downarrow$Expression of VEGF in human multiple myeloma cells	Bhutani et al. (2007)
	$\downarrow$VEGF-induced cell proliferation; $\downarrow$DNA synthesis and capillary-like tube formation in human malignant melanoma cells	Min et al. (2004)
Capsiate	*Antioxidant activity*	Rosa et al. (2002)
	Protects linoleic acid from autooxidation, and iron- or EDTA-mediated oxidation in vitro	
	Induction of apoptosis	
	$\uparrow$Accumulation of ROS; $\downarrow$mitochondrial membrane potential; $\uparrow$caspase-3 activation; arrests cell cycle at S phase in Jurkat cells	Macho et al. (2003b)
	Inhibition of angiogenesis	
	$\downarrow$VEGF-induced proliferation and capillary-like tube formation in primary culture of human endothelial cells; $\downarrow$VEGF-induced formation of new blood vessels, and activation of Src kinase; $\downarrow$sprouting of endothelial cells in the rat aorta	Pyun et al. (2008)
Nordihydrocapsiate	$\downarrow$NF-κB DNA binding, IKK activity and IκBα degradation in PMA plus PHA-stimulated Jurkat cells; $\downarrow$DSS-induced bowel inflammation in Balb/c mice	Sancho et al. (2002)

α-hydroxylation by microsomal mixed function oxidases. The α-carbon hydroxylation of NNK was inhibited after in vitro incubation of NNK with hepatic or pulmonary microsomes isolated from Golden Syrian hamster treated with capsaicin by gavage (Zhang et al. 1997). Moreover, capsaicin inhibited the mutagenicity of NNK in *Salmonella typhimurium* TA1535 by blocking its metabolic activation (Miller et al. 1993; Zhang et al. 1997). Capsaicin diminished the activity of epidermal arylhydrocarbon hydroxylase, thereby attenuating the activation and subsequent DNA binding of BP in human and murine keratinocytes (Modly et al. 1986). Furthermore, capsaicin inhibited the activity of CYP 2E1, thereby attenuating VC- or *N*-nitrosodimethylamine (NDMA)-induced mutagenesis in the *S. typhimurium* TA100 tester strain (Surh et al. 1995).

Besides blocking the metabolic activation of carcinogens, capsaicin enhanced the expression and/or activities of phase II detoxifying enzymes. Capsaicin, given by gavage, elevated the levels of GST and quinone reductase, in the liver, tongue and colon of male F344 rats (Tanaka et al. 2002), which may account for the inhibitory effects of capsaicin on chemically induced colon and tongue carcinogenesis.

6.3.2 Antioxidant Effects

Oxidative stress-induced damage of cellular macromolecules such as DNA or abnormal transmission of intracellular signals contributes to malignant transformation of cells. In order for cells to survive under oxidative stress, a precise control of cellular redox balance should be maintained by effective elimination or scavenging of reactive oxygen species (ROS). Dietary phytochemicals with antioxidant properties exert chemopreventive activity by blocking oxidative DNA damage or by suppressing ROS-mediated abnormal cellular proliferation. The chemopreventive activities of capsicinoids may partly be ascribed to their antioxidant properties (Salimath et al. 1986; Surh et al. 1998).

Excessive lipid peroxidation and subsequent generation of reactive aldehydes cause massive oxidative damage (Nair et al. 2007). Capsaicin attenuated ultraviolet (UV) radiation-induced lipid peroxidation in liposomal membrane (De and Ghosh 1989) and ameliorated the peroxidative changes in rat hepatic and pulmonary tissues induced by various noxious stimuli, such as chloroform, carbon tetrachloride and dichloromethane (De and Ghosh 1992). Capsaicin also inhibited ethanol-induced lipid peroxidation and the myeloperoxidase activity in gastric mucosa of Sprague-Dawley rats (Park et al. 2000). Furthermore, intraperitoneal administration of capsaicin protected against lipid peroxidation and restored the activities of antioxidant enzymes, such as superoxide dismutase (SOD), catalase (CAT), glutathione peroxidase (GPx), glutathione reductase (GR), glucose-6-phosphate dehydrogenase (G6PD), and GST in pulmonary tissues and lung mitochondria of Swiss albino mice treated with BP (Anandakumar et al. 2008a, b).

Treatment of human hepatoma HepG2 cells with capsaicin resulted in the marked elevation of the protein and mRNA levels of heme oxygenase-1 (HO-1), a key antioxidant enzyme involved in maintaining the cellular redox balance

(Joung et al. 2007). According to this study, capsaicin induced ROS generation in HepG2 cells by downregulating the expression and the activity of NAD(P)H:quinone oxidoreductase-1 (NQO1), thereby resulting in the activation of the stress-responsive transcription factor, nuclear factor erythroid related factor-2 (Nrf2). Thus, a mild oxidative stress associated with pro-oxidant potential of capsaicin may account for its upregulation of HO-1 expression in these cells (Joung et al. 2007). The nonpungent vanilloids, such as capsiate and its analogs were shown to protect linoleic acid from auto-oxidation or from iron- or ethylenediamine tetraacetic acid-mediated oxidation in vitro (Rosa et al. 2002).

6.3.3 Anti-inflammatory Effects

The multifaceted role of chronic inflammation in cancer is now a generally accepted paradigm in understanding the molecular basis of carcinogenesis. Thus, dietary phytochemicals that retain pronounced anti-inflammatory properties are expected to hold chemopreventive potential (Kundu and Surh 2008). The evaluation of anti-inflammatory activities of capsaicinoids has largely been focused on that of capsaicin. Although topical application of capsaicin initially causes neurogenic inflammation in human skin (Tafler et al. 1993) and produces mouse ear edema (Gabor and Razga 1992; Inoue et al. 1995), repeated administration of the compound attenuates the progressive inflammatory response (Gabor and Razga 1992; Jancso et al. 1967) by depleting the pro-inflammatory mediator 'substance P' from sensory nerve terminals.

Abnormally elevated expression of cyclooxygenase-2 (COX-2) and inducible nitric oxide synthase (iNOS), two representative pro-inflammatory enzymes, have been implicated in carcinogenesis (Kundu and Surh 2008). While COX-2 catalyzes the breakdown of arachidonic acid to produce prostaglandins (PGs), iNOS is responsible for the oxidative deamination of L-arginine to produce nitric oxide (NO). Both PGs and NO are pro-inflammatory mediators reported to play a pivotal role in malignant transformation of cells (Kundu and Surh 2008). Capsaicin, given by gavage, attenuated ethanol-induced expression of COX-2 in rat gastric mucosal lesion (Park et al. 2000). The compound also inhibited the expression of COX-2 protein and its mRNA transcript, and suppressed the production of PGE_2 in Raw 264.7 cells stimulated with lipopolysaccharide (LPS)- or TPA (Chen et al. 2003). Capsaicin suppressed LPS-induced PGE_2 production without affecting the expression of COX-2 protein and mRNA (Kim et al. 2003). Although capsaicin acts as an agonist of VR1/TRPV1, the lack of this vanilloid receptor expression in murine macrophages suggests that the inhibitory effects of capsaicin on LPS-induced COX-2 activity (Kim et al. 2003) and iNOS expression are VR1/TRPV1-independent (Chen et al. 2003). In contrast, capsaicin elevated the expression of COX-2 and IL-8, and increased the production of PGE_2 in human keratinocytes (HaCaT), which express the VR1/TRPV1. Co-treatment of HaCaT cells with a VR1 antagonist capsazepine abrogated capsaicin-induced expression of COX-2 (Southall et al. 2003). Thus, capsaicin induces COX-2 expression in cells expressing a functional VR1/TRPV1, while it suppresses the induced COX-2 expression in cells lacking this receptor. Capsaicin attenuated the expression of iNOS and the production of NO in Raw 264.7 macrophage cells treated with LPS or interferon-γ (IFN-γ) (Chen et al. 2003) and cultured murine peritoneal macrophage cells stimulated with LPS (Kim et al. 2003).

Over amplification of cellular signaling mediated via upstream kinases and their downstream transcription factors, such as nuclear factor-kappaB (NF-κB) and activator protein-1 (AP-1), results in the elevated expression of COX-2 and iNOS (Surh et al. 2001). Some capsaicinoids have been reported to attenuate inappropriate activation of upstream kinases and transcription factors involved in inflammatory signaling. Capsaicin inhibited the activation of extracellular signal-regulated kinase (ERK), c-Jun-N-terminal kinase (JNK) and IκB kinase (IKK), and suppressed the DNA binding of NF-κB, AP-1 and signal transducer and activator of transcription (STAT)-1 in LPS-stimulated Raw 264.7 macrophage cells (Chen et al. 2003). Treatment of murine peritoneal macrophages with capsaicin attenuated LPS-induced NF-κB activation by blocking IκBα degradation, thereby suppressing iNOS expression and NO production (Kim et al. 2003). Capsaicin inhibited constitutive or IL-1β-induced activation of NF-κB in malignant melanoma cells (Patel et al. 2002a). According to this study, capsaicin significantly reduced the production of IL-8, a pro-inflammatory cytokine involved in tumor promotion and progression. Capsaicin inhibited the activation of NF-κB in human myeloid (ML-1a) cells stimulated with TNF-α by blocking the degradation of IκBα and subsequent nuclear translocation of p65 (Singh et al. 1996). This study also revealed that capsaicin treatment attenuated the TNFα-dependent promoter activity of IκBα that contains NF-κB binding sites (Singh et al. 1996). Likewise, capsaicin diminished the activation of NF-κB by blocking its nuclear migration through inhibition of proteasomal degradation of IκBα in TNFα-stimulated human prostate cancer (PC3) cells (Mori et al. 2006). In another study, intraperitoneal administration of a nonpungent vanilloid, nor-dihydrocapsiate markedly reduced dextran sulfate sodium-induced inflammatory tissue damage in mouse colon (Sancho et al. 2002).

Topical application of capsaicin blunted the activation of both NF-κB and AP-1 in mouse skin stimulated with TPA (Han et al. 2001). Capsaicin also diminished the activation of these transcription factors in cultured human promyelocytic leukemia (HL-60) cells treated with TPA (Surh et al. 2000) and human leukemia (K562 and U937) cells incubated with TNFα or TPA (Duvoix et al. 2004). The inhibition of NF-κB in TPA-treated HL-60 cells was associated with the blockade of IκBα degradation and p65 nuclear translocation, which was abolished when the phenolic hydroxyl group of capsaicin was methylated, suggesting that the presence of a phenolic hydroxyl group is essential for the inhibitory effect of capsaicin on NF-κB activation (Han et al. 2002).

6.3.4 Effects on Tumor Cell Proliferation

Capsaicinoids have been shown to exert antiproliferative and growth inhibitory effects in cancerous cells. Capsaicin attenuated the growth of human esophageal epidermoid carcinoma (CE 81T/VGH) cells (Wu et al. 2006) and human leukemia cells (Ito et al. 2004). According to the former study, capsaicin arrested the cell cycle at the G1 phase and downregulated the expression of cell cycle regulatory proteins cyclin E and cyclin dependent kinase (Cdk)-4 and -6. Moreover, capsaicin induced the expression of the Cdk inhibitor p21 and diminished the expression of E2F in human esophageal epidermoid carcinoma (CE 81T/VGH) cells (Wu et al. 2006). Capsaicin also inhibited proliferation of human multiple myeloma cells by arresting these cells at the G1 phase (Bhutani et al. 2007). This study also revealed that capsaicin abrogated the constitutive as well as IL-6-induced activation of STAT3 by blocking Janus kinase-1 and c-Src kinase. Capsaicin elicited an anti-proliferative effect in these cells partly by downregulating the expression of cyclin D1 and survivin, which are STAT3-regulated gene products. Moreover, capsaicin suppressed the proliferation of immortalized endometriotic cells, suggesting that the compound may have a therapeutic potential for the treatment of endometriosis (Wu et al. 2008), an inflammatory condition that often turns into endometrial adenocarcinomas (Jones et al. 2002).

Intratumoral administration of capsaicin together with *tert*-butylhydroperoxide inhibited the growth of B16 mouse melanoma cells transplanted in C57BL/6 mice (Morre et al. 1996). The compound also reduced the growth of human promyelocytic leukemia (NB4) cells inoculated subcutaneously into non obese diabetic (NOD)/severe combined immunodeficiency (SCID) mice (Ito et al. 2004). In another study, the growth of human prostate cancer xenograft in nude mice was inhibited by capsaicin administered either orally (Mori et al. 2006) or subcutaneously (Sanchez et al. 2006). Likewise, intraperitoneal administration of capsaicin to mice transplanted with multiple myeloma cells resulted in the reduced growth of xenograft tumors (Bhutani et al. 2007).

6.3.5 Effects on Cancer Cell Apoptosis

Capsaicinoids have been reported to exert chemopreventive activities through induction of apoptosis in various cancerous or transformed cells (Chow et al. 2007; Kang et al. 2003). Several mechanisms of capsaicin-induced apoptosis include: (i) generation of ROS and reactive nitrogen species (Qiao et al. 2005; Sanchez et al. 2006; Wu et al. 2006), (ii) inhibition of plasma membrane NADH-oxidoreductase (Morre et al. 1997, 1995, 1996; Wolvetang et al. 1996), (iii) the disruption of mitochondrial membrane permeability transition (Hail and Lotan 2002), (iv) intracellular accumulation of ceramide (Sanchez et al. 2007), (v) increase in the intracellular Ca^{2+} level (Wu et al. 2006), (vi) proteolytic cleavage and increased activity of caspase-3 (Wu et al. 2006), (vii) increased p53 expression (Mori et al. 2006) and phosphorylation of p53 at serine 15 residue (Ito et al. 2004), and (viii) amplified signal transduction through upstream mitogen-activated protein (MAP) kinases (e.g., p38 MAP kinase and JNK) (Chow et al. 2007; Kang et al. 2003).

ROS generation by capsaicin is partly mediated through its antagonistic effects on the coenzyme Q binding to the mitochondrial respiratory chain (Surh 2002). The disruption of the mitochondrial respiratory system by capsaicin results in a pro-oxidant state that may lead to the induction of apoptosis. Capsaicin induced apoptosis in human cutaneous squamous cell carcinomas by suppressing mitochondrial respiration, especially at complex I, and the disruption of mitochondrial membrane permeability transition (Hail and Lotan 2002). Nor-dihydrocapsiate induced apoptosis in Jurkat cells in a ROS-dependent manner (Macho et al. 2003b). The accumulation of intracellular ROS in capsiate-treated cells was diminished when cells were co-treated with ferricyanide as an external electron acceptor or with rotenone, an inhibitor of complex I of mitochondrial respiratory chain. The inhibition of capsiate-induced ROS generation was several fold stronger with ferricyanide as compared to that of rotenone, suggesting that the compound generates ROS from both mitochondrial and extramitochondrial sources. Methylation of the phenolic hydroxyl group of nor-dihydrocapsiate completely abolished its ability to generate ROS and to induce apoptosis, suggesting that the presence of a free phenolic hydroxyl group is essential for the pro-oxidant properties of capsaicinoids (Macho et al. 2003b). Macho and colleagues also demonstrated that capsiate-induced apoptosis in Jurkat cells was initiated at the S phase of the cell cycle and was mediated through disruption of mitochondrial membrane potential and the activation of caspase-3 (Macho et al. 2003a, b).

Likewise, capsaicin induced apoptosis in human prostate cancer (PC3) cells (Sanchez et al. 2006), human esophageal epidermoid carcinoma (CE 81T/VGH) cells (Wu et al. 2006) and human pancreatic cancer (AsPC-1 and BxPC-3) cells (Zhang et al. 2008) through the generation of ROS and dissipation of the mitochondrial inner transmembrane potential. Capsaicin-induced apoptosis in CE 81T/VGH cells was accompanied by increase in the release of intracellular Ca^{2+} and treatment of cells with a Ca^{2+} chelator 1,2-bis(2-aminophenoxy)ethane-N,N,N',N'-tetraacetic acid (BAPTA) abrogated capsaicin-induced apoptosis (Wu et al. 2006). The induction of apoptosis in AsPC-1 and BxPC-3 cells with capsaicin was associated with increased expression of Bax, downregulation of Bcl-2 and survivin, and the release of cytochrome c and apoptosis inducing factor (AIF) into the cytosol (Zhang et al. 2008). In contrast, capsaicin did not induce apoptosis in normal pancreatic acinar cells, suggesting that the compound induces apoptosis selectively in cancer cells (Zhang et al. 2008). The induction of apoptosis in cultured C6 glioma cells by capsaicin was associated not only with the generation of superoxides but also an elevated expression of iNOS and generation of peroxynitrite. Pretreatment of cells with ebselen, a peroxynitrite scavenger, abrogated capsaicin-induced apoptosis in these cells (Qiao et al. 2005).

A p53-dependent mechanism of apoptosis induction by capsaicin has also been reported. Treatment of androgen receptor (AR)-positive (LNCaP) and -negative (PC3, DU-145) human prostate cancer cells (Mori et al. 2006) and human esophageal epidermoid carcinoma (CE 81T/VGH) cells (Wu et al. 2006) with capsaicin caused apoptotic cell death through the induction of p53, p21, and Bax. Likewise, capsaicin induced apoptosis in cultured human gastric cancer (SNU-1) cells through upregulation of p53 (Kim et al. 1997). Capsaicin caused human leukemic cell death partly by phosphorylating p53 at serine 15 residue (Ito et al. 2004). Inactivation of p53 by antisense oligonucleotide significantly attenuated capsaicin-induced cell cycle arrest and apoptosis (Ito et al. 2004).

Capsaicin-induced apoptosis was associated with the upregulation of proapoptotic proteins and downregulation of antiapoptoic proteins. For example, capsaicin induced apoptosis in human gastric adenocarcinoma (Lo et al. 2005), murine B16-F10 melanoma (Jun et al. 2007) and human multiple myeloma (Bhutani et al. 2007) cells by downregulating the expression of ant-apoptotic protein Bcl-2. Overexpression of Bcl-2 abrogated capsaicin-induced apoptosis in human B-cell and mouse myeloid cell lines (Wolvetang et al. 1996). A decrease in the ratio of Bcl-2/Bax and an increase in caspase-3 activation accounted for the induction of apoptosis in capsaicin-treated human hepatocellular carcinoma (SK-Hep-1) cells (Jung et al. 2001).

Roles of several upstream kinases in mediating capsaicin-induced death signals have been reported. Increased phosphorylation of ERK and JNK by capsaicin led to the induction of apoptosis in PC3 cells (Sanchez et al. 2007). In addition, capsaicin elevated the expression of prostate apoptosis response-4 (par-4) and intracellular accumulation of ceramide, thereby contributing to induction of apoptosis in PC3 cells (Sanchez et al. 2007). Capsaicin caused apoptosis in H-*ras*-transformed human mammary epithelial cells through the activation of JNK and p38 MAP kinase (Kang et al. 2003). The compound also decreased mitochondrial membrane permeability and induced apoptosis in gastric cancer cells through activation of Bax and p53 in a JNK-dependent manner (Chow et al. 2007). Likewise, capsaicin activated JNK in AsPC-1 and BxPC-3 human pancreatic cancer cells (Zhang et al. 2008) and pharmacological inhibition of JNK abrogated capsaicin-induced apoptosis in these cells (Zhang et al. 2008). Moreover, oral administration of capsaicin inhibited the growth of AsPC-1 pancreatic cancer xenograft in athymic nude mice partly by inducing apoptosis as characterized by increased phosphorylation of JNK, elevated cytoplasmic levels of Bax, release of cytochrome c, and cleavage of caspase-3 (Zhang et al. 2008). In addition, the activation of adenosine monophosphate-activated protein kinase (AMPK), an enzyme that is usually activated during ATP-depleting metabolic stress, was associated with capsaicin-induced apoptosis in human colon cancer (HT-29) cells (Kim et al. 2007).

A recent study revealed the involvement of TRPV1 in capsaicin-induced cell death (Amantini et al. 2007). Capsaicin induced apoptosis in glioma U373 cells through the increase of Ca^{2+} influx, phosphorylation of p38 MAP kinase, lowering of mitochondrial transmembrane potential, and proteolytic cleavage of caspase-3. Co-treatment of cells with capsazepine, a VR1/TRPV1 antagonist, abrogated capsaicin-induced apoptotic events (Amantini et al. 2007). In contrast, induction of apoptosis in capsaicin-treated human colon cancer (HT-29) (Kim et al. 2004), human glioblastoma (A172) (Lee et al. 2000), and human hepatoma (HepG2) (Kim et al. 2005) cells was independent of VR1/TRPV1. Another vanilloid receptor subtype, TRPV6, was also involved in capsaicin-induced apoptosis. Thus, overexpression of TRPV6 sensitized cancer cells to capsaicin-induced apoptosis, while knockdown of TRPV6 abolished this action (Chow et al. 2007).

Several other molecular mechanisms underlying capsaicin-induced apoptosis in various cancer cells involve the activation of peroxisome proliferator activated receptor (PPAR)-γ (Kim et al. 2004) and the induction of DNA damage-inducible gene 153 (GADD153)/CHOP, an endoplasmic reticulum stress-induced gene (Sanchez et al. 2008). Treatment of HT-29 cells with a specific PPAR-γ antagonist bisphenol A diglycidyl ether (Kim et al. 2004) or the blockade of GADD153/CHOP by RNA interference in PC3 cells (Sanchez et al. 2008) abrogated capsaicin-induced cell death.

6.3.6 Effects on Tumor Angiogenesis

The inhibition of tumor angiogenesis is one of the rational chemoprevention strategies. The chemopreventive activities of capsaicinoids have been attributed to their antiangiogenic potential. Vascular endothelial growth factor (VEGF) is a key molecular switch in tumor angiogenesis. Capsaicinoids inhibited the expression as well as secretion of VEGF and attenuated VEGF-mediated angiogenesis in some cancer models. Capsaicin suppressed the growth of human multiple myeloma cells xenografted in athymic nude mice by downregulating the expression of VEGF through the blockade of both constitutive and IL-6-induced activation of STAT3 (Bhutani et al. 2007). Capsaicin inhibited VEGF-induced proliferation, DNA synthesis, chemotactic motility, and capillary-like tube formation in primary cultures of human endothelial cells (Min et al. 2004). Capsaicin also inhibited VEGF-induced vessel sprouting and vessel formation in the rat aortic ring assay and the mouse matrigel plug assay, respectively (Min et al. 2004). In contrast to its inhibitory effects on VEGF-mediated tumor angiogenesis, Patel and colleagues (2002b) demonstrated that capsaicin upregulated VEGF production in human malignant melanoma (A375P and A375SM) cells by increasing the DNA binding activity of hypoxia inducible factor-1α (HIF-1α).

Capsiate and dihydrocapsiate attenuated VEGF-induced proliferation and capillary-like tube formation in primary cultures of human endothelial cells (Pyun et al. 2008). These nonpungent vanilloids also inhibited sprouting of endothelial cells in the rat aorta and the formation of new blood vessels in response to VEGF. Capsiate suppressed VEGF-induced activation of Src kinase, preferentially by docking at the ATP-binding site of the enzyme, and phosphorylation of its downstream substrates, such as p125/focal adhesion kinase and vascular endothelial cadherin, without affecting autophosphorylation of the VEGF receptor (Pyun et al. 2008).

6.4 Pharmacokinetics of Capsaicinoids

Despite extensive use of capsaicin and related compounds as food additives and in medicine, very limited information is available about the pharmacokinetics of capsaicinoids. In an ex vivo experiment, incubation of everted sacs of rat intestine with 10–500 μg capsaicin revealed that about 82–88% of the compound was absorbed at a lower concentration. However, the rate of absorption was not proportional to the increase in concentration of capsaicin (Suresh and Srinivasan 2007). It has been reported that intragastrically administered [^{3}H]-dihydrocapsaicin and unlabelled capsaicin in rats are readily absorbed from the gastrointestinal tract but are almost completely metabolized before reaching the general circulation. This indicates that capsaicin undergoes a saturable absorption and degradation process in the gastrointestinal tract and a very effective metabolism in the liver (Donnerer et al. 1990).

Chanda and colleagues (2008) studied the metabolism of radio-labeled capsaicin ([^{14}C]-capsaicin) by incubating it with rat, dog and human liver microsomes as well as in S9 fractions. The radiolabeled capsaicin was rapidly metabolized by rat and human microsomes, but the metabolism was relatively slow with S9 fractions as compared to microsomes. Metabolism of [^{14}C]-capsaicin with dog microsomes and S9 fractions were less extensive. Unchanged [^{14}C]-capsaicin (1 μM) was not detected after 20-min incubation with rat S9 fractions. Major metabolites detected were vanillin, vanillylamine, 16-hydroxycapsaicin, 17-hydroxycapsaicin and 16,17-dehydrocapsaicin. [^{14}C]-Capsaicin was slowly metabolized in human skin for over 20 h, yielding vanillylamine and vanillic acid as major metabolites. About 99–100% of radiolabeled capsaicin was found to remain unchanged in mouse skin tissue following topical application (Chanda et al. 2008). In another study, Beaudry and Vachon (2009) reported similar findings on capsaicin metabolism with rat, dog and mouse microsomes as detected by using liquid chromatography-ion trap mass spectrometry. According to this study, the half-life ($t_{1/2}$) of capsaicin was in the range of 2.3–4.1 min, indicative of relatively rapid degradation of capsaicin by microsomes. Only 0.8, 6.9 and 3.5% of capsaicin remained unchanged after 20 min incubation with rat, dog and mouse microsomes, respectively, suggesting rapid clearance of the compound. Vanillylamine, hydroxycapsaiaicn and 16,17-dehydrocapsaicin were detected as major metabolites.

In a recent study, the pharmacokinetic properties of capsaicin after application of a high-concentration capsaicin patch to patients with neuropathic pain have been reported (Babbar et al. 2009). Using a one-compartment model with first-order absorption and linear elimination, Babbar et al. (2009) showed that the maximum plasma concentration observed in any patient was 17.8 ng/ml. After a 60-min application, the mean area under the curve and the C_{max} values were noted as 7.42 ng × h/ml and 1.86 ng/ml, respectively. The elimination half-life of 1.64 h indicated the rapid decline in the systemic capsaicin level. Additional studies will be necessary to provide valuable information about the bioavailability of capsaicinoids given by different routes of administration.

6.5 Conclusion

Many spices as a whole or their chemical constituents, especially secondary metabolites, are effective in the prevention of various human ailments including cancer. Chili peppers and capsaicinoids, particularly the pungent ingredient capsaicin, have long been debated for carcinogenic, co-carcinogenic or anticarcinogenic effects (Surh and Lee 1996). The purity grade and the source of capsaicin used in different studies presumably underly these contrasting results. The European Commission's Scientific Committee on Food has published a report (2002) on the safety of capsaicin consumption and concluded that the review of available data and literature does not allow it to establish a safe maximum exposure to capsaicinoids in foods (http://ec.europa.eu/food/fs/sc/scf/out120_en.pdf). However, the United State Food and Drug Administration (US-FDA) has defined capsaicin as 'generally recognized as safe' (GRAS). Although many investigators have demonstrated the chemopreventive properties of capsaicin, others have reported pro-inflammatory, pro-angiogenic and metastatic potential of the compound. As noted earlier, the activation of VR1/TRPV1 in epidermal HaCaT keratinocytes by capsaicin results in increased Ca^{2+} influx, elevated expression of COX-2 and the release of PGE_2 and IL-8, which are attenuated by the VR1 antagonist capsazepine (Southall et al. 2003). These findings raise the potential of capsaicin to provoke inflammatory responses. Moreover, capsaicin induced VEGF production in malignant melanoma cells, thereby suggesting its pro-angiogenic effects (Patel et al. 2002b). A subsequent study also demonstrated that capsaicin-induced sensory denervation favors lung metastasis of murine 4T1 breast cancer cells transplanted in mice (Erin et al. 2004). Analysis of primary breast tumors from mice treated with capsaicin revealed that the expression of casapse-7, a disintegrin and matrixmetalloproteinase-10 and Elk3 was significantly decreased as compared to those from untreated animals (Erin et al. 2006), thereby leading to the development of more aggressive phenotype of breast cancer (Erin et al. 2006). Contrary to these few studies, capsaicin has largely been reported to elicit anti-inflammatory and anti-angiogenic effects. Thus, more studies with capsaicin and related vanilloids should be carried out in a broad range of experimental models to ascertain their role in modulating various cancer-attributes, such as inflammation, angiogenesis and metastasis.

In contrast to capsaicin, nonpungent vanilloids, such as capsiate and dihydrocapsiate lack the ability to activate VR1/TRPV1, but share many of the biological effects of capsaicin (Sancho et al. 2002). These nonpungent vanilloids are potent anti-oxidants and can inhibit inflammation (Sancho et al. 2002) and angiogenesis (Pyun et al. 2008). A synthetic analog of capsaite, nordihydrocapsiate, attenuated chemically induced skin tumorigenesis (Macho et al. 2003a). Capsiate and dihydrocapsiate have also been included in the US-FDA GRAS list (www.accessdata.fda.gov/scripts/fcn/gras_notices/804880A.PDF). Therefore, attention may also be extended to nonpungent vanilloids lacking the TRPV1 agonistic property as promising chemopreventive agents.

Acknowledgements This work was supported by the Biofoods Research Program, Ministry of Education, Science and Technology, Republic of Korea.

References

Akagi A, Sano N, Uehara H, Minami T, Otsuka H, Izumi K (1998) Non-carcinogenicity of capsaicinoids in B6C3F1 mice. Food Chem Toxicol 36:1065–1071

Amantini C, Mosca M, Nabissi M, Lucciarini R, Caprodossi S, Arcella A et al (2007) Capsaicin-induced apoptosis of glioma cells is mediated by TRPV1 vanilloid receptor and requires p38 MAPK activation. J Neurochem 102:977–990

Anandakumar P, Jagan S, Kamaraj S, Ramakrishnan G, Titto AA, Devaki T (2008a) Beneficial influence of capsaicin on lipid peroxidation, membrane-bound enzymes and glycoprotein profile during experimental lung carcinogenesis. J Pharm Pharmacol 60:803–808

Anandakumar P, Kamaraj S, Jagan S, Ramakrishnan G, Vinodhkumar R, Devaki T (2008b) Capsaicin modulates pulmonary antioxidant defense system during benzo(α)pyrene-induced lung cancer in Swiss albino mice. Phytother Res 22:529–533

Anandakumar P, Kamaraj S, Jagan S, Ramakrishnan G, Vinodhkumar R, Devaki T (2008c) Stabilization of pulmonary mitochondrial enzyme system by capsaicin during benzo(al.)pyrene induced experimental lung cancer. Biomed Pharmacother 62:390–394

Babbar S, Marier JF, Mouksassi MS, Beliveau M, Vanhove GF, Chanda S et al (2009) Pharmacokinetic analysis of capsaicin after topical administration of a high-concentration capsaicin patch to patients with peripheral neuropathic pain. Ther Drug Monit 31: 502–510

Beaudry F, Vachon P (2009) Quantitative determination of capsaicin, a transient receptor potential channel vanilloid 1 agonist, by liquid chromatography quadrupole ion trap mass spectrometry: evaluation of in vitro metabolic stability. Biomed Chromatogr 23:204–211

Bhutani M, Pathak AK, Nair AS, Kunnumakkara AB, Guha S, Sethi G et al (2007) Capsaicin is a novel blocker of constitutive and interleukin-6-inducible STAT3 activation. Clin Cancer Res 13:3024–3032

Bode AM, Cho YY, Zheng D, Zhu F, Ericson ME, Ma WY et al (2009) Transient receptor potential type vanilloid 1 suppresses skin carcinogenesis. Cancer Res 69:905–913

Chanda S, Bashir M, Babbar S, Koganti A, Bley K (2008) In vitro hepatic and skin metabolism of capsaicin. Drug Metab Dispos 36:670–675

Chanda S, Erexson G, Frost D, Babbar S, Burlew JA, Bley K (2007) 26-Week dermal oncogenicity study evaluating pure trans-capsaicin in Tg.AC hemizygous mice (FBV/N). Int J Toxicol 26:123–133

Chen CW, Lee ST, Wu WT, Fu WM, Ho FM, Lin WW (2003) Signal transduction for inhibition of inducible nitric oxide synthase and cyclooxygenase-2 induction by capsaicin and related analogs in macrophages. Br J Toxicol 140:1077–1087

Chow J, Norng M, Zhang J, Chai J (2007) TRPV6 mediates capsaicin-induced apoptosis in gastric cancer cells-Mechanisms behind a possible new 'hot' cancer treatment. Biochim Biophys Acta 1773:565–576

De AK, Ghosh JJ (1989) Capsaicin pretreatment protects free radical induced rat lung damage on exposure to gaseous chemical lung irritants. Phytother Res 3:159–161

De AK, Ghosh JJ (1992) Studies on capsaicin inhibition of chemically induced lipid peroxidation in the lung and liver tissues of rat. Phytother Res 6:34–37

Donnerer J, Amann R, Schuligoi R, Lembeck F (1990) Absorption and metabolism of capsaicinoids following intragastric administration in rats. Naunyn Schmiedebergs Arch Pharmacol 342:357–361

Duvoix A, Delhalle S, Blasius R, Schnekenburger M, Morceau F, Fougere M et al (2004) Effect of chemopreventive agents on glutathione S-transferase P1-1 gene expression mechanisms via activating protein 1 and nuclear factor kappaB inhibition. Biochem Pharmacol 68:1101–1111

Erin N, Boyer PJ, Bonneau RH, Clawson GA, Welch DR (2004) Capsaicin-mediated denervation of sensory neurons promotes mammary tumor metastasis to lung and heart. Anticancer Res 24: 1003–1009

Erin N, Zhao W, Bylander J, Chase G, Clawson G (2006) Capsaicin-induced inactivation of sensory neurons promotes a more aggressive gene expression phenotype in breast cancer cells. Breast Cancer Res Treat 99:351–364

Gabor M, Razga Z (1992) Development and inhibition of mouse ear oedema induced with capsaicin. Agents Actions 36:83–86

Hail N Jr, Lotan R (2002) Examining the role of mitochondrial respiration in vanilloid-induced apoptosis. J Natl Cancer Inst 94:1281–1292

Han SS, Keum YS, Chun KS, Surh Y-J (2002) Suppression of phorbol ester-induced NF-kappaB activation by capsaicin in cultured human promyelocytic leukemia cells. Arch Pharm Res 25: 475–479

Han SS, Keum YS, Seo HJ, Chun KS, Lee SS, Surh Y-J (2001) Capsaicin suppresses phorbol ester-induced activation of NF-κB/Rel and AP-1 transcription factors in mouse epidermis. Cancer Lett 164:119–126

Inoue H, Nagata N, Koshihara Y (1995) Involvement of substance P as a mediator in capsaicin-induced mouse ear oedema. Inflamm Res 44: 470–474

Ito K, Nakazato T, Yamato K, Miyakawa Y, Yamada T, Hozumi N et al (2004) Induction of apoptosis in leukemic cells by homovanillic acid derivative, capsaicin, through oxidative stress: implication of phosphorylation of p53 at Ser-15 residue by reactive oxygen species. Cancer Res 64:1071–1078

Jancso N, Jancso-Gabor A, Szolcsanyi J (1967) Direct evidence for neurogenic inflammation and its prevention by denervation and by pretreatment with capsaicin. Br J Pharmacol Chemother 31:138–151

Jang JJ, Cho KJ, Lee YS, Bae JH (1991) Different modifying responses of capsaicin in a wide-spectrum initiation model of F344 rat. J Korean Med Sci 6:31–36

Jang JJ, Kim SH, Yun TK (1989) Inhibitory effect of capsaicin on mouse lung tumor development. In Vivo 3:49–53

Jones KD, Owen E, Berresford A, Sutton C (2002) Endometrial adenocarcinoma arising from endometriosis of the rectosigmoid colon. Gynecol Oncol 86:220–222

Joung EJ, Li MH, Lee HG, Somparn N, Jung YS, Na HK et al (2007) Capsaicin induces heme oxygenase-1 expression in HepG2 cells via activation of PI3K-Nrf2 signaling: NAD(P)H:quinone oxidoreductase as a potential target. Antioxid Redox Signal 9:2087–2098

Jun HS, Park T, Lee CK, Kang MK, Park MS, Kang HI et al (2007) Capsaicin induced apoptosis of B16-F10 melanoma cells through down-regulation of Bcl-2. Food Chem Toxicol 45:708–715

Jung MY, Kang HJ, Moon A (2001) Capsaicin-induced apoptosis in SK-Hep-1 hepatocarcinoma cells involves Bcl-2 downregulation and caspase-3 activation. Cancer Lett 165:139–145

Kang HJ, Soh Y, Kim MS, Lee EJ, Surh Y-J, Kim HR et al (2003) Roles of JNK-1 and p38 in selective induction of apoptosis by capsaicin in ras-transformed human breast epithelial cells. Int J Cancer 103:475–482

Kim CS, Kawada T, Kim BS, Han IS, Choe SY, Kurata T et al (2003) Capsaicin exhibits anti-inflammatory property by inhibiting IκBα degradation in LPS-stimulated peritoneal macrophages. Cell Signal 15:299–306

Kim CS, Park WH, Park JY, Kang JH, Kim MO, Kawada T et al (2004) Capsaicin, a spicy component of hot pepper, induces apoptosis by activation of the peroxisome proliferator-activated receptor gamma in HT-29 human colon cancer cells. J Med Food 7:267–273

Kim JA, Kang YS, Lee YS (2005) A phospholipase C-dependent intracellular Ca^{2+} release pathway mediates the capsaicin-induced apoptosis in HepG2 human hepatoma cells. Arch Pharm Res 28:73–80

Kim JD, Kim JM, Pyo JO, Kim SY, Kim BS, Yu R et al (1997) Capsaicin can alter the expression of tumor forming-related genes which might be followed by induction of apoptosis of a Korean stomach cancer cell line, SNU-1. Cancer Lett 120:235–241

Kim JP, Park JG, Lee MD, Han MD, Park ST, Lee BH et al (1985) Co-carcinogenic effects of several Korean foods on gastric cancer induced by N-methyl-N'-nitro-N-nitrosoguanidine in rats. Jpn J Surg 15:427–437

Kim YM, Hwang JT, Kwak DW, Lee YK, Park OJ (2007) Involvement of AMPK signaling cascade in capsaicin-induced apoptosis of HT-29 colon cancer cells. Ann N Y Acad Sci 1095:496–503

Kundu JK, Na H-K, Surh Y-J (2008) Intracellular signaling molecules as targets of selected dietary chemopreventive agents. In: Dietary Modulation of Cell Signaling Pathways. Surh Y-J, Packer L, Cadenas E, Dong Z (eds) CRC Press, Taylor & Francis Group, USA. pp 1–44

Kundu JK, Surh Y-J (2008) Inflammation: gearing the journey to cancer. Mutat Res 659:15–30

Lee YS, Nam DH, Kim JA (2000) Induction of apoptosis by capsaicin in A172 human glioblastoma cells. Cancer Lett 161:121–130

Lo YC, Yang YC, Wu IC, Kuo FC, Liu CM, Wang HW et al (2005) Capsaicin-induced cell death in a human gastric adenocarcinoma cell line. World J Gastroenterol 11:6254–6257

Lopez-Carrillo L, Lopez-Cervantes M, Robles-Diaz G, Ramirez-Espitia A, Mohar-Betancourt A, Meneses-Garcia A et al (2003) Capsaicin consumption, Helicobacter pylori positivity and gastric cancer in Mexico. Int J Cancer 106:277–282

Macho A, Lucena C, Sancho R, Daddario N, Minassi A, Munoz E et al (2003a) Non-pungent capsaicinoids from sweet pepper synthesis and evaluation of the chemopreventive and anticancer potential. Eur J Nutr 42:2–9

Macho A, Sancho R, Minassi A, Appendino G, Lawen A, Munoz E (2003b) Involvement of reactive oxygen species in capsaicinoid-induced apoptosis in transformed cells. Free Radic Res 37:611–619

Miller CH, Zhang Z, Hamilton SM, Teel RW (1993) Effects of capsaicin on liver microsomal metabolism of the tobacco-specific nitrosamine NNK. Cancer Lett 75:45–52

Min JK, Han KY, Kim EC, Kim YM, Lee SW, Kim OH et al (2004) Capsaicin inhibits in vitro and in vivo angiogenesis. Cancer Res 64:644–651

Modly CE, Das M, Don PS, Marcelo CL, Mukhtar H, Bickers DR (1986) Capsaicin as an in vitro inhibitor of benzo(a)pyrene metabolism and its DNA binding in human and murine keratinocytes. Drug Metab Dispos 14:413–416

Mori A, Lehmann S, O'Kelly J, Kumagai T, Desmond JC, Pervan M et al (2006) Capsaicin, a component of red peppers, inhibits the growth of androgen-independent, p53 mutant prostate cancer cells. Cancer Res 66:3222–3229

Morre DJ, Caldwell S, Mayorga A, Wu LY, Morre DM (1997) NADH oxidase activity from sera altered by capsaicin is widely distributed among cancer patients. Arch Biochem Biophys 342:224–230

Morre DJ, Chueh PJ, Morre DM (1995) Capsaicin inhibits preferentially the NADH oxidase and growth of transformed cells in culture. Proc Natl Acad Sci U S A 92:1831–1835

Morre DJ, Sun E, Geilen C, Wu LY, de Cabo R, Krasagakis K et al (1996) Capsaicin inhibits plasma membrane NADH oxidase and growth of human and mouse melanoma lines. Eur J Cancer 32A: 1995–2003

Nair U, Bartsch H, Nair J (2007) Lipid peroxidation-induced DNA damage in cancer-prone inflammatory diseases: a review of published adduct types and levels in humans. Free Radic Biol Med 43:1109–1120

Park JS, Choi MA, Kim BS, Han IS, Kurata T, Yu R (2000) Capsaicin protects against ethanol-induced oxidative injury in the gastric mucosa of rats. Life Sci 67:3087–3093

Park KK, Chun KS, Yook JI, Surh Y-J (1998) Lack of tumor promoting activity of capsaicin, a principal pungent ingredient of red pepper, in mouse skin carcinogenesis. Anticancer Res 18:4201–4205

Park KK, Surh Y-J (1997) Effects of capsaicin on chemically-induced two-stage mouse skin carcinogenesis. Cancer Lett 114:183–184

Patel PS, Varney ML, Dave BJ, Singh RK (2002a) Regulation of constitutive and induced NF-κB activation in malignant melanoma cells by capsaicin modulates interleukin-8 production and cell proliferation. J Interferon Cytokine Res 22:427–235

Patel PS, Yang S, Li A, Varney ML, Singh RK (2002b) Capsaicin regulates vascular endothelial cell growth factor expression by modulation of hypoxia inducing factor-1alpha in human malignant melanoma cells. J Cancer Res Clin Oncol 128:461–468

Pyun BJ, Choi S, Lee Y, Kim TW, Min JK, Kim Y et al (2008) Capsiate, a nonpungent capsaicin-like compound, inhibits angiogenesis and vascular permeability via a direct inhibition of Src kinase activity. Cancer Res 68:227–235

Qiao S, Li W, Tsubouchi R, Haneda M, Murakami K, Yoshino M (2005) Involvement of peroxynitrite in capsaicin-induced apoptosis of C6 glioma cells. Neurosci Res 51:175–183

Reilly CA, Crouc DJ, Yost GS, Fatah AA (2001a) Determination of capsaicin, dihydrocapsaicin, and nonivamide in self-defense weapons by liquid chromatography-mass spectrometry and liquid chromatography-tandem mass spectrometry. J Chromatogr A 912:259–267

Reilly CA, Crouch DJ, Yost GS (2001b) Quantitative analysis of capsaicinoids in fresh peppers, oleoresin capsicum and pepper spray products. J Forensic Sci 46:502–509

Rosa A, Deiana M, Casu V, Paccagnini S, Appendino G, Ballero M et al (2002) Antioxidant activity of capsinoids. J Agric Food Chem 50:7396–7401

Salimath BP, Sundaresh CS, Srinivas L (1986) Dietary components inhibit lipid peroxidation in erythrocyte membrane. Nutr Res 6:1171–1178

Sanchez AM, Malagarie-Cazenave S, Olea N, Vara D, Chiloeches A, Diaz-Laviada I (2007) Apoptosis induced by capsaicin in prostate PC-3 cells involves ceramide accumulation, neutral sphingomyelinase, and JNK activation. Apoptosis 12:2013–2024

Sanchez AM, Martinez-Botas J, Malagarie-Cazenave S, Olea N, Vara D, Lasuncion MA et al (2008) Induction of the endoplasmic reticulum stress protein GADD153/CHOP by capsaicin in prostate PC-3 cells: a microarray study. Biochem Biophys Res Commun 372: 785–791

Sanchez AM, Sanchez MG, Malagarie-Cazenave S, Olea N, Diaz-Laviada I (2006) Induction of apoptosis in prostate tumor PC-3 cells and inhibition of xenograft prostate tumor growth by the vanilloid capsaicin. Apoptosis 11:89–99

Sancho R, Lucena C, Macho A, Calzado MA, Blanco-Molina M, Minassi A et al (2002) Immunosuppressive activity of capsaicinoids: capsiate derived from sweet peppers inhibits NF-κB activation and is a potent antiinflammatory compound in vivo. Eur J Immunol 32:1753–1763

Singh S, Natarajan K, Aggarwal BB (1996) Capsaicin (8-methyl-N-vanillyl-6-nonenamide) is a potent inhibitor of nuclear transcription factor-kappa B activation by diverse agents. J Immunol 157:4412–4420

Southall MD, Li T, Gharibova LS, Pei Y, Nicol GD, Travers JB (2003) Activation of epidermal vanilloid receptor-1 induces release of proinflammatory mediators in human keratinocytes. J Pharmacol Exp Ther 304:217–222

Sporn MB (1976) Approaches to prevention of epithelial cancer during the preneoplastic period. Cancer Res 36:2699–2702

Suresh D, Srinivasan K (2007) Studies on the al. absorption of spice principles – curcumin, capsaicin and piperine in rat intestines. Food Chem Toxicol 45:1437–1442

Surh Y-J (2002) More than spice: capsaicin in hot chili peppers makes tumor cells commit suicide. J Natl Cancer Inst 94:1263–1265

Surh Y-J (2003) Cancer chemoprevention with dietary phytochemicals. Nature Rev Cancer 3:768–780

Surh Y-J, Chun KS, Cha HH, Han SS, Keum YS, Park KK et al (2001) Molecular mechanisms underlying chemopreventive activities of anti-inflammatory phytochemicals: down-regulation of COX-2 and iNOS through suppression of NF-κB activation. Mutat Res 480–481:243–268

Surh Y-J, Han SS, Keum YS, Seo HJ, Lee SS (2000) Inhibitory effects of curcumin and capsaicin on phorbol ester-induced activation of eukaryotic transcription factors, NF-κB and AP-1. Biofactors 12:107–112

Surh Y-J, Lee E, Lee JM (1998) Chemoprotective properties of some pungent ingredients present in red pepper and ginger. Mutat Res 402:259–267

Surh Y-J, Lee RC, Park KK, Mayne ST, Liem A, Miller JA (1995) Chemoprotective effects of capsaicin and diallyl sulfide against mutagenesis or tumorigenesis by vinyl carbamate andal.-nitrosodimethylamine. Carcinogenesis 16:2467–2471

Surh Y-J, Lee SS (1996) Capsaicin in hot chili pepper: carcinogen, co-carcinogen or anticarcinogen? Food Chem Toxicol 34:313–316

Tafler R, Herbert MK, Schmidt RF, Weis KH (1993) Small reduction of capsaicin-induced neurogenic inflammation in human forearm skin by the glucocorticoid prednicarbate. Agents Actions 38(Spec No):C31–C34

Tanaka T, Kohno H, Sakata K, Yamada Y, Hirose Y, Sugie S et al (2002) Modifying effects of dietary capsaicin and rotenone on 4-nitroquinoline-1-oxide-induced rat tongue carcinogenesis. Carcinogenesis 23:1361–1367

Teel RW, Huynh HT (1999) Lack of the inhibitory effect of intragastrically administered capsaicin on NNK-induced lung tumor formation in the A.J mouse. In Vivo 13:231–234

Toth B, Gannett P (1992) Carcinogenicity of lifelong administration of capsaicin of hot pepper in mice. In Vivo 6:59–63

Wolvetang EJ, Larm JA, Moutsoulas P, Lawen A (1996) Apoptosis induced by inhibitors of the plasma membrane NADH-oxidase involves Bcl-2 and calcineurin. Cell Growth Differ 7: 1315–1325

Wu CC, Lin JP, Yang JS, Chou ST, Chen SC, Lin YT et al (2006) Capsaicin induced cell cycle arrest and apoptosis in human esophagus epidermoid carcinoma CE 81T/VGH cells through the elevation of intracellular reactive oxygen species and Ca^{2+} productions and caspase-3 activation. Mutat Res 601:71–82

Wu Y, Starzinski-Powitz A, Guo SW (2008) Capsaicin inhibits proliferation of endometriotic cells in vitro. Gynecol Obstet Invest 66:59–62

Yoshitani SI, Tanaka T, Kohno H, Takashima S (2001) Chemoprevention of azoxymethane-induced rat colon carcinogenesis by dietary capsaicin and rotenone. Int J Oncol 19:929–939

Zhang R, Humphreys I, Sahu RP, Shi Y, Srivastava SK (2008) In vitro and in vivo induction of apoptosis by capsaicin in pancreatic cancer cells is mediated through ROS generation and mitochondrial death pathway. Apoptosis 13:1465–1478

Zhang Z, Hamilton SM, Stewart C, Strother A, Teel RW (1993) Inhibition of liver microsomal cytochrome P450 activity and metabolism of the tobacco-specific nitrosamine NNK by capsaicin and ellagic acid. Anticancer Res 13:2341–2346

Zhang Z, Huynh H, Teel RW (1997) Effects of orally administered capsaicin, the principal component of capsicum fruits, on the in vitro metabolism of the tobacco-specific nitrosamine NNK in hamster lung and liver microsomes. Anticancer Res 17:1093–1098

Chapter 7
Influence of dietary Soy Isoflavones Genistein and Daidzein on Genotoxicity and Mammary Carcinogenicity in Rats Exposed to the Model Carcinogen 7,12-Dimethylbenz[a]anthracene (DMBA)

Anane Aidoo and Mugimane G. Manjanatha

Abstract Epidemiological studies provide evidence for the possibility of preventing cancer and/or forestalling the complications of menopause through the consumption of foods containing phytoestrogens such as soy isoflavones. Lifestyle changes in technologically advanced societies, however, limit the consumption of adequate foods to meet health needs; thus supplements of phytoestrogen including soy isoflavones daidzein (DZ) and genistein (GE), considered to be compounds in soy that impart beneficial effects, are ingested in large quantities on a regular basis. This raises health concern since isoflavones are structurally similar to steroidal hormones, and it is possible that they may alter endogenous hormone metabolism and influence the pathogenesis of steroid-dependent diseases such as breast and prostate cancer. Equally important, humans are consistently exposed to mutagenic carcinogens whose toxicities could be enhanced by interaction with ingested isoflavones. Recent report indicates that DZ and GE are not only mutagenic, but also they enhance chemical carcinogenesis in animal models. Here, we report the results of feeding rats with DZ and GE to determine whether the genotoxicity and mammary carcinogenesis induced by the potent rodent mammary carcinogen dimethylbenz[a]anthracene (DMBA) could be altered. The data obtained suggest that DZ and GE diets given separately did not significantly alter DMBA-induced mutagenicity in lymphocytes, liver, mammary and heart, and carcinogenicity in the mammary. The mixture of DZ and GE was effective in reducing DMBA effects, suggesting that consuming diets containing more than one soy isoflavones as opposed to taking supplements in isolation, could impart some benefits; these results are discussed together with other animal studies reported on soy isoflavones.

A. Aidoo (✉)
FDA Jefferson Laboratories, National Center for Toxicological Research, Division of Genetic & Reproductive Toxicology, Jefferson, AR 72079, USA
e-mail: anane.aidoo@fda.hhs.gov

Disclaimer: The views presented in this article do not necessarily reflect those of the Food and Drug Administration.

M. Mutanen, A.-M. Pajari (eds.), *Vegetables, Whole Grains, and Their Derivatives in Cancer Prevention*, Diet and Cancer 2, DOI 10.1007/978-90-481-9800-9_7, © Springer Science+Business Media B.V. 2011

Keywords Estrogen replacement therapy · Phytoestrogens · Soy isoflavones – genistein and daidzein · Genotoxicity · Carcinogenicity · 7,12-dimethylbenz[a]anthracene

Contents

7.1 Introduction

The undesirable symptoms of menopause and other health problems such as cardiovascular disease, cancer and osteoporosis are linked to decreased levels of estrogen (Anderson et al. 1999; Herrington et al. 2000; Hulley et al. 1998). To alleviate these problems, hormone replacement therapy (HRT) is often administered to menopausal women. However, in light of recent studies that call into question the safety of HRT (Herrington et al. 2000; Hulley et al. 1998), many women are switching to naturally occurring estrogens such as soy isoflavones believed to exhibit beneficial effects in the prevention of menopausal symptoms and other related disorders (Anderson et al. 1999; Ramsey et al. 1999). Daidzein (DZ) and Genistein (GE), the major components of soy isoflavones are structurally related to steroidal estrogens (Fig. 7.1), thus they exhibit similar properties for receptor affinity (Tham et al. 1998), but like tamoxifen, these isoflavones appear to be selective estrogen modulators without untoward estrogenic side effects (Messina et al. 1994). These attributes make isoflavones attractive and effective chemopreventive agents for certain types of cancer, particularly breast and prostate cancers (Barnes et al. 1995; Kennedy 1995; Messina et al. 1994). Evidence also points to the beneficial effects of isoflavones in preventing cardiovascular disease and osteoporosis (Arjmandi et al. 1996; Gooderham et al. 1996). In addition, there are other constituents of soy, including lignans, protease inhibitors, saponins, phytosterols, coumestans

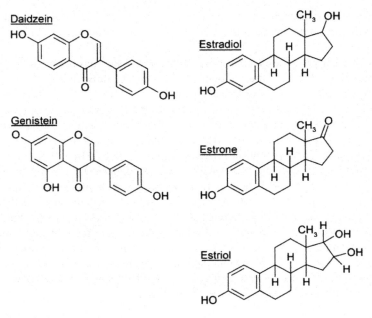

Fig. 7.1 Structures of estrogens and isoflavones

and phytates that might also possess health-promoting benefits (Knight and Eden 1996).

Given the potential role of soy isoflavones in decreasing the risk of certain hormone-dependent cancers and ameliorating menopausal symptoms, it is not surprising that isoflavones are ingested on a daily basis as nutritional supplements or as constituents of other preparations, including tofu, soy milk, tempeh and textured soy protein. The isoflavones can exert their effects by genomic mechanism involving estrogen receptors or through a variety of nongenomic mechanisms, including tyrosine kinase and topoisomerase inhibition (Barnes et al. 1995; Markovits et al. 1989; Okura et al. 1988). Genistein is reported to be a potent inhibitor of topoisomerase II by stabilizing a cleavable complex that results in DNA strand breaks (Metzler et al. 1998). Thus it is conceivable that the biological effects of DZ or GE may also be associated with DNA damage and potentiate the carcinogenesis process (Abe 1999) instead of preventing it. Studies indicate that isoflavones are clastogenic both in vitro and in vivo (Kulling and Metzler 1997; Misra et al. 2002; Morris et al. 1998) and are genotoxic in vivo (Giri and Lu 1995; Misra et al. 2002). Furthermore, dietary genistein has been shown to enhance chemical carcinogenesis in the colon and in mammary glands of rodents (Allred et al. 2004; Day et al. 2001; Rao et al. 1997). Administration of an isoflavone mixture to a p53-deficient mouse that develops early spontaneous tumors, however, showed no effect on the incidence and types of tumors produced (Misra et al. 2002). Unlike the consumption of whole soy products in Asian countries where soybean intake is associated with decreased breast cancer risk (Arai et al. 2000; Chen et al. 1999; Wu et al. 2002), in Western countries, isoflavones are consumed as supplements which may not impart similar health benefits, suggesting a need to determine whether isoflavones taken as dietary supplements could modify the effects of carcinogens in a laboratory setting.

Chemical carcinogenesis in hormone-dependent tissues has been extensively pursued using the rodent mammary model carcinogen 7,12-dimethylbenz(a)anthracene (DMBA) (Bradley et al. 1976; Ip and Ip 1981; Leung et al. 1975). DMBA is a synthetic polycyclic aromatic hydrocarbon (PAH). Major target organs of this agent in rodents are the skin and mammary gland. Many other tissues are susceptible to DMBA insult (Buters et al. 2003). Because mutation induction is positively associated with tumor development, in this report transgenic Big Blue® (BB) rats were treated with a single dose of DMBA with or without dietary DZ, GE or 17β-estradiol (E2) as positive control, and conducted mutagenesis and carcinogenesis experiments in the mammary and uterus. BB rats harbor mutational target that permits the analysis of mutations in any tissue where DNA can be isolated (Manjanatha et al. 1998). The heart and liver were included to better evaluate the effects of the isoflavones on chemical mutagenesis in other estrogen target tissues, the lymphocytes were added as a surrogate tissue for evaluating mutagenic responses in non-estrogenic tissue. Due to the existence of estrogen deficiency at menopause, both ovariectomized (OVX) and intact (INT) rats were used in the study.

7.2 Animals, Diets, and Carcinogen Treatment

The experiments were conducted in female BB transgenic rats obtained from Taconic Farm (Germantown, N.Y.). They were acclimatized in our animal facilities for two weeks before treatment. The Institutional Animal Care and Use Committee at NCTR approved animal handling, maintenance and the study protocol. Starting at five weeks of age rats were fed ad libitum isoflavone-free diet (NIH-31C) and had free access to water. NIH-31C diet has the same basic formulation as standard NIH-31 except that the protein contributed by soy meal and alfalfa was replaced by casein and the soy oil by corn oil. The feed was analyzed by LC/MS and shown to be free of isoflavones at the detection limit of 0.5 μg. Beginning at 7 weeks of age, animals were fed ad libitum either NIH-31C or NIH-31C containing either 0.25 or 1.0 g/kg of the diet isoflavones: DZ and GE, respectively or a mixture (DZG) containing 1.0 g/kg of diet DZ and 1.0 g/kg of diet GE. Other rats received 0.005 g/kg E2 as positive control in some experiments. The doses of the isoflavones used were biologically active, as evidenced by an increase in uterine cell proliferation as determined by proliferating cell nuclear antigen (PCNA) immunohistochemistry in the OVX rats. Also, in a similar experiment, 0.25 g/kg intake of GE increased the expression of Bcl$_2$ gene while 1.0 g/kg decreased this response in the pancreatic endocrine tissue of intact rats (Lyn-Cook LE, meeting abstract). At postnatal day 50 (PND50), the rats were gavaged with a single dose of 80 mg/kg DMBA suspended in sesame oil (Fig. 7.2). This dose of DMBA has been shown to produce tumors in female Fischer 344 rats that are infrequently used for DMBA carcinogenesis compared to female Sprague-Dawley rats. The PND50 treatment was based on carcinogenesis studies indicating that rats at this age have a high density of terminal end buds: ductal

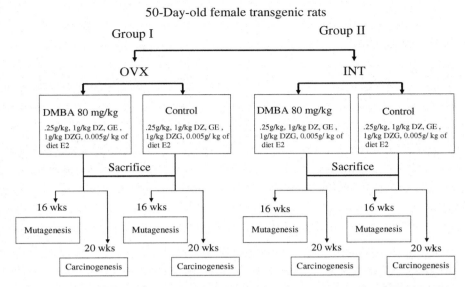

Fig. 7.2 Experimental design used to study the effects of isoflavones, DZ and GE or E2 on DMBA-induced mutagenicity and carcinogenicity in OVX and INT female BB rats. Animals were exposed to the carcinogen for 16 or 20 weeks

structures that are more sensitive to chemically-induced mammary tumors (Russo et al. 1990). The animals were maintained on isoflavone/estradiol-supplement or the isoflavone/estradiol-free diets until the experiments were terminated.

Animals were divided into two groups 2 weeks after DMBA treatment (Fig. 7.2). Group I rats were bilaterally ovariectomized (OVX) under ketamine/xylazine (100 and 15 mg/kg, respectively), anesthesia. Group II were kept intact (INT). The rationale for treating the animals two weeks prior to ovariectomy is based on the fact that sensitivity of the rat to mammary tumor induction by DMBA is in part dependent on the hormonal state of the animal (Dao 1962; Welsch 1985). Animals continued to have free access to food and water. Food consumption and body weight were recorded weekly. Animals were killed at 16 or 20 weeks following DMBA treatment by CO_2 anesthesia and tissues or organs were aseptically harvested. The spleens were used immediately for *Hprt* mutagenesis assay according to previously published methods (Aidoo et al. 1991, 1007), portions of other tissues were either frozen in liquid nitrogen and stored at $-80°C$ for the *lacI* or *cII* mutagenesis assay or preserved in 10% neutral buffered formalin for histopathological analysis.

For the mammary and uterus histopathology, tissues were examined grossly, removed and preserved in 10% neutral buffered formalin. Lesion descriptions were recorded on the IANR form (Individual Animal Necropsy Record). Tissues were trimmed, processed and embedded in Tissue Prep II, sectioned at 4–6 microns, and stained with hematoxylin and eosin. Slides were microscopically examined, and when applicable, non-neoplastic lesions were graded for severity.

7.3 Results

7.3.1 Mortality

In the OVX group, two animals died early in the study (DMBA plus 0.25 and
1.0 g/kg DZ), the cause of death was due to either surgery or gavage error and
the animals were excluded from the study. In ovary-intact animals, one rat in the
group treated with DMBA and fed E2 died early in the study, but the cause of death
was undetermined. Six other animals from the INT group treated with DMBA were
found to be moribund between the 11th and 16th week after DMBA treatment and
therefore euthanized. All of these DMBA-treated INT rats bore mammary gland
adenocarcinomas and were included in the analysis of tumor-bearing animals.

7.3.2 Isoflavone Levels Detected in Serum

Isoflavones undergo extensive metabolism in the intestinal tract prior to absorption
(Welsch 1985). Following absorption, the metabolites and/or the parent compounds
are transported to the liver where they are removed from the portal blood. However,
a percentage of the isoflavones in the portal blood can escape uptake by the liver
and enter the peripheral circulation. The effectiveness of hepatic first-pass clearance influences the amount which reaches peripheral tissues (Barnes et al. 1996).
To ensure bioavailability of the isoflavones, serum concentrations were measured by
HPLC/MS. Table 7.1 shows the mean serum concentrations of DZ, GE, and equol,
a metabolite of DZ 16 weeks after the commencement of isoflavone feeding. The
levels detected in the serum illustrate biological activity because they were within
the range of isoflavone concentrations that significantly modify clinical markers of
cardiovascular disease and osteoporosis (Scheiber et al. 2001). The physiological

Table 7.1 Mean values of serum isoflavones (nM)

Treatment groups	Daidzein	Genistein	Equol
Control diet	0.0	0.0	0.0
DZ 0.25 g/kg diet	13	0.0	1,260
GE 0.25 g/kg diet	0.0	10	0.0
DZ 1.0 g/kg diet	100	0.0	5,240
GE 1.0 g/kg diet	10	600	0.0
DZG 1.0 g/kg diet	13	30	1,510
E2 0.005 g/kg diet	0.0	0.0	0.0
DMBA 80 mg/kg diet	0.0	0.0	0.0
DMBA+DZ 0.25 g/kg diet	100	0.0	1,050
DMBA+GE 0.25 g/kg diet	0.0	0.0	0.0
DMBA+DZ 1.0 g/kg diet	270	0.0	6,300
DMBA+GE 1.0 g/kg diet	0.0	120	0.0
DMBA+DZG 1.0 g/kg diet	600	0.6	2,300
DMBA+E2 0.005 g/kg diet	10	0.0	0.0

relevance or the biological activity of the isoflavone levels in the serum was further demonstrated by an increase in cell proliferation and a reduction in the severity of atrophy seen in low estrogen environment of the OVX rats fed DZ or GE (further discussed below under histopathological changes).

7.3.3 Food Intake, Body and Organ Weights

Food intake and body weight were measured weekly during the course of the study. DZ or GE supplementation alone had no effect on body weight gain (Fig. 7.3). However, the body weight gains of E2-fed rats in both OVX (Fig. 7.3a) and INT (Fig. 7.3b) groups with or without DMBA treatment were markedly reduced. The E2-mediated reduction in body weight gain was not statistically significant. However, it is intriguing to note that this response by E2 has been associated with the suppression of the expression of neuropeptide-Y in the hypothalamus that regulates appetite in rats (Bonavera et al. 1994; Butera and Beikirch 1989). We did not investigate this brain substance in the present study, however we observed that the amount of food consumed per rat was essentially similar in all the treatment groups, and it is possible that the suppression of the neuropeptide may not be the sole determinant of E2-mediated decrease in body weight gain.

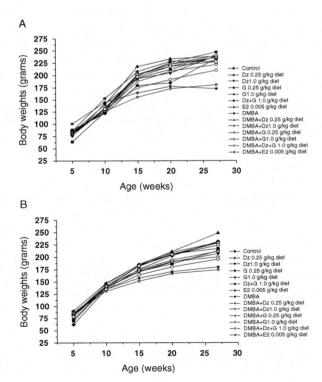

Fig. 7.3 Mean body weights

At necropsy, livers, kidneys, hearts, brains, uteri, thymuses and adrenal glands were removed, examined and weighed wet as soon as possible after dissection, while the thyroid/parathyroid and pituitary glands were weighed after fixation. In the OVX rats, the only gross observation other than decreased uterine weight was the occurrence of mammary gland (lymph node) and clitoral gland adenomas in rats fed the E2 diet. Table 7.2 shows the mean organ weights. While most of the treatment groups, including daidzein and genistein demonstrated organ weights comparable to the control diet group, E2 treatment markedly increased uterine weight of OVX rats (Table 7.2). The E2 related effects in the OVX group suggest exogenous estrogen-mediated induction of dysplasia (discussed below under uterus). In the INT animals, the organ weights including uterine were essentially similar in all the treatment groups (Table 7.3).

7.3.4 Effect of GE on DMBA Mutagenesis in the Heart

Heart disease among women increases at menopause. Relatively little is known about the role of gene mutations in heart disease, probably due to the fact that the heart is a post-mitotic tissue and mutations are generally thought to be associated with mitotic processes of DNA replication. Recent findings, however, indicate that mutations may be involved in cardiovascular disease. A gene mutation has been detected in the LDL receptor in a patient with familial hypercholesterolemia, a condition associated with coronary artery disease (Yu et al. 1999). Researchers at the Cleveland Cardiovascular Clinic have reported that a deletion mutation in MEF2A gene is linked to coronary artery disease (Wang et al. 2003). Also, a mutation in the cholesteryl ester transfer protein gene has been shown to increase coronary heart disease in Japanese-American men (Zhong et al. 1996), Moreover, chemically induced mutation has been demonstrated in the heart tissue of laboratory mice (Cruz-Munoz et al. 2000). These findings suggest that genetic mutations may be directly or indirectly involved in the development of heart disease. Bearing in mind the increase of heart disease in women after menopause due to estrogen decline, we decided to determine the mutagenic activity of the potent carcinogen DMBA in the heart and whether the response could be modified by dietary GE or E2 in OVX rats

The procedure for the BB $lacI$ assay as applied to the heart and other tissues is briefly described here. DNA extraction, lambda packaging, and plating for $lacI$ mutant plaques were carried out in a 'blocked' manner in order to minimize bias from day-to-day variations in experimental procedures. The $lacI$ containing lambda shuttle vector was recovered by mixing the genomic DNA extracted from different tissues such as liver, mammary gland, uterus, heart with Transpack^{TM} in vitro lambda phage packaging extract as described previously (Manjanatha et al. 1998). The resulting phages were preadsorbed to E. coli SCS-8 cells for 20 min at 37°C, mixed with prewarmed NZY top agar containing 1.5 mg/ml of X-gal, and poured into 250-mm assay trays containing Big Blue media. The plates were incubated overnight at 37°C and scored for mutant blue plaques. Color control mutants were included in all plating, and the results were accepted only if mutant CMI could be

Table 7.2 Mean organ weights of OVX rats in grams. All organ weights were essentially similar with the exception of E2-treated rats where the uterine weight was increased

Group	Organs: Brain	Liver	Heart	Spleen	Thymus	Adrenal	Kidney	Pituitary	Thyroid	Uterus
Control diet	1.9	4.6	0.7	0.5	0.2	0.06	1.5	0.01	0.03	0.2
DZ 0.25 g/kg diet	1.9	5.0	0.7	0.5	0.2	0.07	1.5	0.01	0.02	0.2
GE 0.25 g/kg diet	1.9	5.2	0.7	0.5	0.2	0.05	1.4	0.01	0.03	0.2
DZ 1.0 /kg diet	2.0	5.2	0.6	0.5	0.2	0.07	1.5	0.01	0.02	0.1
GE1.0 g/kg diet	2.0	5.1	0.7	0.5	0.3	0.07	1.3	0.01	0.02	0.2
DZ/GE 1.0 g/kg diet	2.1	5.4	0.7	0.5	0.2	0.06	1.4	0.01	0.03	0.2
E2 0.005 g/kg diet	1.9	5.6	0.7	0.5	0.2	0.06	1.4	0.02	0.02	0.4
DMBA 80 mg/kg	2.0	5.0	0.8	0.5	0.3	0.05	1.4	0.01	0.02	0.1
DMBA+DZ 0.25 g/kg diet	1.9	4.9	0.7	0.5	0.3	0.05	1.4	0.01	0.02	0.2
DMBA+GE 0.2 g/kg diet	1.9	5.1	0.7	0.5	0.3	0.05	1.4	0.01	0.03	0.1
DMBA+DZ 1.0 g/ kg diet	1.9	4.6	0.7	0.5	0.2	0.05	1.3	0.01	0.02	0.2
DMBA+ GE1.0 g/ kg diet	2.0	5.0	0.7	0.5	0.3	0.05	1.4	0.01	0.02	0.1
DMBA+DZ/ GE 1.0 g/ kg diet	1.9	4.7	0.7	0.5	0.2	0.05	1.3	0.02	0.02	0.2
DMBA+E2 0.005 g/kg diet	1.9	5.5	0.7	0.5	0.2	0.05	1.4	0.02	0.02	0.5

Table 7.3 Mean organ weights of INT rats in grams. Organ weights were essentially similar for all treatment groups

Group	Organs:									
	Brain	Liver	Heart	Spleen	Thymus	Adrenal	Kidney	Pituitary	Thyroid	Uterus
Control diet	1.9	5.4	0.7	0.5	0.2	0.06	1.4	0.02	0.03	0.5
DZ 0.25 g/kg diet	1.9	5.6	0.7	0.5	0.2	0.05	1.4	0.02	0.02	0.5
GE 0.25 g/kg diet	1.9	5.3	0.7	0.5	0.2	0.07	1.4	0.02	0.03	0.5
DZ1.0 g/kg diet	1.9	5.0	0.7	0.5	0.2	0.06	1.3	0.01	0.03	0.5
GE1.0 g/kg diet	2.0	5.2	0.7	0.5	0.2	0.06	1.5	0.02	0.03	0.6
DZ/GE 1.0 g/kg diet	1.9	5.4	0.6	0.5	0.2	0.05	1.4	0.01	0.03	0.5
E2 0.005 g/kg diet	1.9	5.2	0.7	0.4	0.3	0.05	1.3	0.02	0.02	0.5
DMBA 80 mg/kg	2.0	5.6	0.5	0.5	0.2	0.07	1.4	0.02	0.02	0.6
DMBA+DZ 0.25 g/kg diet	2.0	5.9	0.7	0.5	0.2	0.07	1.5	0.02	0.02	0.6
DMBA+GE 0.25 g/kg diet	1.9	5.8	0.7	0.5	0.2	0.07	1.5	0.02	0.02	0.5
DMBA+DZ 1.0 g/kg diet	2.0	5.6	0.7	0.6	0.2	0.06	1.4	0.02	0.02	0.5
DMBA+GE 1.0 g/kg diet	2.0	5.6	0.7	0.5	0.2	0.06	1.4	0.02	0.02	0.6
DMBA+DZ/ GE1.0 g/ kg diet	2.0	5.2	0.7	0.4	0.2	0.07	1.4	0.02	0.02	0.5
DMBA+E2 0.005 g/kg diet	1.7	5.4	0.6	0.5	0.2	0.06	1.2	0.02	0.02	0.5

detected. Packaging and plating were repeated for the DNA samples until at least 2×10^5 plaques were scored for each data point.

The mutant blue plaques were picked into individual tubes containing 0.5 ml of SM buffer and 50 µl of chloroform. To confirm the mutant phenotypes, and for future use in DNA sequence analysis, all recovered putative mutant phages from the 250-mm assay plates were diluted 1:100 and re-plated on 100-mm plates with 3.5 ml of top agarose containing 1.5 mg/ml of X-gal. The sectored plaques were also verified for their phenotype as specified in previous experiments (Manjanatha et al. 2000), the confirmed sectored plaques were separately scored. The *lac*I mutant frequency was calculated by dividing the number of verified mutant plaques by the total number of plaques analyzed.

DMBA treatment caused an eight-fold increase in MF in the heart ($p < 0.001$) compared to the response seen in the control diet (Fig. 7.4). GE or E2 intake alone did not produce significant *lac*I MF in the heart, although 0.25 and 1.0 g/kg doses of GE induced higher *lac*I MFs relative to control diet. Our results and those of Cruz-Munoz et al. (Cruz-Munoz et al. 2000), indicating that carcinogens induce mutations in a generally nonreplicative tissue suggest that post-mitotic tissues like the heart tend to accumulate mutations probably due to errors associated with mismatch repair. Although gene mutations in the heart may not cause cancer, they

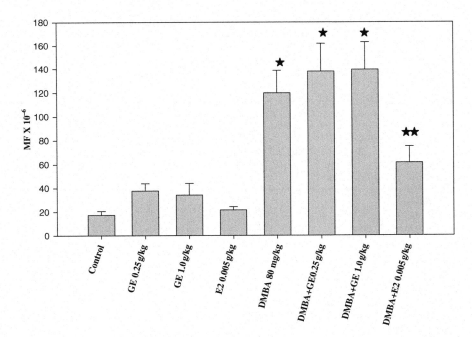

Fig. 7.4 Mean *lac*I MFs measured in the heart of OVX BB rats fed control diet containing GE 0.25, 1.00 g/kg GE, or E2 0.005 g/kg in the presence or absence of DMBA treatment. Each point represents the mean± S.E.M of five rats. ★ Significantly different from control ($p < 0.05$), ★★ significantly different from control and DMBA treated rats

can change the genetic code for amino acid sequence in proteins, thus introducing biochemical errors that lead to disease (Wang et al. 2003; Yu et al. 1999; Zhong et al. 1996). Feeding GE diet to rats treated with DMBA did not significantly affect DMBA mutagenicity, however, dietary E2 resulted in a significant reduction in DMBA mutagenic response ($p < 0.05$), suggesting that E2 is protective. If this response could be extrapolated to the human setting, one would assume that the apparent protective effect of E2 in the heart stands strikingly at variance with the report from the Women's Health Initiative Study that suggested increased risk for cardiovascular disease among women taking HRT (Hulley et al. 1998).

The unexpected reduction in the *lacI* MF seen in rats fed the E2 diet and treated with the potent mutagen prompted us to determine the molecular nature of the mutations. DNA sequence analysis of the mutants revealed that the majority of DMBA-induced mutations which are consistent with DMBA-dA and DMBA-dG adducts reported in mammary gland (Manjanatha et al. 2000), were A:T→T:A (40%) and G:C → T:A (25%) transversions. Interestingly, E2 plus DMBA treatment altered the levels of signature mutations associated with DMBA mutagenesis (Aidoo et al. 1997). We observed A:T → T:A and G:C → T:A transversions reduced from 42 to 23% and 19 to 13%, respectively, whereas A:T → G:C transitions were increased from 8% to 21% in the E2 plus DMBA rats compared to rats treated with only DMBA (Table 7.4). Dietary GE did not have an effect on the types of mutations induced in the heart by DMBA. Although the isoflavone did not have any significant effect on DMBA-induced mutagenicity in the heart of OVX rats, the ability of E2 to alter the DMBA mutant frequency and spectra in the heart appears intriguing and suggests the potential benefit of E2 in conditions of ovariectomy or menopause

Table 7.4 Summary of types of *lacI* independent mutations in heart of OVX rats fed control diet containing 0.25 g/kg GE, or 0.005 g/kg E2 in the presence or absence of DMBA, 80 mg/kg

Types of mutations	Control No. of mutations (% total mutations)	GE 0.25 g/kg No. of mutations (% total mutations)	DMBA No. of mutations (% total mutations)	DMBA+E2 No. of mutations (% total mutations)
Transitions				
G:C → A:T	9 (50)	19 (54)	7 (13)	13 (24)
(CpG sites)	6 (65)	9 (47)	2 (28)	8 (61)
A:T → G:C	1 (5.5)	1 (3)	4 (8)	11 (21)
Transversions				
G:C → T:A	1 (5.5)	2 (6)	10 (19)	7 (13)
G:C → C:G	2 (11)	1 (3)	0 (0)	0 (0)
A:T → C:G	1 (5.5)	1 (3)	3 (6)	4 (7)
A:T → T:A	1 (5.5)	1 (3)	22 (42)	12 (23)
−1 frameshifts	1 (5.5)	3 (9)	3 (6)	0 (0)
+1 frameshifts	2 (11)	5 (14)	0 (0)	2 (4)
Deletion	0 (0)	1 (3)	2 (4)	2 (4)
Insertion	0 (0)	1 (3)	1 (2)	2 (4)
Total	18 (100)	35 (100)	52 (100)	53 (100)

when estrogen levels are low. Nonetheless, this experiment was conducted in the OVX rats only, thus further studies in the heart of rats with intact ovaries could explain why the isoflavones did not produce significant changes in DMBA mutagenicity and also elucidate the underlying mechanism associated with decreased DMBA mutagenic response in OVX rats fed the E2 diet.

7.3.5 Effect of GE on DMBA Mutagenesis in the Liver

The liver is the major organ of drug/chemical metabolism and it is widely accepted that the metabolic activation of DMBA and other polycyclic aromatic hydrocarbons (PAHs) is an essential step in the initiation of cancer by PAHs. However, hepatic metabolism in the rat is known to be influenced by sex hormones and other factors (Colby et al. 1980; Kato and Kamataki 1982). Estrogen also has been suggested as a promoter of liver carcinogenesis in rats (Cameron et al. 1982; Taper 1978; Yager and Yager 1980). It is also suggested that phytoestrogens could act as hormone agonists and elicit hormone-dependent effects (Allred et al. 2001; Casanova et al. 1999). It is therefore conceivable that isoflavones may act as antagonists in premenopausal women in whom circulating levels or endogenous estrogen are high and they may act as agonists in postmenopausal women with lower estrogen levels (Adlercreutz and Mazur 1997). Given the multi-step processes involved in carcinogenesis wherein the accumulation of multiple genetic alterations or mutations in critical genes play a large role, understanding the effect of steroidal estrogens and plant-derived estrogen such as genistein on chemical mutagenesis in liver could be important.

We evaluated DMBA mutagenic activity in this tissue to determine if the response would be influenced by dietary isoflavones in OVX and INT rats. For liver, we evaluated the MF in transgenic rats fed diets containing GE or E2. No significant difference in hepatic MF was found between the control and the GE diet groups in either the OVX or the INT rats, although in the OVX rats, the MF for GE alone appeared to be lower than that of control diet (Fig. 7.5). DMBA-treated rats showed a significant increase in MF ($p < 0.01$) relative to that of controls in both OVX and INT rats. GE did not have an effect on DMBA-induced mutagenicity. Paradoxically, DMBA mutagenic response was significantly higher in OVX rats compared to the INT group. The increase in DMBA-induced MF in the liver of OVX rats relative to the INT group irrespective of GE supplementation (Fig. 7.5) is little understood. It should be noted, however, that the mutagenic response to DMBA seen in the present study is consistent with the chemically induced hepatic DNA adduct levels previously reported in OVX rats (Tokumo et al. 1993).

The observation that DMBA-induced mutagenic response was relatively higher in OVX rats, led us to the analysis of the mutants to determine if differences exist between the types of mutations induced by DMBA in the OVX and in the INT groups. Molecular analysis of the mutants recovered from DMBA alone and DMBA+GE (OVX and INT) showed no significant difference in MFs between any two groups for paired comparison among the four DMBA treatment groups (Table 7.5). However, the spectrum of mutations from any group of the four

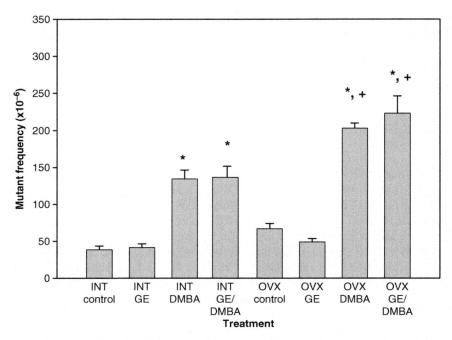

Fig. 7.5 Mutant frequencies (MFs) measured in the liver of OVX and INT rats treated with DMBA or vehicle control with or without GE supplement. * Indicates that the treatment group is significantly different from its concurrent control group ($p < 0.001$); + Indicates that the OVX treatment group is significantly different than the comparable INT treatment group ($p < 0.001$)

Table 7.5 Summary of independent mutations induced by DMBA in the liver of control or genistein-fed intact and ovariectomized rats

	Number (%) of independent mutations				
	Intact		Ovariectomized		
Type of mutation	DMBA	DMBA+GE	DMBA	DMBA+GE	Control[a]
Transitions					
G:C → A:T	15 (21)	8 (14)	2 (6)	4 (9)	27 (42)
% at CpG	67%	63%	100%	50%	74%
A:T → G:C	12 (16)	18 (32)	7 (21)	11 (25)	8 (12)
Transversions					
G:C → T:A	17 (23)	13 (23)	11 (32)	13 (30)	10 (15)
G:C → C:G	5 (7)	7 (12)	6 (18)	4 (9)	7 (11)
A:T → T:A	16 (22)	5 (9)	6 (18)	10 (23)	0 (0)
A:T → C:G	2 (3)	1 (2)	0	0	5 (8)
Frameshifts	5 (7)	5 (9)	2 (6)	2 (5)	8 (12)
Others	1 (1)	0 (0)	0	0	0 (0)
Total mutations	73 (100)	57 (100)	34 (100)	44 (100)	65 (100)

[a]Control data from Harbach et al. (1999)

DMBA-treated groups (INT DMBA alone, INT DMBA+GE, OVX DMBA alone, OVX DMBA+GE) was significantly different from that of the controls. The common types of mutations induced by DMBA were G:C → T:A transversions, A:T → G:C transitions, and A:T → T:A transversions, and these types of mutations are consistent with DNA adduct formation associated with DMBA genotoxic effects. A G:C → A:T transition mutation predominated in the control group (Table 7.5). Over all, the results demonstrate that DMBA is significantly mutagenic in the liver of both OVX and INT rats with higher response seen in the OVX rats compared to the INT group. The DMBA-induced mutation spectra were significantly different from those of control animals, and dietary genistein did not modify these responses.

7.3.6 Effect of DZ and GE on DMBA Mutagenesis and Carcinogenesis in the Mammary Gland

Breast cancer is the most common cancer and possibly the second-leading cause of cancer mortality in women, with approximately one in nine affected in their lifetime (Alberg and Helzlsouer 1997). Populations consuming soy beans have reduced rates of breast and other cancers possibly due, in part, to the presence of isoflavones, DZ and GE. However, GE has been shown to enhance mammary tumor growth in rats (Allred et al. 2004; Day et al. 2001). Therefore, we investigated the effects of DZ and GE or E2 as positive control on DMBA-induced mutagenicity and carcinogenicity in the mammary tissues.

The results obtained from the mutagenesis experiments indicated that DMBA treatment significantly increased *lac*I MFs compared to those seen in the animals fed the control diet without DMBA and that feeding BB rats with low and high doses of DZ, GE, or 0.005 g/kg E2 separately did not alter either spontaneous or chemically-induced *lac*I MFs in rat mammary gland (Table 7.6). The responses in the *lac*I gene were consistent with that of endogenous *Hprt* gene measured in splenic lymphocytes (Table 7.8). However, feeding the animals with a diet containing the mixture (DZG, 1 g/kg GE + 1 g/kg DZ) resulted in a significant reduction in the DMBA-induced *lac*I MF in the mammary glands of the OVX rats ($p < 0.05$, Table 7.6). The *lac*I MFs in the DMBA-treated groups with or without isoflavone supplements were significantly higher in the INT rats compared to the OVX group ($p < 0.05$), indicating a significant enhancement by endogenous estrogens on the MF induced by DMBA, ovariectomy did not significantly alter the MFs of any of the diet groups not receiving DMBA.

Mild atrophy was detected in 10 of the 14 treatment groups in the OVX animals (Fig. 7.6), however atrophy is nonneoplastic and the condition appeared to be attributable to ovariectomy and not to dietary treatment. Animals exposed to a high dose of DZ or DZG and treated with DMBA had a mildly reduced severity in mammary gland atrophy. Since atrophy was absent in animals fed the E2 diet, the reduction seen with the phytoestrogens clearly suggests an enhanced estrogenic action of DZ and GE when administered as a mixture. Also, the incidence of mammary gland ductal hyperplasia (defined here as a relative increase per unit area

Table 7.6 Mutant frequencies (MFs) measured in the mammary gland of OVX and INT rats fed DZ, GE, and mixture (DZG), or E2 in the presence or absence of DMBA

Treatment and dose	Mutant frequency ($\times 10^{-6}$)[a]			
	OVX[b]		INT[b]	
	Vehicle	DMBA	Vehicle	DMBA
Control	22.5 ± 3[b]	201.7 ± 34*	29.5 ± 2 [b]	263.5 ± 18*
DZ 0.25 g/kg diet	33.7 ± 7	140 ± 42*, $\neq$	33 ± 6	215 ± 42*
GE 0.25 g/kg diet	30 ± 10	227.6 ± 66 *	34.2 ± 6	295.7 ± 42*
DZ 1.0 g/kg diet	24 ± 19	149.4 ± 43*, $\neq$	27 ± 7	264.5 ± 17*
GE 1.0 g/kg diet	27.5 ± 9	197.5 ± 39*	41.5 ± 4	307.5 ± 32*
DZG 1.0 g/kg diet	21.2 ± 6	127.4 ± 31**	27.5 ± 6	247.5 ± 39*
E2 0.005 g/kg diet	40 ± 10	186.6 ± 98*	39.5 ± 11	288.4 ± 33* #

[a]Values are means $\pm$ SEM of five rats for all treatment groups except those marked '$\neq$' which had only four rats per group
[b]Significant difference between OVX and INT groups ($p < 0.05$)
*Significant differences were found between rats treated with DMBA and those exposed to isoflavones or vehicle only ($p < 0.01$), **significant changes were found among the groups treated with DMBA and among group treated with vehicle ($p < 0.05$)

of hypodermis of branching intralobular and/or interlobular ducts), was highest in OVX rats fed the 1.0 g/kg DZ or the DZG diet without DMBA treatment (Fig. 7.6). However, ductal hyperplasia was absent in OVX animals fed the control diet, the low dose DZ and GE diets, and the high dose GE diet, DMBA treatment reduced the hyperplasia seen in the high dose DZ and the DZG diets. Ductal hyperplasia of the mammary can be considered as a precursor to the development of ductal carcinoma in situ (Harvell et al. 2000; Mehta et al. 2001), it is not clear why the incidence was high in animals treated with isoflavone alone. Hyperplasia is generally initiated by hormonal stimuli or other factors and even though it reflects non-neoplastic cellular proliferation with neoplastic transformation potential, it also can serve as a physiologic and adaptive response useful to organisms. Thus, ductal hyperplasia seen in OVX rats fed control diet containing isoflavones alone may relate to a physiologic or adaptive response to the estrogenic action of DZ and GE in ovariectomy (compare with ductal hyperplasia in INT rats discussed below).

Despite the significant DMBA mutagenic response seen in *lac*I gene in the mammary and endogenous *Hprt* gene in lymphocytes in the OVX group (Tables 7.7 and 7.8), histopathological examination of the mammary tissues in this group revealed that DMBA exposure was not associated with significant mammary tumor induction (Fig. 7.6). The lack of DMBA tumorigenicity in the mammary gland of OVX rats was not surprising because previous studies have indicated that the development and growth of mammary tumors by DMBA is greatly influenced by the presence or absence of estrogen (Bradley et al. 1976; Leung et al. 1975; McCormick et al. 1982; Teller et al. 1969). This finding is consistent with the demonstration that exposure to exogenous estrogen is accompanied with mammary tumor development in OVX

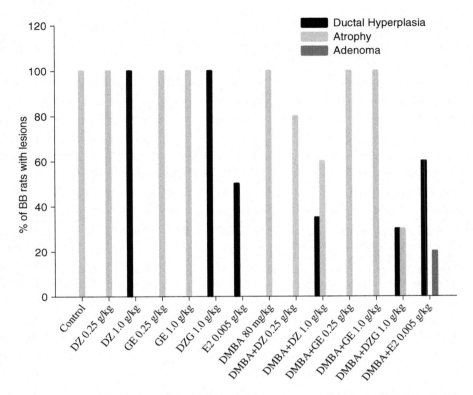

Fig. 7.6 Neoplastic and non-neoplastic changes in the mammary glands of OVX BB rats fed control diets containing DZ, GE, and mixture (DZG) or E2. Animals were sacrificed 20 weeks following DMBA treatment

rats exposed to DMBA (Teller et al. 1969). Furthermore, feeding DMBA-treated rats with E2 in the present study resulted in adenoma (20%) in the mammary of OVX rats, whereas in the DMBA-treated rats fed DZ or GE no tumors were seen (Fig. 7.6). The virtual absence of neoplasia in the DMBA-treated OVX rats also fed DZ and GE suggests that isoflavones are strongly estrogen receptor competitive weak agonists compared to estradiol, and they may be less toxic in a menopausal condition when estrogen levels are low (Adlercreutz and Mazur 1997).

Consistent with the occurrence of ductal hyperplasia observed in the isoflavone-treated animals in the OVX group, in the INT rats similar response was noted in the animals receiving isoflavones with or without DMBA exposure (Fig. 7.7). However, contrary to the lack of DMBA-induced tumors in the OVX rats, a majority of rats in the INT group treated with DMBA developed mammary tumors by 20 weeks following carcinogen treatment (Fig. 7.7). These mammary pathologic lesions, classified as either adenoma or adenocarcinoma were combined and their percentages are presented in Fig. 7.7. Among the DMBA-treated animals, 40% developed adenocarcinoma while the rest displayed ductal hyperplasia (Fig. 7.7).

Table 7.7 Mutant frequencies (MFs) in the uterus measured 16 weeks following DMBA treatment in OVX and INT BB rats fed control diet containing DZ, GE, mixture (DZG), or E2

| Treatment | Mutant frequency ($\times 10^{-6}$)[a] | | | |
| | OVX[b] | | INT[b] | |
	Vehicle	DMBA	Vehicle	DMBA
Control diet	13.3 ± 2.9[b]	83 ± 12.5*	15.3 ± 3.6[b]	100.0 ± 37*
DZ 0.25 g/kg diet	16 ± 6.5	64 ± 47*, $\neq$	16.2 ± 5.9	70.0 ± 19.2*
GE 0.25 g/kg diet	17 ± 4.5	94 ± 25*	20.7 ± 11.2	123.7 ± 61*
DZ 1.0 g/kg diet	11.2 ± 4.8	71 ± 11.5*, $\neq$	11.8 ± 5.2	89.7 ± 12.9*
GE 1.0 g/kg diet	18.7 ± 7.5	89.5 ± 16.7*	25.5 ± 6.2	135.5 ± 62*
DZG 1.0 g/kg diet	8.4 ± 2.9	60.5 ± 49*	16.9 ± 5.6	81 ± 42*
E2 0.005 g/kg diet	23.3 ± 2.9	95.7 ± 37.8*	32 ± 9.2	140.0 ± 44*, #

[a]Values are means $\pm$ SEM of five rats for all treatment groups except those marked '$\neq$' which had only four rats per group
[b]No significant difference between OVX and INT groups ($p > 0.14$)
*Significant differences were found between rats treated with DMBA and those treated with vehicle or isoflavone only ($p < 0.05$)

Table 7.8 Mutant frequencies (MFs) in lymphocytes measured 16 weeks following DMBA treatment in OVX and INT BB rats fed control diet containing DZ, GE, mixture (DZG), or E2

| Treatment | Mutant frequency ($\times 10^{-6}$)[a] | | | |
| | OVX[b] | | INT[b] | |
	Vehicle	DMBA	Vehicle	DMBA
Control diet	6.63 ± 1.9	97.8 ± 11.2*	9.6 ± 3.4	147.3 ± 31.8*
DZ 0.25 g/kg diet	8.5 ± 2.5	114.9 ± 15.7*	7.3 ± 2.2	128.7 ± 21.7*
GE 0.25 g/kg diet	14.7 ± 4.7	123.4 ± 28.5*	3.9 ± 0.8	113.3 ± 25.7*
DZ 1.0 g/kg diet	3.9 ± 0.9	84.2 ± 3.9*	11.9 ± 3.1	88.5 ± 19.9*
GE 1.0 g/kg diet	8.9 ± 4.0	68.8 ± 5.3*	5.4 ± 1.7	60.8 ± 11.0*
DZG 1.0 g/kg diet	8.8 ± 3.5	89.5 ± 22.1*	9.4 ± 3.2	59.9 ± 5.1*
E2 0.005 g/kg diet	4.2 ± 1.3	77.0 ± 11.0*	19.9 ± 13.5	98.3 ± 19.0*

[a]Values are means $\pm$ SEM of five rats per a treatment group
[b]No significant difference was observed between OVX rats and the INT group
*Significant differences were found between DMBA-treated rats and those exposed to either isoflavones or vehicle alone ($p < 0.001$)

In the rats fed DZ or GE, the DMBA-induced mammary tumors were increased, but the responses were not statistically significant. Feeding DMBA-treated rats with the mixture resulted in decreased mammary tumor incidence, perhaps due to synergy inherent in mixtures. The carcinogenic potency of DMBA in the INT rats could be due to the presence of endogenous ovarian hormones, including estrogen, which may have augmented the effect of DMBA. Like the OVX rats, the INT rats were

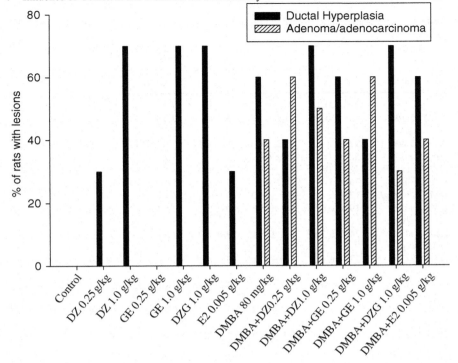

Fig. 7.7 Neoplastic and non neoplastic lesions in the mammary glands of INT BB rats fed control diet containing GE, DZ, mixture (DZG), and E2. Animals were sacrificed 20 weeks following DMBA treatment

also given exogenous E2. Even though 17β-estradiol is considered a weak mutagen (Liehr 2000), its metabolism by cytochrome P450 isoforms has been shown to generate catechol estrogens that can directly or indirectly interact with DNA and may initiate the carcinogenesis process (Nebert 1993). It also has been shown that the metabolites of estrogens can directly or indirectly, through redox cycling processes, generate reactive radical species that cause oxidative DNA damage (Han and Liehr 1994; Liehr and Roy 1990; Liehr et al. 1990). It is likely that these events could overwhelm E2 toxicity in the INT rats compared to the OVX group (Table 7.9).

Although the observed increase in DMBA carcinogenicity by the isoflavones was not significant, it may reflect the intrinsic estrogenic activity of phytoestrogens. The fact that isoflavones can increase DMBA-induced carcinogenicity suggests that, like estrogens, these compounds can act as co-carcinogens or tumor promoters in tissues with pre-existing DNA damage or exposed to carcinogens. An increase in DMBA-induced mammary adenocarcinoma by 1.0 g/kg GE in wild-type, but not in estrogen receptor-α-knockout mice, has been reported (Day et al. 2001). Chronic intake of 0.75 g/kg GE administered six weeks following carcinogen treatment and ovariectomy (when tumors had already developed) increased the growth of these tumors in Sprague-Dawley rats (Allred et al. 2004). In addition, dietary GE at a

Table 7.9 Effect of DZ and GE on cell proliferation and apoptosis in the mammary gland of OVX and INT rats

Treatment Group	OVX			INT		
	S phase	G1	Apoptosis	S phase	G1	Apoptosis
Control diet	4.5 ± 0.7	7.5 ± 0.7	3.5 ± 0.7	7.5 ± 1.4	13.5 ± 2.1	10 ± 2.8
DZ 0.25 g/kg	5.6 ± 0.9	5.0 ± 0.5	4.8 ± 05	7.5 ± 2.1	12.0 ± 1.4	8.5 ± 0.7
DZ 1.0 g/kg	4.0 ± 1.4	6.5 ± 0.7	5.5 ± 0.7	6.0 ± 1.4	11.0 ± 0.0	8.0 ± 4.2
GE 0.25 g/kg	9.5 ± 1.2	7.2 ± 1.0	5.8 ± 0.6	$6.0 \pm 0.1.4$	10.0 ± 1.4	14.5 ± 6.3
GE 1.0 g/kg	5.5 ± 0.7	4.5 ± 0.7	2.5 ± 0.7	16.0 ± 2.8	24.5 ± 3.5	9.5 ± 6.3
DZ/GE 1.0 g/kg	4.3 ± 0.6	10.3 ± 1.5	5.4 ± 0.4	9.5 ± 2.1	15.0 ± 2.8	8.5 ± 4.2
E 0.005 g/kg	7.6 ± 0.9	9.7 ± 0.5	4.9 ± 0.5	12.0 ± 1.4	15.5 ± 2.1	5.5 ± 2.1
DMBA 80 mg/kg	12.4 ± 4.8	20.6 ± 8.0	6.6 ± 4.1	8.8 ± 3.1	14.1 ± 3.7	10.4 ± 2.4
DMBA+DZ 0.25 g/kg	19.4 ± 6.3	28.7 ± 8.6	8.0 ± 3.3	12.3 ± 3.4	19.2 ± 5.2	12.6 ± 3.9
DMBA+DZ 1.0 g/kg	$24.1 \pm 3.6^*$	$33.4 \pm 5.1^*$	7.9 ± 2.7	$17.4 \pm 2.6^*$	$26.3 \pm 5.3^*$	11.6 ± 3.2
DMBA+GE 0.25 g/kg	$23.7 \pm 8.2^*$	$33.0 \pm 9.1^*$	8.5 ± 4.0	13.7 ± 4.3	20.7 ± 4.9	11.1 ± 2.8
DMBA+GE 1.0 g/kg	18.6 ± 4.7	28.3 ± 8.4	9.4 ± 2.4	15.0 ± 5.9	24.8 ± 8.3	10.1 ± 4.1
DMBA+DZGE 1000 ppm	12.5 ± 3.9	22.3 ± 8.6	7.5 ± 2.3	9.4 ± 3.1	16.0 ± 6.0	12.8 ± 3.2
DMBA+E2 0.005 g/kg	18.2 ± 2.3	28.5 ± 3.0	6.5 ± 2.6	$20.6 \pm 1.4^*$	$30.4 \pm 5.8^*$	11.6 ± 4.0

7,12-dimethylbenz[a]anthracene, 80 mg/kg values are mean $\pm$ standard deviation
*Significantly different from DMBA alone at $p < 0.05$

level of 0.25 g/kg fed to female Fischer 344 rats also treated with azoxymethane enhanced colon carcinogenesis (Rao et al. 1997). In contrast, in the present study dietary DZ or GE, starting two weeks before DMBA treatment did not cause significant changes in mammary gland carcinogenesis in the INT rats (Fig. 7.5). Our results suggest that DZ and GE are comparatively weak estrogens since the mixture containing both high dose of DZ and GE slightly decreased DMBA carcinogenicity in the mammary gland compared to E2. Also, differences such as experimental design, duration of treatment, use of transgenic animals, and the weak estrogenic activity of the phytoestrogens may have contributed to a lack of significant effect of the isoflavones on DMBA-induced tumorigenicity in the present study.

7.3.7 Effect of DZ and GE on DMBA Mutagenesis and Carcinogenesis in the Uterus

An association between soy consumption and the risk for endometrial cancer has been discussed (Cline and Hughes 1998; Goodman et al. 1997; Horn-Ross et al. 2003), however, comparatively little is known about the possible action of naturally occurring phytoestrogens in chemical carcinogenesis in the uterus. Since the uterus appears especially sensitive to neoplastic transformation by estrogens (Leavitt et al. 1982), experiments were performed to determine the effects of DZ, GE or E2 on DMBA-induced mutagenicity and carcinogenicity in the uterus of OVX and INT rats. The uterine tissues from rats sacrificed at 16 or 20 weeks following DMBA treatment were processed to assess *lac*I mutant frequencies and histopathological parameters, respectively. As shown in Table 7.7 and Fig. 7.8, the effect of the isoflavones on DMBA-induced mutagenicity in the uterus was similar to that of E2. In both OVX and INT rats, DMBA treatment significantly increased *lac*I MFs compared to the animals that were not exposed to DMBA, however, DZ, GE, or E2 diets did not alter either the DMBA-induced or spontaneous *lac*I MFs in the uterus nor in the endogenous *Hprt* gene in splenic lymphocytes (Tables 7.7 and 7.8). Interestingly,

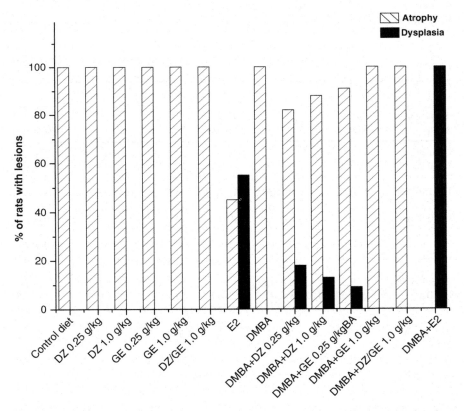

Fig. 7.8 Histopathology of uterine tissues from OVX rats sacrificed at 20 weeks post-DMBA treatment. Atrophy was marked in most of the treatment groups including the control, but the incidence was less marked in rats fed E2 diet alone. Note that atrophy was virtually absent when E2-fed rats were treated with DMBA treatment; however, 100% dysplasia was observed in this group. Compared to E2, exposure of isoflavone-fed diets to DMBA produced a low incidence of dysplasia, 10–18%

the MF of the DMBA-treated INT rats was greater than that seen in the corresponding OVX animals, an effect that could be attributable to endogenous ovarian action.

Histopathology analysis of uterine samples derived from OVX rats revealed no neoplastic transformation, malignant or non-malignant in the uterus of rats exposed to DMBA alone or those fed isoflavone and treated with the carcinogen (Fig. 7.8). DMBA is a multi-organ carcinogen and it is possible that its failure to induce tumors in the uterus may be due, in part, to toxicological factors such as the inefficiency of local or distant metabolism of DMBA, removal of DNA adducts by excision repair, cell proliferation rate or doubling time of initiated cells in the uterus. Besides the latter hypothesis, the other factors appear to be unlikely because DMBA exposure resulted in a significant mutagenicity in uterus, liver and also in a surrogate tissue, lymphocytes (Table 7.8) of OVX rats, with cell proliferation increased in DMBA-treated rats (Table 7.10). Further, the lack of DMBA carcinogenic effect in the uterus may not be due to endogenous estrogen deficiency as a result of ovariectomy. In

Table 7.10 Effect of DZ and GE on cell proliferation and apoptosis in the uterus of OVX and INT rats

Treatment group	OVX			INT		
	S phase	G1	Apoptosis	S phase	G1	Apoptosis
Control diet	6.0 ± 1.4	12.5 ± 0.7	22.0 ± 0.0	57.5 ± 16.3	67.0 ± 19.8	30.5 ± 4.9
DZ 0.25 g/kg	18.9 ± 4.5**	20.4±2.6	15.8 ± 3.2	37.5 ± 18.9	42.0 ± 26.8	37.5 ± 9.2
DZ 1.0 g/kg	27.0 ± 5.7**	50.0±8.5**	9.5 ± 0.7**	45.5 ± 17.7	54.5 ± 19.1	28.5 ± 10.6
GE 0.25 g/kg	21.3 ± 3.9	29.5 ± 9.8**	11.6 ± 1.8	75.0 ± 19.8	73.5 ± 16.3	35.0 ± 1.4
GE 1.0 g/kg	14.0 ± 1.4	24.0 ± 1.4	10.5 ± 0.7	29.5 ± 9.2	39.0 ± 2.8	31.0 ± 2.8
DZ/GE 1.0 g/kg	20.4 ± 2.8**	31.8 ± 8.7**	13.4 ± 2.0	74.0 ± 7.0	76.5 ± 9.2	22.5 ± 6.4
E2 0.005 g/kg	29.5 ± 7.8*	33.8 ± 12.8	9.8 ± 1.6*	55.5 ± 7.8	71.5 ± 7.8	21.0 ± 11.3
DMBA	19.8 ± 10.1	30.3 ± 11.2	29.3 ± 5.9	58.1 ± 18.2	65.0 ± 21.7	28.4 ± 8.2
DMBA+DZ 0.25 g/kg	24.5 ± 7.9	39.5 ± 10.7	25.3 ± 6.6	50.3 ± 22.5	56.7 ± 23.3	27.9 ± 6.3
DMBA+DZ 1.0 g/kg	39.8 ± 10.6*	52.1 ± 14.7*	28.1 ± 5.1	50.0 ± 18.4	56.7 ± 19.9	29.2 ± 6.9
DMBA+GE 0.25 g/kg	31.1 ± 6.9	42.8 ± 9.7	28.0 ± 7.3	51.8 ± 26.6	51.6 ± 18.7	28.9 ± 7.9
DMBA+GE 1.0 g/kg	31.4 ± 7.7	47.1 ± 10.4	28.4 ± 5.6	54.2 ± 16.5	62.2 ± 15.6	32.7 ± 5.7
DMBA+DZ/GE 1.0 g/kg	46.5 ± 8.9*	62.7 ± 12.1*	22.9 ± 9.5	39.9 ± 9.1	44.8 ± 11.3	32.5 ± 6.6
DMBA+E2 0.005 g/kg	59.0 ± 8.0*	84.4 ± 11.4*	24.5 ± 10.5	49.3 ± 23.6	60.9 ± 29.8	32.7 ± 4.4

1,12-Dimethylben[a]anthracene, 80 mg/kg values are mean ± standard deviation
*Significantly different from DMBA alone at $p < 0.05$, **significantly different from control diet at $p < 0.05$

INT rats treated with DMBA alone, only a clitoral gland carcinoma in one rat was induced and no uterine tumors, a response strikingly similar to that shown in rats fed E2 and exposed to DMBA, where only a developmental malformation in the uterus in one rat and a clitoral gland adenoma in another were the only pathologies observed. As shown in Fig. 7.8, uterine atrophy was prominent in the OVX group with or without the supplements or DMBA treatment as expected in ovariectomy. Although the percentage of OVX rats with atrophy as depicted in Fig. 7.8 appears essentially similar in all the treatment groups, except E2, the degree of severity of atrophy (graded as 3–4 high and 2 or below low), was high in rats receiving the control diet and those fed the isoflavones or treated with DMBA alone (data not shown). Interestingly, the degree of severity was only reduced in DMBA-treated rats fed the isoflavones, while it was completely eliminated in E2-fed rats exposed to DMBA, suggesting lower estrogenic activity of the isoflavones compared to E2. This finding is consistent with the absence of uterine dysplasia in rats exposed to the phytoestrogens or DMBA alone in both OVX (Fig. 7.6 and INT not shown) groups. Dietary E2 however caused a high incidence of dysplasia in OVX rats (55% in E2-fed alone and 100% in E2-fed plus DMBA treatment).

The high incidence of dysplasia found in OVX rats fed E2 and treated with DMBA essentially imply that E2 not only induced dysplasia by itself, but also was capable of promoting chemically initiated cells into dysplasia. Dysplasia is an abnormal atypical cellular proliferation, and while it is not a tumor and does not cause health problems, if left untreated, it sometimes can progress to an early form of cancer. These findings have important health implications due to the fact that one of the major adverse effects of estrogen replacement therapy among menopausal women is endometrial cancer (Kelsey and Whittemore 1994). In contrast, in the INT group dysplasia was not detected, but asynchronistic growth pattern was observed in the uterus possibly due to exposure to the isoflavones or E2, uterine hemangiosarcoma also was detected in one rat from the INT group fed 1.0 g/kg DZ and treated with DMBA. In addition, isolated incidences of mild to marked dilatations were seen in some animals exposed to DMBA with or without the isoflavones. No incidence of dilatation, mild or marked, was seen in E2-fed rats in this group. The incidence of these pathologic lesions was sporadic and too low to be interpreted as treatment-related.

Dietary DZ and GE combined with DMBA treatment also produced dysplasia in the uterus of OVX rats (Fig. 7.8), but the incidence was relatively low (ranging from 10 to 18%). The low incidence of dysplasia in this group illustrates the relatively weak estrogenic potency of phytoestrogens and indicates that they may be safer than estradiol. However, under the conditions of these experiments, the period of isoflavone administration was not long enough to actually determine whether they were carcinogenic by themselves. Nonetheless, their ability to induce dysplasia even on a small scale, when a carcinogen is present clearly indicates that they can potentially influence the growth of initiated cells in rat uterus. The underlying mechanism of action of isoflavones is not clearly understood, however, they can function both as estrogen agonists and antagonists (Diel et al. 2001; Markiewicz et al. 1993), depending on many factors including hormonal milieu, or receptor occupancy, treatment regimen, and tissues under investigation. From a genotoxic perspective, this result may imply that when estrogen levels are low as they tend to be in ovariectomy or menopause, isoflavones can substitute for the organism's own estrogen and act as co-carcinogens (already discussed above).

Since DZ, GE and E2 did not increase DMBA-induced MFs and DMBA alone did not induce uterine dysplasia in OVX rats, it is possible that the mechanism of action for the induction of dysplasia by E2 and/or the phytoestrogens results from their ability to increase cell proliferation. The most widely established role of estrogen in carcinogenesis involves increased cell proliferation (Ethier 1995; Nandi et al. 1995; Preston-Martin et al. 1990), therefore, we assessed cell proliferation by PCNA immunochemistry. As expected, the percentage of PCNA-positive cells in S-phase and G1-phase of the cell cycle in the uterus of OVX rats fed E2 diet and treated with DMBA was significantly higher than the other groups (Table 7.10, $p < 0.05$). There also was a corresponding increase in uterine weight in E2-fed animals treated with DMBA (Table 7.2), this finding was in contrast to the atrophy seen in the OVX rats fed the isoflavone and the control diets. Cell proliferation also was increased in the isoflavone-fed animals treated with DMBA in the OVX group (Table 7.10). In the INT rats, no significant changes in G1- and S-phases were observed in any of the treatment groups (Table 7.10). These results suggest that cell proliferation is partly responsible for the induction of dysplasia in the uterus of OVX rats by dietary E2 and by the isoflavones and that DMBA-induced cytolethality also contributes to the observed pathologic lesion.

Considering the fact that prolonged exposure to synthetic or endogenous steroidal hormones or their metabolites is causally linked to several human cancers, including endometrial cancer (Henderson and Bernstein 1991; Henderson et al. 1988; Preston-Martin et al. 1990), it was unexpected that dysplasia was virtually absent in the uterus of INT rats treated with DMBA and fed E2 or the phytoestrogens. One possible explanation for this phenomenon is hormone balance. It has been shown that postmenopausal hormone replacement therapy using unopposed estrogen significantly increases endometrial cancer risk. This risk, however, is markedly reduced when estrogen is administered in conjunction with progestin (Barnes et al. 1995). Also, E2 is metabolized along two competing pathways to form 2-hydroxylated and 16α-hydroxylated metabolites. Because of their different biological activities, the ratio of these metabolites, 2-hydroxyestrogen:16α-hydroxyestrone has been used as a biomarker for breast cancer risk (Hankinson et al. 1998; Ho et al. 1998). Since the ovary produces many other hormones in addition to E2, it is also possible that some of these hormones or their metabolites may function against estrogenic action and inhibit cell proliferation in the uterus of INT rats (Kelsey and Whittemore 1994).

7.3.8 Effect of DZ and GE on Histopathological Lesions in Other Organs/Tissues

In addition to the mammary gland and the uterus, other tissues were examined for the presence of pathologic lesions in rats killed 20 weeks after DMBA treatment. In the OVX rats treated with DMBA alone, no neoplastic lesion was seen except a mild duct dilatation in the clitoral gland. However, a neural crest tumor was observed in the ear of one rat fed 0.25 g/kg DZ diet and treated with DMBA, another rat in the DMBA-treated group fed E2 had clitoral gland adenoma. In the INT group, ovarian cysts were seen in all the treatment groups, including those fed the control diet. Also, GE feeding caused cellular infiltration in lymph node in one rat and abscess in the oral mucosa in another. DMBA treatment resulted only in clitoral gland tumor in one rat, and nonneoplastic lesions such as fibrosis in the liver and marked hematopoietic cell proliferation in the spleen. In rats treated with DMBA and fed 1.0 g/kg DZ diet, lung carcinoma in one rat and skin carcinoma in another was detected. It should be noted, however that these pathological lesions seen in 27 weeks old rats were low and sporadic, and could represent background alterations in female rats of this age rather than the treatment related effects.

7.4 Summary and Conclusions

Phytoestrogens such as soy isoflavones, DZ and GE are naturally occurring estrogens that are believed to exhibit health benefits in a variety of human ailments or conditions, including heart disease, menopause, osteoporosis, and cancer. Many women are using these compounds as an alternative to hormone replacement therapy that has been suggested to play a role in heart disease, cancer and stroke. However, the structural similarity of the isoflavones to that of estrogens suggests that they may interfere with estrogen receptors and influence steroid-dependent diseases, such as prostate or breast cancer. Thus, this study evaluated the effects of DZ, GE, or E2 on chemical mutagenesis in heart, liver, lymphocytes, mammary glands and uterus of OVX and INT rats. Mammary glands and uterus were also used to evaluate carcinogenic responses. Dietary isoflavones were bioavailable and acted like estrogens especially in the uterus where increased cell proliferation and decreased atrophy were seen in the OVX rats While dietary E2 (alone or combined with DMBA induced a high incidence of dysplasia in the uterus of OVX rats, the incident was very low in the isoflavones-treated group, and occurred only when DZ or GE was combined with DMBA exposure. This finding suggests weak estrogenic effects of the isoflavones relative to E2, and that DZ or GE may be safer compared to E2. DMBA treatment caused tumors in the mammary glands of the INT rats, and these responses were non-significantly increased by the isoflavones. However, the combined exposure of DZ and GE slightly reduced DMBA carcinogenicity compared to E2. Feeding both OVX and INT rats control diets containing the isoflavones did not significantly alter the mutagenicity of DMBA in the hormone-responsive tissues (heart, liver, mammary, and uterus). Interestingly, feeding E2 to rats effectively reduced DMBA-induced mutagenicity in the heart of OVX rats and molecular analysis of the mutants also showed a shift in the mutational spectra of DMBA from the common type, A:T $\rightarrow$ T:A to G:C $\rightarrow$ A:T and A:T$\rightarrow$ G:C, suggesting the importance of E2 in low estrogen environment as existed in the OVX rats. The data presented here demonstrate that DZ and GE have weak estrogenic activity and would be less toxic in low estrogen environment as occurs in menopause. The positive responses seen with DZ and GE mixture also suggest the potential health benefit of eating soy products containing the isoflavones and perhaps, other health promising compounds, as opposed to taking them separately as dietary supplements. This study serves as a useful prototype for further exploration of the effects of isoflavones on environmental chemicals or drugs to which humans are consistently exposed.

Acknowledgments This study was funded in part by the FDA Office of Women's Health, Rockville, MD, USA.

References

Abe T (1999) Infantile leukemia and soybeans – a hypothesis. Leukemia 13:317–320

Adlercreutz H, Mazur W (1997) Phyto-oestrogens and Western diseases. Ann Med 29:95–120

Aidoo A, Lyn-Cook LE, Mittelstaedt RA et al (1991) Induction of 6-thioguanine-resistant lymphocytes in Fischer 344 rats following in vivo exposure to N-ethyl-N-nitrosourea and cyclophosphamide. Environ Mol Mutagen 17:141–151

Aidoo A, Morris SM, Casciano DA (1997) Development and utilization of the rat lymphocyte hprt mutation assay. Mutat Res 387:69–88

Alberg AJ, Helzlsouer KJ (1997) Epidemiology, prevention, and early detection of breast cancer. Curr Opin Oncol 9:505–511

Allred CD, Allred KF, Ju YH et al (2001) Soy diets containing varying amounts of genistein stimulate growth of estrogen-dependent (MCF-7) tumors in a dose-dependent manner. Cancer Res 61:5045–5050

Allred CD, Allred KF, Ju YH et al (2004) Dietary genistein results in larger MNU-induced, estrogen-dependent mammary tumors following ovariectomy of Sprague-Dawley rats. Carcinogenesis 25:211–218

Anderson JJ, Anthony MS, Cline JM et al (1999) Health potential of soy isoflavones for menopausal women. Public Health Nutr 2:489–450

Arai Y, Uehara M, Sato Y et al (2000) Comparison of isoflavones among dietary intake, plasma concentration and urinary excretion for accurate estimation of phytoestrogen intake. J Epidemiol 10:127–135

Arjmandi BH, Alekel L, Hollis BW et al (1996) Dietary soybean protein prevents bone loss in an ovariectomized rat model of osteoporosis. J Nutr 126:161–167

Barnes S, Peterson TG, Coward L (1995) Rationale for the use of genistein-containing soy matrices in chemoprevention trials for breast and prostate cancer. J Cell Biochem Suppl 22: 181–187

Barnes S, Sfakianos J, Coward L et al (1996) Soy isoflavonoids and cancer prevention. Underlying biochemical and pharmacological issues. Adv Exp Med Biol 401:87–100

Bonavera JJ, Dube MG, Kalra PS et al (1994) Anorectic effects of estrogen may be mediated by decreased neuropeptide-Y release in the hypothalamic paraventricular nucleus. Endocrinology 134:2367–2370

Bradley CJ, Kledzik GS, Meites J (1976) Prolactin and estrogen dependency of rat mammary cancers at early and late stages of development. Cancer Res 36:319–324

Butera PC, Beikirch RJ (1989) Central implants of diluted estradiol: independent effects on ingestive and reproductive behaviors of ovariectomized rats. Brain Res 491:266–273

Buters J, Quintanilla-Martinez L, Schober W et al (2003) CYP1B1 determines susceptibility to low doses of 7,12-dimethylbenz[a]anthracene-induced ovarian cancers in mice: correlation of CYP1B1-mediated DNA adducts with carcinogenicity. Carcinogenesis 24:327–334

Cameron RG, Imaida K, Tsuda H et al (1982) Promotive effects of steroids and bile acids on hepatocarcinogenesis initiated by diethylnitrosamine. Cancer Res 42:2426–2428

Casanova M, You L, Gaido KW et al (1999) Developmental effects of dietary phytoestrogens in Sprague-Dawley rats and interactions of genistein and daidzein with rat estrogen receptors alpha and beta in vitro. Toxicol Sci 51:236–244

Chen Z, Zheng W, Custer LJ et al (1999) Usual dietary consumption of soy foods and its correlation with the excretion rate of isoflavonoids in overnight urine samples among Chinese women in Shanghai. Nutr Cancer 33:82–87

Cline JM, Hughes CL Jr (1998) Phytochemicals for the prevention of breast and endometrial cancer. Cancer Treat Res 94:107–134

Colby HD, Marquess ML, Johnson PB et al (1980) Effects of steroid hormones in vitro on adrenal xenobiotic metabolism in the guinea pig. Biochem Pharmacol 29:2373–2377

Cruz-Munoz W, Kalair W, Cosentino L et al (2000) ENU induces mutations in the heart of lacZ transgenic mice. Mutat Res 469:23–34

Dao TL (1962) The role of ovarian hormones in initiating the induction of mammary cancer in rats by polynuclear hydrocarbons. Cancer Res 22:973–981

Day JK, Besch-Williford C, McMann TR et al (2001) Dietary genistein increased DMBA-induced mammary adenocarcinoma in wild-type, but not ER alpha KO, mice. Nutr Cancer 39: 226–232

Diel P, Smolnikar K, Schulz T et al (2001) Phytoestrogens and carcinogenesis-differential effects of genistein in experimental models of normal and malignant rat endometrium. Hum Reprod 16:997–1006

Ethier SP (1995) Growth factor synthesis and human breast cancer progression. J Natl Cancer Inst 87:964–973

Giri AK, Lu LJ (1995) Genetic damage and the inhibition of 7,12-dimethylbenz[a] anthracene-induced genetic damage by the phytoestrogens, genistein and daidzein, in female ICR mice. Cancer Lett 95:125–133

Gooderham MH, Adlercreutz H, Ojala ST (1996) A soy protein isolate rich in genistein and daidzein and its effects on plasma isoflavone concentrations, platelet aggregation, blood lipids and fatty acid composition of plasma phospholipid in normal men. J Nutr 126:2000–2006

Goodman MT, Wilkens LR, Hankin JH (1997) Association of soy and fiber consumption with the risk of endometrial cancer. Am J Epidemiol 146:294–306

Han X, Liehr JG (1994) 8-Hydroxylation of guanine bases in kidney and liver DNA of hamsters treated with estradiol: role of free radicals in estrogen-induced carcinogenesis. Cancer Res 54:5515–5517

Hankinson SE, Willett WC, Manson JE (1998) Plasma sex steroid hormone levels and risk of breast cancer in postmenopausal women. J Natl Cancer Inst 90:1292–1299

Harbach PR, Zimmer DM, Filipunas AL, Mattes WB, Aaron CS (1999) Spontaneous mutation spectrum at the lambda cII locus in liver, lung, and spleen tissue of Big Blue transgenic mice. Environ Mol Mutagen 33:132–143

Harvell DM, Strecker TE, Tochacek, M (2000) Rat strain-specific actions of 17beta-estradiol in the mammary gland: correlation between estrogen-induced lobuloalveolar hyperplasia and susceptibility to estrogen-induced mammary cancers. Proc Natl Acad Sci USA 97:2779–2784

Henderson BE, Bernstein L (1991) The international variation in breast cancer rates: an epidemiological assessment. Breast Cancer Res Treat 18(Suppl 1):S11–S17

Henderson BE, Ross R, Bernstein L (1988) Estrogens as a cause of human cancer: the Richard and Hinda Rosenthal Foundation award lecture. Cancer Res 48:246–253

Herrington DM, Pusser BE, Riley WA (2000) Cardiovascular effects of droloxifene, a new selective estrogen receptor modulator, in healthy postmenopausal women. Arterioscler Thromb Vasc Biol 20:1606–1612

Ho GH, Luo XW, Ji CY et al (1998) Urinary 2/16 alpha-hydroxyestrone ratio: correlation with serum insulin-like growth factor binding protein-3 and a potential biomarker of breast cancer risk. Ann Acad Med Singapore 27:294–299

Horn-Ross PL, John EM, Canchola AJ (2003) Phytoestrogen intake and endometrial cancer risk. J Natl Cancer Inst 95:1158–1164

Hulley S, Grady D, Bush T (1998) Randomized trial of estrogen plus progestin for secondary prevention of coronary heart disease in postmenopausal women. Heart and Estrogen/progestin Replacement Study (HERS) Research Group. JAMA 280:605–613

Ip C, Ip MM (1981) Serum estrogens and estrogen responsiveness in 7,12-dimethylbenz [a]anthracene-induced mammary tumors as influenced by dietary fat. J Natl Cancer Inst 66:291–295

Kato R, Kamataki T (1982) Cytochrome P-450 as a determinant of sex difference of drug metabolism in the rat. Xenobiotica 12:787–800

Kelsey JL, Whittemore AS (1994) Epidemiology and primary prevention of cancers of the breast, endometrium, and ovary. A brief overview. Ann Epidemiol 4:89–95

Kennedy AR (1995) The evidence for soybean products as cancer preventive agents. J Nutr 125:733S–743S

Knight DC, Eden JA (1996) A review of the clinical effects of phytoestrogens. Obstet Gynecol 87:897–904

Kulling SE, Metzler M (1997) Induction of micronuclei, DNA strand breaks and HPRT mutations in cultured Chinese hamster V79 cells by the phytoestrogen coumoestrol. Food Chem Toxicol 35:605–613

Leavitt W, Evans R, Hendry W, III (1982) Etiology of DES-induced uterine tumors in Syrian hamsters. In: Leavitt W (ed), Hormones and cancer. Plenum, New York, NY 63–86

Leung BS, Sasaki GH, Leung JS (1975) Estrogen-prolactin dependency in 7,12-dimethylbenz(a)anthracene-induced tumors. Cancer Res 35:621–627

Liehr JG (2000) Is estradiol a genotoxic mutagenic carcinogen? Endocr Rev 21:40–54

Liehr JG, Roy D (1990) Free radical generation by redox cycling of estrogens. Free Radic Biol Med 8:415–423

Liehr JG, Roy D, Ari-Ulubelen A et al (1990) Effect of chronic estrogen treatment of Syrian hamsters on microsomal enzymes mediating formation of catecholestrogens and their redox cycling: implications for carcinogenesis. J Steroid Biochem 35:555–560

Manjanatha MG, Shelton SD, Aidoo A et al (1998) Comparison of in vivo mutagenesis in the endogenous Hprt gene and the lacI transgene of Big Blue(R) rats treated with 7, 12- dimethylbenz[a]anthracene. Mutat Res 401:165–178

Manjanatha MG, Shelton SD, Culp SJ et al (2000) DNA adduct formation and molecular analysis of in vivo lacI mutations in the mammary tissue of Big Blue rats treated with 7, 12- dimethylbenz[a]anthracene. Carcinogenesis 21:265–273

Markiewicz L, Garey J, Adlercreutz H et al (1993) In vitro bioassays of non-steroidal phytoestrogens. J Steroid Biochem Mol Biol 45:399–405

Markovits J, Linassier C, Fosse P et al (1989) Inhibitory effects of the tyrosine kinase inhibitor genistein on mammalian DNA topoisomerase II. Cancer Res 49:5111–5117

McCormick DL, Mehta RG, Thompson CA et al (1982) Enhanced inhibition of mammary carcinogenesis by combined treatment with N-(4-hydroxyphenyl) retinamide and ovariectomy. Cancer Res 42:508–512

Mehta RG, Bhat KP, Hawthorne ME (2001) Induction of atypical ductal hyperplasia in mouse mammary gland organ culture. J Natl Cancer Inst 93:1103–1106

Messina MJ, Persky V, Setchell KD (1994) Soy intake and cancer risk: a review of the in vitro and in vivo data. Nutr Cancer 21:113–131

Metzler B, Hu Y, Sturm G et al (1998) Induction of mitogen-activated protein kinase phosphatase-1 by arachidonic acid in vascular smooth muscle cells. J Biol Chem 273:33320–33326

Misra RR, Hursting SD, Perkins SN et al (2002) Genotoxicity and carcinogenicity studies of soy isoflavones. Int J Toxicol 21:277–285

Morris SM, Chen JJ, Domon OE (1998) p53, mutations, and apoptosis in genistein-exposed human lymphoblastoid cells. Mutat Res 405:41–56

Nandi S, Guzman RC, Yang, J (1995) Hormones and mammary carcinogenesis in mice, rats, and humans: a unifying hypothesis. Proc Natl Acad Sci USA 92:3650–3657

Nebert DW (1993) Elevated estrogen 16 alpha-hydroxylase activity: is this a genotoxic or nongenotoxic biomarker in human breast cancer risk? J Natl Cancer Inst 85:1888–1891

Okura A, Arakawa H, Oka H (1988) Effect of genistein on topoisomerase activity and on the growth of [Val 12] Ha-ras-transformed NIH 3T3 cells. Biochem Biophys Res Commun 157:183–189

Preston-Martin S, Pike MC, Ross RK (1990) Increased cell division as a cause of human cancer. Cancer Res 50:7415–7421

Ramsey LA, Ross BS, Fischer RG (1999) Phytoestrogens and the management of menopause. Adv Nurse Pract 7:26–30

Rao CV, Wang CX, Simi B (1997) Enhancement of experimental colon cancer by genistein. Cancer Res 57: 3717–3722

Russo J, Gusterson BA, Rogers AE (1990) Comparative study of human and rat mammary tumorigenesis. Lab Invest 62:244–278

Scheiber MD, Liu JH, Subbiah MT (2001) Dietary inclusion of whole soy foods results in significant reductions in clinical risk factors for osteoporosis and cardiovascular disease in normal postmenopausal women. Menopause 8:384–392

Taper HS (1978) The effect of estradiol-17-phenylpropionate and estradiol benzoate on N-nitrosomorpholine-induced liver carcinogenesis in ovariectomized female rats. Cancer 42: 462–467

Teller MN, Kaufman RJ, Bowie M (1969) Influence of estrogens and endocrine ablation on duration of remission produced by ovariectomy or androgen treatment of 7, 12-dimethylbenz(a)anthracene-induced rat mammary tumors. Cancer Res 29:349–352

Tham DM, Gardner CD, Haskell WL (1998) Clinical review 97: Potential health benefits of dietary phytoestrogens: a review of the clinical, epidemiological, and mechanistic evidence. J Clin Endocrinol Metab 83:2223–2235

Tokumo K, Umemura T, Sirma H (1993) Inhibition by gonadectomy of effects of 2-acetylaminofluorene in livers of male, but not female rats. Carcinogenesis 14:1747–1750

Wang L, Fan C, Topol SE (2003) Mutation of MEF2A in an inherited disorder with features of coronary artery disease. Science 302:1578–1581

Welsch CW (1985) Host factors affecting the growth of carcinogen-induced rat mammary carcinomas: a review and tribute to Charles Brenton Huggins. Cancer Res 45:3415–3443

Wu AH, Wan P, Hankin, J et al (2002) Adolescent and adult soy intake and risk of breast cancer in Asian-Americans. Carcinogenesis 23:1491–1496

Yager JD Jr, Yager R (1980) Oral contraceptive steroids as promoters of hepatocarcinogenesis in female Sprague-Dawley rats. Cancer Res 40:3680–3685

Yu L, Heere-Ress E, Boucher B (1999) Familial hypercholesterolemia. Acceptor splice site (G-->C) mutation in intron 7 of the LDL-R gene: alternate RNA editing causes exon 8 skipping or a premature stop codon in exon 8. LDL-R(Honduras-1) [LDL-R1061(-1) G-->C]. Atherosclerosis 146:125–131

Zhong S, Sharp DS, Grove JS (1996) Increased coronary heart disease in Japanese-American men with mutation in the cholesteryl ester transfer protein gene despite increased HDL levels. J Clin Invest 97:2917–2923

Chapter 8
The Potential Roles of Seeds and Seed Bioactives on the Prevention and Treatment of Breast and Prostate Cancer

Krista A. Power and Lilian U. Thompson

Abstract Several seeds have been suggested to play a role in the prevention and treatment of cancer. These include flaxseed, grape seed, sesame seed, pomegranate seed, caper seed, black cumin seed, and adlay seed. This chapter describes the research to date on the determination of their anticancer effects using different experimental models (in vitro, animal, clinical), the findings identifying the active seed components, and mechanisms of action which may mediate the anticancer effects. Of the above seeds, more extensive studies have been conducted on flaxseed and grape seed particularly in relation to breast and prostate cancer; therefore they are discussed in greater detail than the others.

Keywords Chemoprevention · Flaxseed · Grape seed · Breast cancer · Prostate cancer

Abbreviations

ALA	α-linolenic acid
AR	androgen receptor
BD	basal diet
BW	body weight
DMBA	9,10-dimethyl-1,2-benzanthracene
E2	estradiol
EDC	endocrine disrupting chemicals
EGF	epidermal growth factor
END	enterodiol
ENL	enterolactone
ER	estrogen receptor
FS	flaxseed
GSE	grape seed extract
HER2	human epidermal growth factor receptor 2

K.A. Power (✉)
Guelph Food Research Centre, Agriculture and Agri-food Canada, Guelph, ON, Canada
e-mail: krista.power@agr.gc.ca

M. Mutanen, A.-M. Pajari (eds.), *Vegetables, Whole Grains, and Their Derivatives in Cancer Prevention*, Diet and Cancer 2, DOI 10.1007/978-90-481-9800-9_8,
© Springer Science+Business Media B.V. 2011

HIF	hypoxia-inducible factor
IGF	insulin-like growth factor
IGFBP3	insulin-like growth factor binding protein 3
MAPK	mitogen activated protein kinases
MMP	matrix metalloproteinase
MNU	N-methyl-N-nitrosourea
OVX	ovariectomized
PARP	poly (ADP-ribose) polymerase
PIN	prostatic intraepithelial neoplasia
PND	postnatal day
PR	progesterone receptor
PSA	prostate specific antigen
PUFA	polyunsaturated fatty acid
SDG	secoisolariciresinol diglycoside
TAM	tamoxifen
TRAMP	transgenic adenocarcinoma of mouse prostate
VEGF	vascular endothelial growth factor

Contents

8.1 Introduction

Cancer incidence and mortality continues to increase and thus the prevention and reduction of the progression of cancers remain to be an important public health concern. In particular in Canada, breast cancer is the most prevalent malignancy and the second leading cause of cancer-related deaths among women. The incidence rates for breast cancer have increased steadily since 1981, and the majority of women with breast cancer are between the ages of 50 and 69. In men however, prostate cancer is the most commonly diagnosed cancer and the third leading cause of cancer-related deaths (Canadian Cancer Society 2009).

It is well known that the development and treatment of certain cancers can be influenced by life-style factors, such as diet (World Cancer Research Fund 2007); thus much research has been focused on determining the anti-cancer effects of various foods and food components. Many seeds including flaxseed, grape, pomegranate, sesame, adlay, black cumin, and caper have demonstrated some anti-cancer effects and therefore will be described in this chapter. However, two seeds that have received much attention, i.e. flaxseed (FS) and grape seed, particularly with regards to breast and prostate cancers, will be discussed in greater detail here. Since epidemiological studies have not been conducted to demonstrate a link between specific seed consumption and cancer risk, this chapter will discuss the evidence from experimental studies (in vitro, animal and human models) on the preventive and therapeutic effects of the seeds, as well as their components, on breast and prostate cancer, and the cellular and molecular mechanisms through which these seeds induce their effects.

8.2 Flaxseed

FS is an oilseed, which has recently gained a lot of attention as a component in foods with health promoting effects. FS is composed of approximately 30% fiber, 20% protein, and 40% oil, of which greater than 50% is the n-3 polyunsaturated fatty acid (PUFA) α-linolenic acid (ALA). FS is also the richest dietary source of the plant lignan, secoisolariciresinol diglycoside (SDG), and contains other lignans namely matairesinol, isolariciresinol, and pinoresinol (Thompson et al. 2006). Both the lignans and the ALA-rich components of FS are suggested to be major bioactives responsible for the health promoting effects of FS. Conversion of ALA to eicosapentaenoic acid (EPA), although limited, is thought to mediate anti-inflammatory responses thereby reducing the risk of various chronic diseases (Simopoulos 2002). Upon ingestion, the FS lignans are converted to mammalian lignans, enterolactone (ENL) and enterodiol (END), by the colonic microflora. Since they are the major lignan metabolites detected in serum after consumption of flaxseed (Nesbitt et al. 1999), they are thought to also play a major role in the health effects of FS. FS and mammalian lignans have demonstrated anti-oxidant activities (Hu et al. 2007; Prasad 1997, 2000). Furthermore, because of their structural similarity to estrogen, they may modulate estrogen signaling depending on the hormonal milieu of the experimental model used (i.e. induce estrogenic effects in the absence of estrogen or induce antiestrogenic effects in the presence of estrogen (Wang 2002). As will be described in this chapter, many experimental studies have shown that FS, and its oil and lignan components can modulate the prevention and treatment of breast and prostate cancers.

8.2.1 Flaxseed and Breast Cancer

8.2.1.1 Modulation of Mammary Gland Development

It is hypothesized that exposures to certain dietary factors early in life may result in epigenetic changes to the developing mammary gland, which then can alter breast cancer risk during adulthood (Hilakivi-Clarke 2007; Russo et al. 1983) The mammary gland undergoes extensive remodelling during embryonic and pubertal life stages, and these remodelling events are highly susceptible to hormonal stimuli. The rodent mammary gland has been used for decades as a model of human breast development and carcinogenesis. In the mouse, the mammary gland starts to develop around embryonic day (E) 11, as five lens-shaped ectodermal structures that appear along the mammary line. At E 16, mammary epithelial buds elongate and sprout into the primitive mammary fat pad and the mesenchyme. By E 18, branching has occurred and the ductal lumen starts to be formed. From birth to puberty, the rudimentary mammary gland undergoes little morphological changes as it grows isometrically with body growth. However, at puberty when ovarian hormones such as estrogen are secreted, allometric growth is triggered and the gland undergoes rapid primary duct elongation into the surrounding fat pad (Howlin et al. 2006). Elongation is driven by highly proliferative bulbous-shaped terminal end buds, which bifurcate and continue to elongate until the end of the fat pad is reached. After recurrent estrous cycles, lateral and then tertiary side branches sprout off the primary and secondary ducts until the mammary fat pad is occupied by an extensively branched and complex ductal tree (Sternlicht et al. 2006). Once the gland reaches the outer limits of the fat pad, terminal end buds regress and the differentiated alveolar buds develop at the ductal ends; these await hormonal signals associated with pregnancy and lactation to prepare for the secretory phase of mammary gland development (Brisken 2002). It has been demonstrated that terminal end buds are highly susceptible to carcinogen-induced malignant transformation, while the more differentiated alveolar buds are not (Russo et al. 1983). Thus, dietary components that can modify mammary gland morphogenesis early in life, such that in adulthood terminal end buds numbers are reduced and alveolar buds are enhanced, may result in a more mature mammary gland that is less susceptible to cancer development.

Although estrogen is required for normal mammary gland development, increased exposure to estrogens throughout life has been associated with increased breast cancer risk (Brekelmans 2003; Ruder et al. 2008; Russo and Russo 1998; Yager and Davidson 2006). The mechanisms by which enhanced estrogen exposure increases breast cancer risk are not fully understood, however it has been shown that depending on the developmental stage in which estrogen exposure occurs, different effects on breast cancer risk may result. For example, fetal estrogen exposure increases breast cancer risk later in life (Soto et al. 2008), while prepubertal exposure reduces risk (Murrill et al. 1996). In addition, the effects of estrogen on mammary gland development has been shown to be dose dependent, in a non-monotonic manner (i.e. stimulatory at low doses and inhibitory at high doses) (Vandenberg et al. 2006). Thus, both timing and level of exposure are important factors in how estrogens mediate the development of the mammary gland. FS contains high levels of lignan, SDG, and small amounts of matairesinol, isolariciresinol, and pinoresinol (Thompson et al. 2006). Upon consumption, the gut microflora converts flaxseed lignans to mammalian lignans, which can weakly bind and activate estrogen receptor (ER) signalling (Mueller et al. 2004; Penttinen et al. 2007). Therefore, like estrogen, depending on the level and timing of exposure, FS may also induce effects on mammary gland morphogenesis and breast cancer risk.

Several comprehensive studies have been conducted to determine if early life exposure to FS, or its lignan SDG, could mediate estrogen-like effects, modulate mammary gland development, and ultimately breast cancer risk, including exposures in utero only (Khan et al. 2007; Yu et al. 2006), in utero and lactation (Tou et al. 1998; Tou and Thompson 1999), during lactation only and lactation through to adulthood (Bryzgalova et al. 2008; Khan et al. 2007; Tan et al. 2004; Ward et al 2000), or throughout life (Tou and Thompson 1999). The resulting effects on mammary gland and breast cancer risk have been variable and potentially dependent on the FS variety, level of lignans, as well as other FS components consumed, and the timing of exposure. For example, consumption of a 10% FS diet during pregnancy and throughout lactation, resulted in an estrogenic effect in the dams, as indicated by an increased uterine and ovarian weight (Tou et al. 1998), and an estrogenic effect in adult female offspring, as indicated by increased serum estradiol levels, increased ovarian weight, accelerated pubertal onset, and enhanced maturation of the mammary gland (reduced terminal end buds and enhanced alveolar buds) (Tou and Thompson 1999). However, exposure to 5% flaxseed or the equivalent amount of SDG, during the same developmental period, resulted in an antiestrogenic effect, as indicated by a delay in pubertal onset, and a less well developed mammary gland (reduced terminal end buds and alveolar buds) (Tou and Thompson 1999). On the other hand, if exposure to a 10% FS diet is limited to lactation and onward, reproductive indices (reproductive organ weights and pubertal onset) were not affected in the adult female offspring (Ward et al. 2001). However, in a similar manner to that observed during pregnancy and lactational exposure, the effects on mammary gland morphogenesis remained (reduced terminal end buds and enhanced alveolar buds) (Tan et al. 2004; Ward et al. 2000).

From these studies, several important findings can be highlighted. Firstly, mammary gland maturation is enhanced in female offspring exposed to a 10% FS diet during early life, in a manner which may reduce the risk of breast cancer later in life. Secondly, in utero exposure to a 10% FS diet alters reproductive indices in the female offspring, which raises safety concerns, since these effects are also observed when the fetus is exposed to endocrine disrupting chemicals (EDC). The long-term effects of embryonic exposures to EDC can include infertility, reproductive tract abnormalities and cancers, as well as obesity, cardiovascular diseases, and effects on the immune system (Newbold et al. 2007a, b; Uzumcu and Zachow 2007). Thus, FS exposure during this critical developmental period may also induce deleterious long-term health effects, and thus should be avoided. Lastly, since exposure to FS after pregnancy was devoid of effects on reproductive indices, but still had potential beneficial effects on mammary gland development, this may be a safe exposure period that could influence breast cancer risk later in life.

8.2.1.2 Early Life Flaxseed Exposure and Later Breast Cancer Development

To determine whether prepubertal exposure to FS or SDG could modulate breast tumorigenesis, rat dams were fed a basal diet (BD) during pregnancy and then, following birth of the pups, fed diets containing either 10% FS, SDG (equivalent to the amount in 10% FS diet), or remained on the BD until postnatal day (PND) 21 (Chen et al. 2003). At PND 50, the female offspring were administered a breast carcinogen 9,10-dimethyl-1,2-benzanthracene (DMBA) and were sacrificed 21 weeks later. While there were no differences in tumor latency, the FS and SDG treatment groups had lower tumor incidence (proportion of animals with tumors) (31.3% and 42.0%, respectively) and multiplicity (46.9 and 44.8%, respectively) compared to the rats exposed to BD only during lactation. At PND 21, prior to DMBA administration, there was a significant increase in terminal end buds, demonstrating that FS intake during lactation stimulated mammary gland development (Tan et al. 2004). At the time of DMBA administration (PND 50), the number of terminal end buds in the FS- and SDG-treated animals was significantly reduced (Tan et al. 2004). In another study, when 5% FS diet was fed to adolescent mice (PND 21) until the administration of DMBA (PND 50), later tumor incidence and multiplicity were also reduced (Serraino and Thompson 1992). These studies indicate that lactational and pubertal exposures to FS and its lignan can reduce breast carcinogenesis later in life potentially by stimulating mammary gland morphogenesis in the young adult animal.

To add to the complexity of the effects of early FS exposure on carcinogenesis, a more recent study investigated the effects of a 5 and 10% FS diet, fed to either pregnant or lactating dams, on the development of offspring mammary carcinogenesis (Khan et al. 2007). At 8 weeks of age, female offspring were then administered DMBA and the effects of early exposure to the FS diets were assessed 18 weeks later. Although the 5% FS diet did not affect carcinogenesis, exposure to the 10% FS diet in utero or during lactation, significantly reduced mammary tumor latency (week at which the first tumor was recorded) and increased tumor multiplicity (number of tumors per animal). This suggests that early exposure to a 10% FS diet, either during pregnancy or lactation, increases breast cancer development later in life (Khan et al. 2007). These results are in contrast to those described above, at least for the protective effect of 10% FS diet fed during lactation on breast carcinogenesis. However, one important difference in the observed effects should be noted; in this recent study, no effects on mammary gland morphogenesis were observed in the female offspring. The reasons for the lack of effect on mammary gland morphogenesis is yet unknown, but it is possible that different varieties of FS used in the different studies, may account for some of the differences. It is known that depending on the cultivar (Eliasson et al. 2003), soil conditions, and year of harvest, that variations in lignan levels and accumulation of other components (e.g. cadmium, which are known to have estrogenic effect), can occur (Thompson et al. 1997). Thus, before a consensus concerning the effects of early exposure to FS on breast cancer prevention can be made, more studies are required to thoroughly assess the effects of various doses and varieties of FS and other FS components.

8.2.1.3 Adult Flaxseed Exposure and Breast Cancer Growth and Development

Besides modulation of breast cancer risk through early life FS exposure, there is also evidence that FS consumption in adulthood can affect breast cancer development and growth. Since breast carcinogenesis involves multiple steps including initiation, promotion, progression and metastasis, several study designs and experimental models have been implemented in order to identify which steps are affected by FS and its components.

Initiation, Promotion, and Progression of Carcinogen-Induced Breast Cancer

In assessing initiation and early promotional stages of carcinogenesis, a 5% FS diet was fed to rats immediately after DMBA administration and a significant reduction in tumor size was observed (Serraino and Thompson 1992). To determine if the effects on the promotion stage of carcinogenesis was due to the lignan component of FS, 1.5 mg/d SDG (equivalent to the amount of SDG found in 5% FS diet) was given to rats starting 1 week after DMBA administration (Thompson et al. 1996b). After 20 weeks, the SDG group had significantly lower tumor multiplicity and number of tumors per group, demonstrating that the effect of the FS diet may be due to its lignan, SDG. These studies demonstrate that FS can modulate breast carcinogenesis when consumed in adulthood, affecting both the initiation and promotional stages of carcinogenesis.

To determine the effects of FS, and its components, on tumor progression and new tumor formation, 13 weeks after DMBA-administration, rats were fed either control diet, 5% FS diet, or control diet containing FS oil or SDG (levels equivalent to that found in 5% FS diet) (Thompson et al. 1996a). After 7 weeks of treatment, FS and FS oil diets were able to reduce the growth of previously established mammary tumors, while the SDG group had the lowest incidence of new tumor formation. This study suggests that the different bioactives in FS (i.e. ALA and SDG), may have different anti-cancer targets and thus play different roles on breast cancer progression. Since SDG is converted to the mammalian lignan, ENL, it is thought to be one active component responsible for the anti-tumorigenic effects of FS. Thus, ENL was also assessed for its potential to reduce tumor growth (Saarinen et al. 2002). Nine weeks after DMBA administration, tumor bearing rats were given 1 or 10 mg/Kg BW ENL daily for 7 weeks. ENL, 10 mg/Kg BW, significantly reduced total tumor volume, while the lower ENL dose had minimal effects. Although the mechanism for the effect of ENL on tumor progression is unknown, the 10 mg/Kg dose also reduced uterine weight, suggesting a potential anti-estrogenic effect of ENL. However, whether this effect was due to a direct inhibition of ER signaling or an inhibition of estrogen synthesis (i.e. by inhibiting aromatase) is yet to be determined (Saarinen et al. 2002).

Utilizing the N-methyl-N-nitrosourea (MNU)-induced breast cancer rat model, 50 day old rats were given MNU carcinogen and 2 days later (representing early promotion period of carcinogenesis), rats were fed either a BD, 2.5 or 5% FS diet, or given a daily gavage of SDG equivalent to the amount in the 2.5 or 5% FS diet for 22 weeks (Rickard et al. 1999). The results showed that all treatment groups had less invasive tumors, but only the high SDG group had lower tumor multiplicity compared to the BD group. Although the 5% FS-fed rats had tumors that were smaller than the BD group throughout the study, final tumor volume, weight, and incidence were not significantly affected by the FS or lignan treatment. However, all treatments reduced the invasiveness and grade of the MNU tumors, suggesting that tumor progression was reduced by FS and its lignan.

Effects on ER+ Human Breast Cancer

FS and its components have also been investigated for their ability to modulate human breast cancer progression. To determine the effects on ER+ breast cancers, the nude mouse model bearing MCF-7 human tumors has been utilized. As described in Section 8.2.1.1, depending on the dose or timing of exposure, FS can induce either estrogenic or antiestrogenic effects. Since ER+ breast cancers are dependent on estrogen to stimulate growth, it is of interest to determine if the estrogenic or antiestrogenic potential of FS can also modulate the growth of these tumors.

Two experimental designs have been used to determine if the effects of FS are dependent on the animal's circulating estrogen levels. In both cases the mice are ovariectomized (OVX) and implanted with an estradiol (E2) pellet, which stimulates growth of MCF-7 tumors. Once the tumors are established, the E2 pellet is removed, to establish a low circulating estrogen level (mimicking postmenopausal breast patients), or replenished to maintain elevated E2 levels (mimicking premenopausal breast cancer patients). In the postmenopausal model, the ability of FS and its components to modulate tumor regression or to stimulate tumor re-growth thereby inducing estrogenic effects is assessed. In the premenopausal model, FS and its components have been assessed for their ability to modulate the tumor-stimulatory effect of E2, thereby inducing estrogenic or antiestrogenic effects.

Studies using the above mentioned in vivo pre- and postmenopausal models showed that FS has some tumor growth inhibitory effects, suggesting that its consumption by breast cancer patients may yield beneficial effects. For example, in the premenopausal ER+ breast cancer model, feeding a 10% FS diet for 6 weeks resulted in a reduction in E2-stimulated tumor growth, proliferation index, and an increase in tumor cell apoptosis (Chen et al. 2004). When different doses of FS were assessed after 8 weeks of treatment, both a 5 and 10% FS diet reduced E2-stimulated tumor growth to a similar extent, which was accompanied by reductions in tumor cell proliferation and progesterone receptor (PR) expression (Chen et al. 2007c). Since PR is an ER regulated gene product, this result suggests that FS, or some component of FS, may interfere with E2 action through the ER, thereby modulating estrogen signaling; however this mechanism has not yet been fully explored.

Using a similar study design, MCF-7 tumor bearing mice treated with a 10%FS diet, or 15 mg/Kg BW ENL or END, demonstrated that FS or the mammalian lignans induced a decrease in markers of angiogenesis to a similar extent, as indicated by a reduction in vascular endothelial growth factor (VEGF) and tumor blood vessels (Bergman-Jungestrom et al. 2007). This study suggests that the effects of FS on E2-stimulated tumor growth may be due to the conversion of the FS lignans to the mammalian lignans, which can inhibit angiogenesis development.

Using the postmenopausal model, establishing the tumor inhibitory effects of FS has been more difficult, since at the end of the treatment periods, which have ranged from 7 to 25 weeks, tumors in the control and FS groups have regressed to a nearly immeasurable size, have similar cell proliferation levels, and similar numbers of apoptotic cells (Chen et al. 2004, 2007b; Saarinen et al. 2006). However, in one study, treatment with a 10% FS diet resulted in a greater tumor regression rate than in the control group during the first 7 weeks of treatment (Saarinen et al. 2006). Further analysis of tumor growth factor signaling biomarkers after 2 weeks of FS treatment, showed a significant reduction in level of phosphorylated mitogen-activated protein kinase (MAPK), suggesting that FS may reduce the activation of growth factor signaling pathways, and thus may be a mechanism by which it enhances early tumor regression in the postmenopausal model (Power et al. 2008). On the other hand, treatment of tumor bearing mice with ENL or END (10 mg/Kg BW) for 22 weeks resulted in an increase in final tumor cell apoptosis (Power et al. 2006). This may indicate that while the lignans as such can induce apoptosis, when consumed as part of a whole food, other components of FS may interfere with lignan effects. Further studies are currently ongoing to determine the effects of the various FS components on breast cancer growth, the results of which will help establish the modes of action of FS and its components.

The pre- and post-menopausal breast cancer models have also been used to determine if FS and its components can modulate the effects of the breast cancer drug tamoxifen (TAM). TAM has been used for decades as an adjuvant therapy for ER+ breast cancers. However, after prolonged use, some patients experience TAM resistance resulting in tumor growth stimulation, as well as the development of various side effects such as increased menopausal-like symptoms and risk of uterine cancers (Jordan 2004). Therefore, some patients use complimentary treatments to help reduce these problems. In Canada, about 12% of breast cancer patients appear to take FS as complementary therapy (Boon et al. 2007).

Using the premenopausal nude mouse model, MCF-7 tumor bearing mice treated with TAM, alone or in combination with a high fat diet supplemented with 10% FS (TAM+FS) for 6 weeks (Chen et al. 2004), showed a significantly greater reduction in tumor cell proliferation in the TAM+FS group, compared to TAM alone group. In a later study, tumor bearing mice treated with TAM, alone or in combination with a low fat diet supplemented with 5 or 10% FS diet for 8 weeks again showed that FS can enhance the tumor inhibitory effects of TAM, with the 5% FS diet inducing a greater inhibitory effect (Chen et al. 2007c). FS significantly reduced insulin-like growth factor 1 (IGF-1) levels, indicating that the added beneficial effect of FS on the anti-tumor effects of TAM may be through modulation of tumor growth factor signaling.

In the postmenopausal nude mouse model, combining FS and TAM also enhanced the anti-tumor effects of TAM. In one study, tumor bearing mice were treated with TAM, alone or in combination with a high fat diet supplemented with 10% FS diet for 7 weeks (Chen et al. 2004). Although tumors initially regressed, those in the TAM alone group eventually started to re-grow, demonstrating TAM resistance. However, in combination with FS, the tumor stimulatory effect of TAM was negated, resulting in smaller tumors containing less proliferating and more apoptotic cells than those in the TAM alone group. In a further study, the anti-tumor effects of a low fat diet supplemented with 5 or 10% FS diet, alone or in combination with TAM were assessed after 15 weeks (Chen et al. 2007b). Similar to the effects in the previous study, the 10% FS diet combined with TAM enhanced the tumor inhibitory effects of TAM, but the 5% FS diet did not. However, the 5% FS diet with TAM reduced various tumor growth biomarkers (i.e. cyclin D1, ERα, human epidermal growth factor receptor 2 (HER2), and IGF-1R) to a similar extent as the 10% FS diet. This finding may indicate that the effects of FS on the anti-tumorigenic effects of TAM may be dependent on the FS dose, with the higher dose inducing the greater effects. These results are in contrast to those in the previously described premenopausal breast cancer model in which the 5% FS diet was more effective than the 10% FS diet in enhancing the anti-tumor effects of TAM (Chen et al. 2007c). This suggests that the effectiveness of different FS doses may also be dependent on the tumor hormonal milieu.

In the several studies described above, using either the pre- or post-menopausal experimental designs, the results have consistently demonstrated that a 5 or 10% FS diet, or the mammalian lignans (ENL and END), do not stimulate the growth of MCF-7 human breast tumors (Bergman-Jungstrom et al. 2007; Chen et al. 2004, 2007b, c; Power et al. 2006; Saarinen et al. 2006). This finding indicates that in this breast cancer model, FS or the lignans do not induce estrogenic effects. This is also supported by the lack of uterotrophic effects induced by FS or its lignans when consumed by these tumor bearing mice (Chen et al. 2004, 2007c). These findings are in contrast with the estrogenic effects induced by the mammalian lignans in vitro. Several studies have shown that ENL can stimulate MCF-7 cell growth (Cosentino et al. 2007; Mousavi and Adlercreutz 1992; Welshons et al. 1987), bind and activate ERα (Mueller et al. 2004; Penttinen et al. 2007), and modulate the expression of certain genes in a manner similar to that of E2 (Dip et al. 2008). The reasons why lignan-rich FS and the mammalian lignans do not induce estrogen-like effects on MCF-7 tumors in vivo are unknown. One obvious possibility is that in vivo, the lignans may be metabolized in such a way as to render them unable to bind and activate the ER. On the other hand, it has been shown that the flaxseed lignan can reach and accumulate within MCF-7 tumors in these mice, suggesting that they are available to induce direct effects on tumor cells (Saarinen et al. 2008). Despite the contradictory findings when comparing the effects of lignans in vitro and in vivo, the lack of estrogenic effects in vivo highlights the potential safety of consumption of FS by patients with ER+ breast cancer. This is significant because of rising concerns over the safety of consuming phytoestrogens and phytoestrogen-rich foods, due to their potential estrogenic and tumor stimulatory potential.

Effects on ER– Human Breast Cancer

In addition to the effects of FS on estrogen responsive human breast cancer, the effects of FS and its components have been determined using the MDA-MB-435 human breast cancer cell line. This cell line is not responsive to estrogen, does not contain ER, and is highly metastatic, thus it can be used to determine the effect of FS and its components on metastasis and other non-ER mediated mechanisms. Athymic nude mice with established MDA-MB-435 tumors fed a 10% FS diet for 7 weeks had smaller tumors and less incidence of total metastasis (including lung and lymph node) compared to untreated control mice (Chen et al. 2002; Dabrosin et al.

2002). To determine the active components in FS responsible for the induced effects, mice with established MDA-MB-435 tumors were fed diets containing either 10% FS, SDG, FS oil (FO), or SDG+FO (Wang et al. 2005). The levels of SDG and FO were equivalent to that found in the 10% FS diet. After 6 weeks, the 10% FS and SDG+FO groups had significant reductions in metastasis incidence, suggesting that both the lignan and the ALA-rich oil components contribute to the anti-metastatic effect of FS.

In a later study, tumors were excised prior to randomization into the same five treatment groups as above to determine if FS and its components could reduce the tumor recurrence and metastasis (Chen et al. 2006). After 6 weeks treatment, no significant effect of FS or its components on recurrent tumor incidence was observed compared to the BD control. However, when the treatment groups were subdivided according to the size of the primary tumors that were excised i.e. ≤ 9 g or >9 g, FS and SDG diets significantly lowered the recurrent tumor incidence in mice with tumors ≤ 9 g compared to those with tumors >9 g. No such difference was observed in the BD control, FO, and SDG+FO groups. In addition, all treatment groups reduced the incidence of total metastasis (lymph node, lung, and other organs). This study suggests that FS and its components may affect tumor metastasis to a greater extent than tumor recurrence. However, the results on tumor recurrence incidence indicate that smaller tumors may be more susceptible to the effects of FS and its lignan.

Mechanistically, how FS and its components reduce tumor metastasis is still unclear. It has been shown in mice treated with FS, that tumor growth factors and growth factor receptors such as IGF-1, and epidermal growth factor receptor (EGFR) (Chen et al. 2002), as well as VEGF (Dabrosin et al. 2002) are significantly reduced. Since these growth factors are involved in tumor metastasis, in particular with angiogenesis, reduction of cell signalling cascades to reduce angiogenesis may be a mechanism by which FS and its components reduce ER– tumor growth and metastasis. Furthermore, in vitro analyses of the effects of ENL and END on metastasis processes (cell adhesion, invasion, and migration) were assessed using MDA-MB-435 and MDA-MB-231 cell lines (Chen and Thompson 2003). ENL and END significantly reduced cell adhesion at concentrations of 1 or 5 μM, however, this effect differed between the two cell lines, with END being more effective in the MDA-MB-435 cells. Cell invasion was also reduced by the compounds, with the greatest effect seen at 5 μM, while cell migration was decreased by both lignans (0.1–10 μM). These results suggest that both mammalian lignan metabolites possess the ability to reduce tumor cell metastasis at various stages of the metastatic process. However, mammalian lignans may only be one of the active components responsible for the effects of FS in reducing ER– breast tumor metastasis in vivo.

Effects of Flaxseed on Cancer Biomarkers in Breast Cancer Patients

In a randomized double-blind placebo-controlled clinical trial, postmenopausal women with newly diagnosed breast cancer (mostly ER+PR+) were assigned to eat either a muffin containing 25 g flaxseed or placebo for a mean duration of 32 and 39 days, respectively, to determine if FS could alter tumor growth biomarkers on tumor biopsies taken at diagnosis and at time of surgery (end of treatment period) (Thompson et al. 2005). While the placebo did not cause significant changes in the tumors, FS treatment significantly reduced tumor cell proliferation (34%) (Ki67 labelling index), increased apoptosis (31%), and decreased the expression of c-erbB2 (71%). In addition, urinary lignans increased by 1,300% in the FS treated patients and the intake of FS was significantly correlated with changes in c-erbB2 score and apoptotic index. These results suggest that the lignans, perhaps in combination with other components such as the oil in FS, may in part be responsible for the changes in tumor biomarkers. This study showing the ability of FS to reduce biomarkers of tumor growth in breast cancer patients validates the results obtained in the above described animal models indicating that FS and its components do not have an estrogenic, growth promoting effect on breast cancer.

8.2.2 Flaxseed and Prostate Cancer

As with many cancers, prostate cancer growth arises from uncontrolled proliferative and/or apoptotic cellular events. Prostate cancer initially is androgen sensitive and thus growth is triggered upon androgen binding to the androgen receptor (AR) resulting in the activation of androgen sensitive genes and induction of proliferation. Thus, the first stage of prostate cancer treatment is androgen ablation (Debes and Tindall 2002). As prostate cancer progresses however, the cells become insensitive to androgens, thereby making the ablation therapy ineffective and subsequently a more aggressive prostate cancer results. At this stage, the prostate cancer metastasizes and is ultimately untreatable. This androgen-refractory period is thought to be due to an overproduction of growth factors, such as EGF and IGF-1, an increased activity of growth factor receptors, and/or a mutated AR (Grossmann et al. 2001). Therefore, introducing alternative therapies with various cellular targets (hormone sensitive and hormone resistant) may prove to be beneficial in reducing development or growth of prostate cancer cells.

8.2.2.1 Effects on Prostate Cancer Growth and Development in Experimental Models

Compared to the extensive research conducted on breast cancer, the role of FS on prostate cancer prevention and treatment has been far less studied. Two studies have been conducted to determine the effects of FS exposure during different life stages on prostate development in rodents (Tou et al. 1998, 1999). Exposure to FS during early life (in utero and lactation) resulted in a dose-dependent effect on adult prostate morphology and serum hormone levels. For example, in rats, in utero and lactational exposure to 10% FS resulted in a larger prostate, increased prostate cell proliferation, and higher testosterone and E2 in the adult animal (PND 132), while early life exposure to 5% FS led to reduced prostate growth and serum hormone levels (Tou et al. 1998). Since early exposure to the 10% FS diet enhanced prostate cell proliferation, a potential safety concern of increased FS exposure during early life and prostate cancer risk later in life may exist. However, no further studies have been conducted to examine this risk, and thus it is a research area requiring further attention. On the other hand, exposure to FS after weaning (PND 21) does not result in developmental changes to the rodent adult prostate (Tou et al. 1999). This indicates that the effects of FS on prostate development are dose and time dependent and that post-lactational/pubertal exposure to FS may be safe with regards to prostate cancer risk.

Exposure to FS starting at puberty has demonstrated some beneficial effects on the progression of prostate cancer in the TRAMP (transgenic adenocarcinoma of mouse prostate) model. The TRAMP model bears a minimal rat probasin regulatory element which drives the expression of simian virus 40 early genes in the prostate epithelium (Greenberg et al. 1995). These genes mediate the expression of oncoproteins which abrogates the function of tumor suppressor protein p53 and retinoblastoma (Rb), thereby enhancing cell proliferation. The expression of these genes is evident as early as 4 weeks in the TRAMP mouse and initially androgen dependent. The earliest pathology in these mice is prostatic intraepithelial neoplasia (PIN) lesions which are also early prostate cancer markers in humans. When the animals are castrated, the PIN lesions develop into well differentiated adenocarcinomas followed by the development of more aggressive poorly differentiated tumors, similar to the progression of prostate cancer in men (Gingrich et al. 1999). Therefore, using the TRAMP model, the chemopreventative properties of FS can be tested at various stages of cancer progression, in a model which mimics prostate cancer progression in humans.

TRAMP mice were supplemented with a 5% FS diet, starting at puberty (5–6 weeks of age), for 20 or 30 weeks (Lin et al. 2002). After 30 weeks, FS-treated mice had reduced relative urogenital/tumor weight and significantly fewer poorly differentiated tumors, compared to control mice. Furthermore, FS reduced prostate cell proliferation and enhanced apoptosis. Since there were no differences in the number of well or moderately differentiated tumors, this indicates that 5% FS was unable to prevent early prostate tumor development, however, progression was reduced as indicated by the reduction of poorly differentiated tumors (Lin et al. 2002). In this study, there were no additional measurements conducted (i.e. serum hormones, growth factors, cell signalling biomarkers) to determine the mechanisms as to how FS diet could modulate prostate tumor differentiation; however, several in vitro studies in various prostate cancer cell lines have been conducted and provided some evidence of the anti-cancer effects of FS components.

As discussed previously, it is hypothesized that the mammalian lignans are major bioactives associated with the beneficial effects of FS consumption. Treatment of various prostate cancer cell lines (androgen sensitive (LNCaP) and insensitive (DU145 and PC-3)) with mammalian lignans have demonstrated an antiproliferative effect (Chen et al. 2007a; Lin et al., 2001; McCann et al. 2008) while non-transformed prostate epithelial cells are not affected (Chen et al. 2007a). This suggests that the effects of the mammalian lignans are specific to cancer cells, and may be mediated through both hormonal and non-hormonal mechanisms. ENL has been shown to induce apoptosis, potentially by activating the caspase signalling pathway. Caspases are a family of proteases which exist in an inactive proform or zymogen within the cell. The caspase cascade is initiated by the release of cytochrome c from the mitochondria (D'Amelio et al. 2008). Cytochrome c plays a key role in inducing the activation of the apoptosome, a macromolecular complex comprised of Apaf1 and dATP. Once cytochrome c is released, it induces a conformational change in Apaf1, resulting in the binding and activation of procaspase 9. The active apoptosome then triggers the activation of downstream executioner caspases, such as caspase 3. Once caspase 3 is activated it initiates the cleavage and inactivation of proteins responsible for cell survival including the enzymes involved in DNA repair, poly (ADP-ribose) polymerase (PARP). Caspase-3 also activates the enzymes responsible for degrading DNA such as caspase activated DNase (CAD). ENL significantly enhanced the release of mitochondrial cytochrome c, increased activated caspase 3, as well as PARP in LNCaP cells, and thus activation of the mitochondrial caspase cascade may be one of the molecular mechanisms of the anti-cancer effects of ENL.

ENL has also been shown to be one of the few phytoestrogens with anti-androgenic properties, as indicated by its ability to inhibit androgen stimulated activation of AR signalling (Takeuchi et al. 2009). Therefore, in androgen-sensitive cell lines, ENL may inhibit AR signalling and reduce growth. Furthermore, ENL-treated LNCaP cells induce a down-regulation in genes involved in cell cycle regulation and cell proliferation (i.e. CDK2, CDKN3, BRCA1, and PCNA) (McCann et al. 2008). In androgen-insensitive cells (PC-3), ENL also enhances the expression of insulin-like growth factor binding protein 3 (IGFBP3) (Chen et al. 2009). The role of IGFBP3 is to bind and thus reduce free IGF, which are potent stimulators of proliferation and growth. Thus, ENL may reduce the growth of prostate cancer cells by interfering with IGF signaling. Collectively, these studies indicate that ENL may reduce prostate cancer growth through many mechanisms, however, how these relate to the anti-cancer effects of FS in vivo, remains to be determined.

8.2.2.2 Effects on Prostate Cancer Biomarkers in Humans

To determine the potential role of FS in reducing prostate cancer development and growth in humans, a small pilot study was conducted in 15 men at increased risk of developing prostate cancer (high grade dysplasia or atypical small glands demonstrated from initial biopsy) (Demark-Wahnefried et al. 2004). The men were instructed to consume 30 g ground FS, in addition to restricting their fat intake to 20% of calories for 6 months, at which time a second prostate biopsy was taken as well as serum samples for measurement of prostate specific antigen (PSA), testosterone, and cholesterol. The results showed that prostate cell proliferation and serum PSA (an early biomarker of prostate cancer risk) and cholesterol were significantly reduced, while serum testosterone was unaffected by the FS-supplemented fat restricted diet, compared to the baseline values. This indicates a potential anti-cancer effect of the dietary intervention. However, since there was no control group (low fat diet group) in the study, it is unclear if the effects were due to the FS or low fat diet. On the other hand, this study did provide promising results that led to a larger study in prostate cancer patients who were awaiting prostatectomy (Demark-Wahnefried et al. 2008). The patients were randomly assigned to consume either their usual diets supplemented with 30 g ground FS, a FS-supplemented low fat diet (subjects instructed to consume $\leq$20% energy from fat), or the respective control diets (usual and low-fat diet, respectively), for 1 month. FS consumption increased lignan levels in the seminal fluid, as well as prostatic EPA levels, indicating that the prostate was exposed to the potential bioactive components of the FS diet. Furthermore, tumor cell proliferation was reduced in the FS supplemented cancer patients, compared to the control and low fat groups, suggesting a role of FS in the prevention of prostate cancer progression. On the other hand, there were no effects of FS supplementation on serum PSA, testosterone, steroid hormone binding globulin, total and LDL-cholesterol, C-reactive protein, IGF-1, and IGFBP-3. These results differ from the previously described pilot study in which PSA and cholesterol were reduced, which may simply be due to the shorter intervention time or possibly due to the differences in the stage of prostate cancer development between the two studies (i.e. high risk non-cancerous subjects vs. prostate cancer patients). These clinical studies are in line with the effects of FS on prostate cancer growth observed in vitro and in vivo, and support an anti-cancer effect of FS, and potentially its lignan component, in the prostate.

8.3 Grape Seed

Grape seed is another seed that has received a lot of attention for its potential to enhance health. Unlike FS, it is not common for grape seeds to be consumed as such in our diets, however grape seed extract (GSE) is now commercially available and is promoted as natural health product. Grape seeds contain 7–16% protein; 10–18% oil found mainly in the endosperm and consisting of approximately 70% linoleic acid and 20% oleic acid; 39–44% fiber; and 5–10% polyphenols which are primarily found in the seed epiderm (Fantozzi and Betschart 1979; Tangolar et al. 2007). GSE contains gallic acid, catechin, epicatechin, and procyanidin dimers (i.e B1: Epicatechin-(4$\beta\rightarrow$8)-catechin; B2: Epicatechin-(4$\beta\rightarrow$8)-epicatechin), trimers, and polymerized oligomers, composed of flavan-3-ol units with C4–C8 or C4–C6 interflavan linkages or otherwise called B-type linkages. These compounds can also be present as gallate esters. Procyanadins (polymers of epicatechin and/or catechin) are the most common class of proanthocyanadins (also called condensed tannins) which are second only to lignin as being the most abundant naturally found phenolic in nature. Proanthocyanidins possess antioxidant activities which are thought to be a mechanism for their anticancer effects (Faria et al. 2006); however, as will be described in the following sections, other cellular and molecular mechanisms may also be involved.

8.3.1 Grape Seed and Breast Cancer

8.3.1.1 Effects on Breast Cancer Growth and Development in Experimental Models

Thus far, no studies have been conducted to assess the effects of early life exposure to grape seed and breast cancer risk at adulthood. However, studies have investigated the role of grape seed on the initiation, promotion, and progression of breast cancer in in vivo and in vitro models. Using the carcinogen-induced rodent breast cancer model, starting at 35 days old, female rats were fed diets AIN-76A (purified casein based) or rodent chow (soy protein based), with or without 1.25 or 5% GSE (95% flavanols composed of 86% proanthocyanidins) (Kim et al. 2004). At age 50 days the rodents were administered the DMBA carcinogen and then continued on their respective treatment diets for another 120 days. Although the 5% GSE-supplemented rodent chow diet reduced the number of tumors that developed in each rat (multiplicity) by 45%, the same GSE dose had no effect on tumor multiplicity when supplemented in the AIN-76A diet, compared to their respective control diets. This lack of effect on DMBA tumor growth was also observed in another study in which 0–1% GSE was incorporated into a soy-free basal diet (AIN-93G) (Singletary and Meline 2001). This suggests that the chemopreventative effect of GSE is dependent on the composition of the background diet. Interestingly, the rodent chow diet resulted in elevated levels of serum equol and other daidzein metabolites (>2 μM), as well as genistein ($\sim$400 nM), which are isoflavones with potential chemopreventative properties. Thus, an interactive effect may have occurred between these isoflavones and compounds in the GSE when GSE was supplemented in the rodent chow as opposed to the isoflavone-free AIN-76A diet.

To determine the effects of GSE on breast cancer progression, mice were fed diets containing 0.2 and 0.5% GSE for 2 weeks prior to being inoculated with mouse mammary carcinoma 4T1 cells (highly invasive and metastatic cell line) (Mantena et al. 2006). Both the 0.2 and 0.5% GSE diets delayed primary tumor development and reduced tumor growth by 21 and 49%, respectively. This effect was shown to be due to an increase in apoptosis, triggered by the mitochondrial caspase cascade, as indicated by GSE-induced increase in tumor mitochondrial release of cytochrome c, Apaf-1, and activated caspase 3, as well as a reduction in anti-apoptotic protein Bcl-2 and increase in pro-apoptotic protein Bax. Furthermore, GSE dose dependently reduced cancer cell metastasis, as indicated by a reduction in the number and size of tumors in the lungs.

The effects of GSE on human breast tumor growth have also been studied in mice. In one study, nude mice were treated with 50 mg/Kg BW GSE by gavage for 2 weeks prior to the inoculation of the mice with ER– human breast cancer cell line, MD-MBA-231, and continued for 80 days (Wen et al. 2008). Mice administered GSE had reduced tumor development, MAPK signalling, as well as tumor blood vessel density, suggesting its ability to reduce angiogenesis. GSE also reduced VEGF gene and protein expression in these tumors, potentially by inhibiting hypoxia-inducible factor (HIF)-1α expression (a transcription factor which regulates VEGF expression) (Lu et al. 2009).

The role of GSE on inhibition of aromatase activity was investigated in mice with established MCF-7 aromatase overexpressing (MCF-7aro) tumors. Aromatase is a cytochrome P450 enzyme responsible for converting C19 androgens to aromatic estrogens. In situ over expression of aromatase can lead to excess estrogen production which can induce growth of breast tumors by way of the ER signaling pathway. Thus, one therapeutic approach to reducing breast cancer development is to inhibit the activity and/or expression of aromatase. Androgen-supplemented nude mice were given GSE (500 or 750 μg) orally for 1 week prior to inoculation with MCF-7aro cells, and continued for 30 days. GSE reduced the formation of MCF-7aro tumors which was shown to be due to its ability to inhibit aromatase activity (Kijima et al. 2006). These findings suggest a potential use of GSE as a botanical aromatase inhibitor for breast cancer risk reduction.

GSE dose-dependently also inhibits MCF-7 and MDA-MB-468 cell proliferation in vitro supporting a non-ER dependent mechanism of action (Mantena et al. 2006). To determine the active components of GSE (i.e. catechin or procyanidins) responsible for its anti-cancer effects, various GSE fractions were tested for their ability to modulate the growth of MCF-7 cells (Faria et al. 2006). It was found that the catechin- and procyanidin dimer- containing fractions reduced MCF-7 proliferation, while the more complex procyanidin oligomers had little effect. Although, this suggests that the lower molecular weight compounds can reduce breast cancer cell proliferation, it is unknown if the larger molecules can cross cell membranes to induce cellular effects. Thus, further studies should be conducted to determine the bioavailability of the complex procyanidin oligomers, in order to determine the mechanisms of action of GSE.

8.3.1.2 Effects on Grape Seed on Breast Cancer Biomarkers in Humans

Although the in vitro and in vivo animal studies have indicated that GSE can reduce the growth and progression of breast cancer, thus far, there have been no studies conducted in breast cancer patients to confirm this effect. However, currently a clinical trial is underway at the City of Hope Comprehensive Cancer Center, Duarte, California entitled, "A Phase I Prevention Trial of ACTIVIN Grape Seed Extract as an Aromatase Inhibitor in Healthy High-Risk Post-Menopausal Women" (http://www.clinicaltrials.gov/ct2/show/NCT00100893). This clinical trial's primary objective is to investigate the effectiveness of a GSE in reducing estrogen biosynthesis in women at risk of developing breast cancer.

8.3.2 Grape Seed and Prostate Cancer

Throughout the past decade, much work has been done to determine the preventive and therapeutic properties of grape seed on prostate cancer. The majority of studies conducted to date have investigated the role of GSE on prostate cancer growth and progression in vitro, while few studies have been conducted in vivo. Thus far, there have been no clinical studies conducted in humans. Much effort has been done to determine the specific cellular and molecular mechanisms of effect of GSE and its components. Singh and Agarwal (2006), nicely highlighted the cellular and molecular targets to which dietary components could act on prostate cancer cells to reduce growth (Singh and Agarwal 2006). These targets include those involved in cell signalling (i.e. AR signalling, EGFR signalling, IGF-1R signalling, signal transducer and activator of transcription (STAT) signalling, β-catenin signalling, and toll-like receptor signalling); cell cycle regulation (i.e. cyclins and cyclin dependent kinases and telomerases); cell survival and apoptosis (i.e. nuclear factor κB (NF-κB) pathway and Bcl-2 family proteins), and angiogenesis and metastasis (i.e.VEGF signaling, matrix metalloproteinase (MMP), and HIF-1α) (Singh and Agarwal 2006). The following sections will describe the experimental studies assessing the role of GSE in prostate cancer and highlight the most significant molecular targets involved in the induced effects.

8.3.2.1 Effects on Prostate Cancer Cell Growth and Modulation of Cell Signaling

The DU145 human prostate carcinoma cell line is androgen insensitive and therefore has been used to examine the chemopreventive properties of treatments on the growth of more aggressive and advanced prostate cancers (Alimirah et al. 2006; Singh and Agarwal 2006). Treatment of DU145 cells with GSE (10–100 μg/ml) resulted in a time- and dose-dependent reduction in cell growth and increase in cell death (Agarwal et al. 2000; Vayalil et al. 2004). This effect was accompanied by reductions in MAPK signaling (i.e. decreased phosphorylated ERK1 and ERK2), increases in proteins associated with cell cycle arrest (i.e. p21), and reductions in proteins responsible for cell cycle progression (i.e. cyclin E, and cyclin-dependent kinase 4). A more in-depth mechanistic study of the effects of GSE on prostate cancer cell signaling identified a dose-dependent inhibition of EGF-induced activation of EGFR and activation of its downstream adaptor protein, Shc. GSE also inhibits the activation of nuclear transcription factors, Elk1 and AP1, which are downstream targets of the MAPK signalling pathway (Tyagi et al. 2003).

The cellular and molecular mechanisms involved in the pro-apoptotic effects of GSE, has also been investigated (Agarwal et al. 2000, 2002; Kaur et al. 2006; Neuwirt et al. 2008). GSE time- and dose-dependently enhances the DU145 prostate cancer cell apoptosis through the activation of the caspase signalling pathway. Treatment of DU145 prostate cancer cells with GSE (150–200 μg/ml) results in an increased release of cytochrome c from mitochondria, an increased activity of caspase 9, and an increased level of activated caspase 3 (Agarwal et al. 2002). GSE also increases apoptosis in LNCaP cells which was accompanied by reduction in activated PARP and inhibition of pro-apoptotic protein, Bcl-2 (Neuwirt et al. 2008).

The involvement of the NF-κB signalling pathway has also been suggested in the anti-cancer effects of GSE. NF-κB is a family of dimeric transcription factors which include five members; Rel (c-Rel), RelA (p65), RelB, NF-κB1 (p50/p105) and NF-κB2 (p52/p100), with p50/p65 being the most commonly found heterodimer (Brown et al. 2008). NF-κB lies inactive in the cytoplasm when bound to its inhibitor protein IκB. When IκB is phosphorylated, it dissociates from NF-κB and is then targeted for proteasomal degradation. The activated NF-κB translocates to the nucleus where it binds specific DNA binding sites and activates genes involved in cell survival and apoptosis inhibition. The upstream kinases responsible for the phosphorylation of IκB include IKKα and IKKβ, and these protein kinases have been shown to be activated by a number of factors including proinflammatory cytokine, toll-like receptor (TLR), and tumor necrosis factor α (TNFα) signalling pathways (Brown et al. 2008). The NF-κB signalling pathway is thought to be a major player in the progression of androgen-sensitive prostate cancer to the more aggressive, androgen-resistant cancer. Treatment of DU145 cells with GSE (50–100 µg/ml) results in a decrease in NF-κB nuclear protein levels and DNA binding, a decrease in cytoplasmic IκB phosphorylation, as well as a decrease in IKKα activation (Dhanalakshmi et al. 2003). Furthermore, GSE inhibits TNFα-induced activation of NK-κB signalling pathway and actually sensitizes the cells to the apoptosis inducing effect of TNFα. How GSE modulates these pathways is unclear. However, recent studies have suggested that components of GSE could increase the levels of reactive oxygen or hydrogen peroxide, which could mediate a stress response thereby activating signalling cascades to induce apoptosis (Kaur et al. 2006).

Cancer cell metastasis occurs when cancer cells migrate from the primary tissue origin and invade secondary tissues. MMPs are zinc-dependent proteinases which can selectively degrade extracellular matrix proteins and non-matrix proteins, including collagens, gelatin, laminin, elastin, fibronectin, plasminogen, and E-cadherin and thus, play a crucial role in tumor cell invasion and metastasis (Yoon et al. 2003). Downregulation or inhibition of MMPs can therefore be a target for chemopreventative approaches to reducing prostate cancer invasion, metastasis, and progression. GSE has been shown to cause a dose-dependent (20–80 µg/ml) reduction in growth factor-induced MMP-2 (gelatinase A) and MMP-9 (gelatinase B) extracellular secretion and cellular protein expression in DU145 cells (Vayalil et al. 2004). MMPs are known to be regulated by the activation of MAPK signalling and NF-κB activation, and thus GSE-induced modulation of these cell signaling pathways may be the mechanism by which MMPs are regulated. This effect was also demonstrated in LNCaP cells in which GSE dose dependently inhibited androgen-induced expression of MMP-2 and MMP-9 protein expression. Treatment of DU145 cells with GSE also results in a dose-dependent inhibition of VEGF secretion (Singh et al. 2004), which is an important growth factor ligand in the angiogenesis process.

In another study, the biologically active components in GSE which may be responsible for its anti-cancer effects in the prostate were investigated (Veluri et al. 2006). GSE phenolics were separated into eight fractions which were then individually tested for their anti-cancer potential. It was shown that the GSE fraction containing gallic acid was more effective in reducing DU145 cell growth and increasing cell death, than whole GSE. Gallic acid was further shown to increase active caspases 9 and 3, as well as activated PARP, and thus may be the component of GSE responsible for caspase signalling activation. On the other hand, GSE with gallic acid removed displayed DU145 cell growth inhibitory effects, although its efficiency was reduced. Fractions containing monomers catechin and epicatechin and dimers had no effect on DU145 cell growth, however, fractions containing trimers and gallate esters of dimers and trimers induced growth inhibitory effects, with B2-3,3′-di-O-gallate having the greatest effect (Agarwal et al. 2007). Thus, besides gallic acid, other components, potentially the procyanidins, could also play a role in the chemopreventative effects of GSE. Collectively, these in vitro studies highlight that GSE induces anti-cancer effects in various prostate cancer cell lines through multiple mechanism, which may prove to be beneficial for prostate cancer patients at various stages of carcinogenesis.

8.3.2.2 Effects on Prostate Cancer Growth In Vivo

Pre-clinical mouse studies have been conducted to determine if the anti-cancer effects of GSE displayed in the above described in vitro studies can also be observed in vivo. Starting at 4 weeks of age, GSE (200 mg/Kg BW) administered orally to TRAMP mice for 28 weeks, resulted in a decrease in the progression of PIN lesions to well-differentiated and poorly differentiated prostate tumors (Raina et al. 2007). This was accompanied by a reduction in prostate cell proliferation and an increase in apoptosis. Furthermore, the dorsolateral prostate had reduced biomarkers of cell cycle progression including cyclin B1, A, E, and Cdk2, 4, and 6, in mice treated with GSE. This study demonstrated the potential for GSE to reduce the progression of advanced prostate cancer in vivo, and suggested that modulation of cell cycle regulators is a potential mechanism of action.

A similar study was also conducted using gallic acid supplementation, which is a known active component of GSE (Raina et al. 2008). Like GSE, gallic acid supplementation (0.3 and 1%) also resulted in a decrease in prostate cancer progression to a more aggressive disease in the TRAMP model, accompanied by reduction in prostate cell proliferation and an increase in apoptosis. Similar to the effects of GSE, cell cycle regulatory proteins were also reduced by gallic acid suggesting that it may be a major component of GSE responsible for its chemopreventative effects (Raina et al. 2008).

To investigate the in vivo anti-cancer effects of GSE on human prostate tumors, DU145 cells were injected into the right flank of athymic nu/nu male mice (Singh et al. 2004). After 24 h, mice were gavaged with control (saline), 100, or 200 mg/Kg BW GSE (~2.5 and 5 mg/d) 5 days a week for 7 weeks. During the treatment period, palpable tumor volume was consistently lower in the GSE-treated mice compared to control treated, resulting in a 59–73% tumor growth inhibition by the GSE. GSE reduced tumor cell proliferation and CD31 (endothelial cell antigen – marker of blood vessel formation/angiogenesis) and increased apoptosis. Furthermore, GSE greatly enhanced the secretion of IGFBP-3, binding protein which reduces freely circulating IGF. GSE also reduced tumor expression of VEGF, which indicates a potential mechanism whereby angiogenesis is reduced by GSE. This study demonstrates that GSE administered in vivo, maintains its growth inhibitory properties observed in vitro and thus may prove beneficial for prostate cancer patients with androgen-insensitive tumors.

8.4 Other Seeds and Their Roles in Breast and Prostate Cancer

Studies on other seeds that have been reported to have anticancer effects particularly on breast and prostate are summarized in Table 8.1. The table lists the model systems and research design used in the study of the seeds and their components, the major findings, and the suggested mechanisms of action, where available. Evidently, the studies were done primarily using in vitro or animal models using carcinogen-treated rats or athymic mice with tumor xenografts. Most of the seeds demonstrate

Table 8.1 The effects of seeds on breast and prostate cancer prevention and treatment

Seed source	Potential Seed Bioactives	Cancer and Model	Study Design	Results	Indicated Potential Mechanisms or Targets	Reference
Pomegranate	Oil components: punicic acid, a conjugated linolenic acid isomer; 17-α-estradiol, estrone, estriol, testosterone, β-sitosterol, coumestrol, γ-tocopherol, campesterol, stigmasterol	Prostate cancer cells: DU145, PC-3, LNCaP	Treat cells with cold pressed seed oil	Dose dependent decrease in cell growth, with an ED_{50} of 30, 50, and 20 μg/ml for DU145, PC-3, LNCaP cells, respectively.	Cell cycle arrest inducing apoptosis	Albrecht et al. (2004)
		DMBA-induced mammary cancer in mouse mammary cultures	Treat mammary gland cultures with/without seed oil (1–10 μg/ml) followed by DMBA; observe development of precancerous lesions	The number of precancerous lesions, in the DMBA-induced mammary glands, was reduced when pretreated with seed oil.	Inhibition of prostaglandin synthesis	Mehta and Lansky (2004)
		Human breast cancer cells in vitro: MCF-7 and MDA-MB-435	Treat cells with cold pressed seed oil (1–1,000 μg/ml) for 1–9 days	Dose and time dependent reduction in MCF-7 cell growth and invasion; enhanced apoptosis in MDA-MB-435 cells	Inhibition of prostaglandin synthesis; inhibition of estradiol synthesis	Kim et al. (2002)

Table 8.1 (continued)

Seed source	Potential Seed Bioactives	Cancer and Model	Study Design	Results	Indicated Potential Mechanisms or Targets	Reference
Sesame	Oil components: Sesame lignans sesamin, sesamolin, sesaminol,	DMBA-induced mammary cancer in rat	Feed 0.2% sesamin supplemented diet starting 1 week prior to DMBA administration	Sesamin reduced total breast tumor number by 36%	Antioxidant and mammalian lignan precursor effect; reduce lipid peroxidation in tumors; reduce prostaglandin E2	Hirose et al. (1992)
		MCF-7 xenografts in OVX nude mouse model	Treat mice with MCF-7 tumors with 10% sesame seed diet alone or in combination with TAM for 7 weeks; at low or high circulating E2	At both high and low E2, sesame seed alone did not affect tumor growth but it adversely affected the tumor growth inhibitory effects of TAM	Unknown	Sacco et al. (2008, 2007)
		MCF-7 cells in vitro	Treat cells with sesamin (12.5–100 μM) for 1–3 days	Sesamin induced a dose and time dependent inhibition of MCF-7 cells growth	Cell cycle arrest by reducing cyclin D1 levels	Yokota et al. (2007)
		MCF-7 cells in vitro	Treat cells with sesamol (100 or 250 μM sesamol for 1–3 days	Sesamol inhibited the growth of MCF-7 cells	Cell cycle arrest	Jacklin et al. (2003)

Table 8.1 (continued)

Seed source	Potential Seed Bioactives	Cancer and Model	Study Design	Results	Indicated Potential Mechanisms or Targets	Reference
Black cumin (*Nigella sativa*)	Oil component; thymoquinone	Prostate cancer cells: DU145, PC-3, LNCaP in vitro	Treat cells with thymoquinone (0–100 μmol/l) for 1–3 days	Thymoquinone induced a dose and time dependent decrease in cell proliferation	Blocks cell cycle progression by reducing expression of AR and transcription factor, E2F-1, and its down-stream gene targets	Kaseb et al. (2007)
		C4–2B prostate cancer tumors in nude mouse model	Treat tumor-bearing mice with thymoquinone (20 mg/Kg) daily for 30 days.	Thymoquinone reduced tumor growth	Blocks the expression of AR and E2F-1, and cyclin A1; enhances apoptosis	Kaseb et al. (2007)
		PC-3 human prostate cancer cells in vitro	Treat cells with 0–1 μM thymoquinone	Thymoquinone reduced cell proliferation and migration	Inhibition of angiogenesis to reduce tumor cell growth	Yi et al. (2008)
		SCID mouse model with established PC-3 tumors	Treat mice with thymoquinone (6 mg/kg) for 15 days	Thymoquinone reduced tumor growth and blood vessel formation	Reduced angiogenesis	Yi et al. (2008)
Caper	Protein component	MCF-7 cells in vitro	Treat cells with seed protein extract	Dose dependent decrease in cell growth, $IC_{50} = 60$ μM	unknown	Lam and Ng (2009)

Table 8.1 (continued)

Seed source	Potential Seed Bioactives	Cancer and Model	Study Design	Results	Indicated Potential Mechanisms or Targets	Reference
Adlay (coixseed, Job's Tears)	Oil components	MDA-MB-231 human breast tumor xenografts in vivo	Treat mice with 50 µg seed oil extract daily at time of cell implantation	Coix oil reduced development of tumors	Reduced COX-2 expression	Woo et al. (2007)
		MDA-MB-231 human breast cancer cells in vitro	Treat cells with 0–7.5 mg/ml coix extract	Reduced cell invasion	Reduced COX-2, NF-κB activity, protein kinase C activity, genes related to invasion and metastasis	Woo et al. (2007)

tumor cell growth inhibitory effects, with mechanisms of action including modulation of cell cycle, anti-oxidant, and anti-inflammatory effects. On the other hand, sesame seed, which is also rich in lignans, although different from the SDG found in FS, did not show the same cancer protective effect as FS. In the MCF-7 xenografts model, sesame seed did not modulate the growth of tumors, and for unknown reasons, it interfered with the anti-tumor effects of the breast cancer drug tamoxifen (Sacco et al. 2007, 2008). Further studies should thus be conducted to determine the safety of these seeds with regards to their interaction with cancer drugs. This is of major importance since the majority of cancer patients may take the seeds as alternative complementary medicines with various cancer drugs. Overall, although in many cases, the results showed a cancer protective effect, none of the listed seeds have been tested in prostate or breast cancer clinical trials.

8.5 Conclusions

There is strong evidence in animal models that FS can play a role in breast and prostate cancer prevention and treatment. Some clinical evidence are also available suggesting that FS can reduce the progression of breast and prostate cancer in humans and thus may serve as an alternative or complementary therapeutic for cancer patients. Both the ALA-rich oil and lignans have been suggested to be the components responsible for the health promoting effects of FS. FS oil and lignans are now commercially available and have been shown to produce similar effects as FS, but there is yet no clear evidence in humans suggesting that these FS components as such, can mitigate carcinogenesis. The mechanisms of their tumor reducing effects appear to involve both the reduction of tumor cell proliferation and angiogenesis and increasing apoptosis through modulation of the ER– and growth factor-mediated cell signaling pathways. In 2009, the US FDA has given GRAS (generally regarded as safe) status to high linolenic FS oil (http://www.accessdata.fda.gov/scripts/fcn/fcnDetailNavigation.cfm?rpt=grasListing&id=256), as well as to whole and milled flax (http://www.accessdata.fda.gov/scripts/fcn/fcnDetailNavigation.cfm?rpt=grasListing&id=280). This indicates its safe use by adult humans. In the in vivo studies described in this chapter, FS does not have tumor promoting effects nor does it adversely interfere with the action of the drug tamoxifen; in fact it increases the effectiveness of tamoxifen. However this FS-drug interaction has yet to be established in clinical trials. Furthermore, the timing of FS exposure deserves further attention, since there are conflicting data in animal models on the effect of early exposure to FS on breast cancer risk.

GSE has been shown to be a strong inhibitor of cancer growth in various experimental models of breast and prostate cancer however clinical studies have yet to be completed in cancer patients. The suggested major components of GSE responsible for its anti-cancer effects include the phenolics, namely gallic acid and the procyanidins. The mechanisms of action are multi-targeted ranging from anti-oxidant activities to direct effects on cell signalling pathways. Thus, GSE may prove to be a beneficial anti-cancer dietary component in humans at various stages of cancer development. The US FDA has approved GRAS status for GSE (http://www.accessdata.fda.gov/scripts/fcn/fcnDetailNavigation.cfm?rpt=grasListing&id =125), however, as a relatively new food-derived extract, its physiological effects after long-term consumption by humans still have to be assessed. The effects of GSE in cancer patients should also be studied in the future.

Overall, all the seeds described in this chapter have displayed some anti-cancer effects with regards to prostate and/or breast cancer in experimental models. More research is required for pomegranate, sesame, adlay, caper, and black cumin seeds to determine their mechanisms of action and anti-cancer potential in experimental models and in humans. Furthermore, the potential for the seeds to modulate the activity of anti-cancer drugs must be assessed to ensure safe use as complementary treatments for cancer patients.

References

Agarwal C, Sharma Y, Agarwal R (2000) Anticarcinogenic effect of a polyphenolic fraction isolated from grape seeds in human prostate carcinoma DU145 cells: modulation of mitogenic signaling and cell-cycle regulators and induction of G1 arrest and apoptosis. Mol Carcinog 28:129–138

Agarwal C, Singh RP, Agarwal R (2002) Grape seed extract induces apoptotic death of human prostate carcinoma DU145 cells via caspases activation accompanied by dissipation of mitochondrial membrane potential and cytochrome c release. Carcinogenesis 23: 1869–1876

Agarwal C, Veluri R, Kaur M et al (2007) Fractionation of high molecular weight tannins in grape seed extract and identification of procyanidin B2-3,3'-di-O-gallate as a major active constituent causing growth inhibition and apoptotic death of DU145 human prostate carcinoma cells. Carcinogenesis 28:1478–1484

Albrecht M, Jiang W, Kumi-Diaka J et al (2004) Pomegranate extracts potently suppress proliferation, xenograft growth, and invasion of human prostate cancer cells. J Med Food 7:274–283

Alimirah F, Chen J, Basrawala Z et al (2006) DU-145 and PC-3 human prostate cancer cell lines express androgen receptor: implications for the androgen receptor functions and regulation. FEBS Lett 580:2294–2300

Bergman-Jungestrom M, Thompson LU, Dabrosin C (2007) Flaxseed and its lignans inhibit estradiol-induced growth, angiogenesis, and secretion of vascular endothelial growth factor in human breast cancer xenografts in vivo. Clin Cancer Res 13:1061–1067

Boon HS, Olatunde F, Zick SM (2007) Trends in complementary/alternative medicine use by breast cancer survivors: comparing survey data from 1998 and 2005. BMC Womens Health 7:4

Brekelmans CT (2003) Risk factors and risk reduction of breast and ovarian cancer. Curr Opin Obstet Gynecol 15:63–68

Brisken C (2002) Hormonal control of alveolar development and its implications for breast carcinogenesis. J Mammary Gland Biol Neoplasia 7:39–48

Brown KD, Claudio E, Siebenlist U (2008) The roles of the classical and alternative nuclear factor-kappaB pathways: potential implications for autoimmunity and rheumatoid arthritis. Arthritis Res Ther 10:212

Bryzgalova G, Lundholm L, Portwood N et al (2008) Mechanisms of antidiabetogenic and body weight-lowering effects of estrogen in high fat diet-fed mice. Am J Physiol Endocrinol Metab 295:E904–E912

Canadian Cancer Society (2009) Canadian cancer statistics: Canadian cancer society's steering committee

Chen LH, Fang J, Li H et al (2007a) Enterolactone induces apoptosis in human prostate carci- noma LNCaP cells via a mitochondrial-mediated, caspase-dependent pathway. Mol Cancer Ther 6:2581–2590

Chen LH, Fang J, Sun Z et al (2009) Enterolactone Inhibits Insulin-Like Growth Factor-1 Receptor Signaling in Human Prostatic Carcinoma PC-3 Cells. J Nutr 139:653–659

Chen J, Hui E, Ip T et al (2004) Dietary flaxseed enhances the inhibitory effect of tamoxifen on the growth of estrogen-dependent human breast cancer (mcf-7) in nude mice. Clin Cancer Res 10:7703–7711

Chen J, Power KA, Mann J et al (2007b) Dietary flaxseed interaction with tamoxifen induced tumor regression in athymic mice with MCF-7 xenografts by downregulating the expression of estrogen related gene products and signal transduction pathways. Nutr Cancer 58:162–170

Chen J, Power KA, Mann J et al (2007c) Flaxseed alone or in combination with tamoxifen inhibits MCF-7 breast tumor growth in ovariectomized athymic mice with high circulating levels of estrogen. Exp Biol Med (Maywood) 232:1071–1080

Chen J, Stavro PM, Thompson LU (2002) Dietary flaxseed inhibits human breast cancer growth and metastasis and downregulates expression of insulin-like growth factor and epidermal growth factor receptor. Nutr Cancer 43:187–192

Chen J, Tan KP, Ward WE et al (2003) Exposure to flaxseed or its purified lignan during suck- ling inhibits chemically induced rat mammary tumorigenesis. Exp Biol Med (Maywood) 228: 951–958

Chen J, Thompson LU (2003) Lignans and tamoxifen, alone or in combination, reduce human breast cancer cell adhesion, invasion and migration in vitro. Breast Cancer Res Treat 80: 163–170

Chen J, Wang L, Thompson LU (2006) Flaxseed and its components reduce metastasis after surgical excision of solid human breast tumor in nude mice. Cancer Lett 234: 168–175

Cosentino M, Marino F, Ferrari M et al (2007) Estrogenic activity of 7-hydroxymatairesinol potas- sium acetate (HMR/lignan) from Norway spruce (*Picea abies*) knots and of its active metabolite enterolactone in MCF-7 cells. Pharmacol Res 56:140–147

D'Amelio M, Tino E, Cecconi F (2008) The apoptosome: emerging insights and new potential targets for drug design. Pharmacol Res 25:740–751

Dabrosin C, Chen J, Wang L et al (2002) Flaxseed inhibits metastasis and decreases extracellular vascular endothelial growth factor in human breast cancer xenografts. Cancer Lett 185:31–37

Debes JD, Tindall DJ (2002) The role of androgens and the androgen receptor in prostate cancer. Cancer Lett 187:1–7

Demark-Wahnefried W, Polascik TJ, George SL et al (2008) Flaxseed supplementation (not dietary fat restriction) reduces prostate cancer proliferation rates in men presurgery. Cancer Epidemiol Biomarkers Prev 17:3577–3587

Demark-Wahnefried W, Robertson CN, Walther PJ et al (2004) Pilot study to explore effects of low-fat, flaxseed-supplemented diet on proliferation of benign prostatic epithelium and prostate-specific antigen. Urology 63:900–904

Dhanalakshmi S, Agarwal R, Agarwal C (2003) Inhibition of NF-kappaB pathway in grape seed extract-induced apoptotic death of human prostate carcinoma DU145 cells. Int J Oncol 23: 721–727

Dip R, Lenz S, Antignac JP et al (2008) Global gene expression profiles induced by phytoestrogens in human breast cancer cells. Endocr Relat Cancer 15:161–173

Eliasson C, Kamal-Eldin A, Andersson R et al (2003) High-performance liquid chromatographic analysis of secoisolariciresinol diglucoside and hydroxycinnamic acid glucosides in flaxseed by alkaline extraction. J Chromatogr A 1012:151–159

Fantozzi P, Betschart AA (1979) Development of Grapeseed Protein. J Am Oil Chemists' Soc 56:457–459

Faria A, Calhau C, de Freitas V et al (2006) Procyanidins as antioxidants and tumor cell growth modulators. J Agric Food Chem 54:2392–2397

Gingrich JR, Barrios RJ, Foster BA et al (1999) Pathologic progression of autochthonous prostate cancer in the TRAMP model. Prostate Cancer Prostatic Dis 2:70–75

Greenberg NM, DeMayo F, Finegold MJ et al (1995) Prostate cancer in a transgenic mouse. Proc Natl Acad Sci USA 92:3439–3443

Grossmann ME, Huang H, Tindall DJ (2001) Androgen receptor signaling in androgen-refractory prostate cancer. J Natl Cancer Inst 93:1687–1697

Hilakivi-Clarke L (2007) Nutritional modulation of terminal end buds: its relevance to breast cancer prevention. Curr Cancer Drug Targets 7:465–474

Hirose N, Doi F, Ueki T et al (1992) Suppressive effect of sesamin against 7,12-dimethylbenz[a]-anthracene induced rat mammary carcinogenesis. Anticancer Res 12:1259–1265

Howlin J, McBryan J, Martin F (2006) Pubertal mammary gland development: insights from mouse models. J Mammary Gland Biol Neoplasia 11:283–297

Hu C, Yuan YV, Kitts DD (2007) Antioxidant activities of the flaxseed lignan secoisolari-ciresinol diglucoside, its aglycone secoisolariciresinol and the mammalian lignans enterodiol and enterolactone in vitro. Food Chem Toxicol 45:2219–2227

Jacklin A, Ratledge C, Welham K et al (2003) The sesame seed oil constituent, sesamol, induces growth arrest and apoptosis of cancer and cardiovascular cells. Ann N Y Acad Sci 1010: 374–380

Jordan VC (2004) Selective estrogen receptor modulation: concept and consequences in cancer. Cancer Cell 5:207–213

Kaseb AO, Chinnakannu K, Chen D et al (2007) Androgen receptor and E2F-1 targeted thymoquinone therapy for hormone-refractory prostate cancer. Cancer Res 67:7782–7788

Kaur M, Agarwal R, Agarwal C (2006) Grape seed extract induces anoikis and caspase-mediated apoptosis in human prostate carcinoma LNCaP cells: possible role of ataxia telangiectasia mutated-p53 activation. Mol Cancer Ther 5:1265–1274

Khan G, Penttinen P, Cabanes A et al (2007) Maternal flaxseed diet during pregnancy or lactation increases female rat offspring's susceptibility to carcinogen-induced mammary tumorigenesis. Reprod Toxicol 23:397–406

Kijima I, Phung S, Hur G et al (2006) Grape seed extract is an aromatase inhibitor and a suppressor of aromatase expression. Cancer Res 66:5960–5967

Kim H, Hall P, Smith M et al (2004) Chemoprevention by grape seed extract and genistein in carcinogen-induced mammary cancer in rats is diet dependent. J Nutr 134:3445S–3452S

Kim ND, Mehta R, Yu W et al (2002) Chemopreventive and adjuvant therapeutic potential of pomegranate (*Punica granatum*) for human breast cancer. Breast Cancer Res Treat 71:203–217

Lam SK, Ng TB (2009) A protein with antiproliferative, antifungal and HIV-1 reverse transcriptase inhibitory activities from caper (*Capparis spinosa*) seeds. Phytomedicine 16:444–450

Lin X, Gingrich JR, Bao W et al (2002) Effect of flaxseed supplementation on prostatic carcinoma in transgenic mice. Urology 60:919–924

Lin X, Switzer BR, Demark-Wahnefried W (2001) Effect of mammalian lignans on the growth of prostate cancer cell lines. Anticancer Res 21:3995–3999

Lu J, Zhang K, Chen S et al (2009) Grape seed extract inhibits VEGF expression via reducing HIF-1{alpha} protein expression. Carcinogenesis 30:636–644

Mantena SK, Baliga MS, Katiyar SK (2006) Grape seed proanthocyanidins induce apoptosis and inhibit metastasis of highly metastatic breast carcinoma cells. Carcinogenesis 27:1682–1691

McCann MJ, Gill CI, Linton T et al (2008) Enterolactone restricts the proliferation of the LNCaP human prostate cancer cell line in vitro. Mol Nutr Food Res 52:567–580

Mehta R, Lansky EP (2004) Breast cancer chemopreventive properties of pomegranate (Punica granatum) fruit extracts in a mouse mammary organ culture. Eur J Cancer Prev 13:345–348

Mousavi Y, Adlercreutz H (1992) Enterolactone and estradiol inhibit each other's proliferative effect on MCF-7 breast cancer cells in culture. J Steroid Biochem Mol Biol 41:615–619

Mueller SO, Simon S, Chae K et al (2004) Phytoestrogens and their human metabolites show distinct agonistic and antagonistic properties on estrogen receptor alpha (ERalpha) and ERbeta in human cells. Toxicol Sci 80:14–25

Murrill WB, Brown NM, Zhang JX et al (1996) Prepubertal genistein exposure suppresses mammary cancer and enhances gland differentiation in rats. Carcinogenesis 17:1451–1457

Nesbitt PD, Lam Y, Thompson LU (1999) Human metabolism of mammalian lignan precursors in raw and processed flaxseed. Am J Clin Nutr 69:549–555

Neuwirt H, Arias MC, Puhr M et al (2008) Oligomeric proanthocyanidin complexes (OPC) exert anti-proliferative and pro-apoptotic effects on prostate cancer cells. Prostate 68:1647–1654

Newbold RR, Jefferson WN, Padilla-Banks E (2007a) Long-term adverse effects of neonatal exposure to bisphenol A on the murine female reproductive tract. Reprod Toxicol 24:253–258.

Newbold RR, Padilla-Banks E, Snyder RJ et al (2007b) Developmental exposure to endocrine disruptors and the obesity epidemic. Reprod Toxicol 23:290–296

Penttinen P, Jaehrling J, Damdimopoulos AE et al (2007) Diet-derived polyphenol metabolite enterolactone is a tissue-specific estrogen receptor activator. Endocrinology 148:4875–4886

Power KA, Chen JM, Saarinen NM et al (2008) Changes in biomarkers of estrogen receptor and growth factor signaling pathways in MCF-7 tumors after short- and long-term treatment with soy and flaxseed. J Steroid Biochem Mol Biol 112:13–19

Power KA, Saarinen NM, Chen JM et al (2006) Mammalian lignans enterolactone and enterodiol, alone and in combination with the isoflavone genistein, do not promote the growth of MCF-7 xenografts in ovariectomized athymic nude mice. Int J Cancer 118:1316–1320

Prasad K (2000) Antioxidant activity of secoisolariciresinol diglucoside-derived metabolites, secoisolariciresinol, enterodiol, and enterolactone. Int J Angiol 9:220–225

Prasad K (1997) Hydroxyl radical-scavenging property of secoisolariciresinol diglucoside (SDG) isolated from flax-seed. Mol Cell Biochem 168:117–123

Raina K, Rajamanickam S, Deep G et al (2008) Chemopreventive effects of oral gallic acid feeding on tumor growth and progression in TRAMP mice. Mol Cancer Ther 7:1258–1267

Raina K, Singh RP, Agarwal R et al (2007) Oral grape seed extract inhibits prostate tumor growth and progression in TRAMP mice. Cancer Res 67:5976–5982

Rickard SE, Yuan YV, Chen J et al (1999) Dose effects of flaxseed and its lignan on N-methyl-N-nitrosourea-induced mammary tumorigenesis in rats. Nutr Cancer 35:50–57

Ruder EH, Dorgan JF, Kranz S et al (2008) Examining breast cancer growth and lifestyle risk factors: early life, childhood, and adolescence. Clin Breast Cancer 8:334–342

Russo IH, Russo J (1998) Role of hormones in mammary cancer initiation and progression. J Mammary Gland Biol Neoplasia 3:49–61

Russo J, Tait L, Russo IH (1983) Susceptibility of the mammary gland to carcinogenesis. III. The cell of origin of rat mammary carcinoma. Am J Pathol 113:50–66

Saarinen NM, Huovinen R, Warri A et al (2002) Enterolactone inhibits the growth of 7,12-dimethylbenz(a) anthracene-induced mammary carcinomas in the rat. Mol Cancer Ther 1:869–876

Saarinen NM, Power K, Chen J et al (2006) Flaxseed attenuates the tumor growth stimulating effect of soy protein in ovariectomized athymic mice with MCF-7 human breast cancer xenografts. Int J Cancer 119:925–931

Saarinen NM, Power KA, Chen J et al (2008) Lignans are accessible to human breast cancer xenografts in athymic mice. Nutr Cancer 60:245–250.

Sacco SM, Chen J, Power KA et al (2008) Lignan-rich sesame seed negates the tumor-inhibitory effect of tamoxifen but maintains bone health in a postmenopausal athymic mouse model with estrogen-responsive breast tumors. Menopause 15:171–179

Sacco SM, Power KA, Chen J et al (2007) Interaction of sesame seed and tamoxifen on tumor growth and bone health in athymic mice. Exp Biol Med (Maywood) 232:754–761

Serraino M, Thompson LU (1992) The effect of flaxseed supplementation on the initiation and promotional stages of mammary tumorigenesis. Nutr Cancer 17:153–159

Simopoulos AP (2002) Omega-3 fatty acids in inflammation and autoimmune diseases. J Am Coll Nutr 21:495–505

Singh RP, Agarwal R (2006) Mechanisms of action of novel agents for prostate cancer chemoprevention. Endocr Relat Cancer 13:751–778

Singh RP, Tyagi AK, Dhanalakshmi S et al (2004) Grape seed extract inhibits advanced human prostate tumor growth and angiogenesis and upregulates insulin-like growth factor binding protein-3. Int J Cancer 108:733–740

Singletary KW, Meline B (2001) Effect of grape seed proanthocyanidins on colon aberrant crypts and breast tumors in a rat dual-organ tumor model. Nutr Cancer 39:252–258

Soto AM, Vandenberg LN, Maffini MV et al (2008) Does breast cancer start in the womb? Basic Clin Pharmacol Toxicol 102:125–133

Sternlicht MD, Kouros-Mehr H, Lu P et al (2006) Hormonal and local control of mammary branching morphogenesis. Differentiation 74:365–381

Takeuchi S, Takahashi T, Sawada Y et al (2009) Comparative study on the nuclear hormone receptor activity of various phytochemicals and their metabolites by reporter gene assays using Chinese hamster ovary cells. Biol Pharm Bull 32:195–202

Tan KP, Chen J, Ward WE et al (2004) Mammary gland morphogenesis is enhanced by exposure to flaxseed or its major lignan during suckling in rats. Exp Biol Med (Maywood) 229:147–157

Tangolar SG, Ozogul Y, Tangolar S et al (2007) Evaluation of fatty acid profiles and mineral content of grape seed oil of some grape genotypes. Int J Food Sci Nutr 19:1–8

Thompson LU, Boucher BA, Liu Z et al (2006) Phytoestrogen content of foods consumed in Canada, including isoflavones, lignans, and coumestan. Nutr Cancer 54:184–201

Thompson LU, Chen JM, Li T et al (2005) Dietary flaxseed alters tumor biological markers in postmenopausal breast cancer. Clin Cancer Res 11:3828–3835

Thompson LU, Rickard SE, Cheung F et al (1997) Variability in anticancer lignan levels in flaxseed. Nutr Cancer 27:26–30

Thompson LU, Rickard SE, Orcheson LJ et al (1996a) Flaxseed and its lignan and oil components reduce mammary tumor growth at a late stage of carcinogenesis. Carcinogenesis 17:1373–1376

Thompson LU, Seidl MM, Rickard SE et al (1996b) Antitumorigenic effect of a mammalian lignan precursor from flaxseed. Nutr Cancer 26:159–165

Tou JC, Thompson LU (1999) Exposure to flaxseed or its lignan component during different developmental stages influences rat mammary gland structures. Carcinogenesis 20:1831–1835

Tou JC, Chen J, Thompson LU (1998) Flaxseed and its lignan precursor, secoisolariciresinol diglycoside, affect pregnancy outcome and reproductive development in rats. J Nutr 128:1861–1868

Tou JC, Chen J, Thompson LU (1999) Dose, timing, and duration of flaxseed exposure affect reproductive indices and sex hormone levels in rats. J Toxicol Environ Health A 56:555–570

Tyagi A, Agarwal R, Agarwal C (2003) Grape seed extract inhibits EGF-induced and constitutively active mitogenic signaling but activates JNK in human prostate carcinoma DU145 cells: possible role in antiproliferation and apoptosis. Oncogene 22:1302–1316

Uzumcu M, Zachow R (2007) Developmental exposure to environmental endocrine disruptors: consequences within the ovary and on female reproductive function. Reprod Toxicol 23:337–352

Vandenberg LN, Wadia PR, Schaeberle CM et al (2006) The mammary gland response to estradiol: monotonic at the cellular level, non-monotonic at the tissue-level of organization? J Steroid Biochem Mol Biol 101:263–274

Vayalil PK, Mittal A, Katiyar SK (2004) Proanthocyanidins from grape seeds inhibit expression of matrix metalloproteinases in human prostate carcinoma cells, which is associated with the inhibition of activation of MAPK and NF kappa B. Carcinogenesis 25:987–999.

Veluri R, Singh RP, Liu Z et al (2006) Fractionation of grape seed extract and identification of gallic acid as one of the major active constituents causing growth inhibition and apoptotic death of DU145 human prostate carcinoma cells. Carcinogenesis 27:1445–1453

Wang LQ (2002) Mammalian phytoestrogens: enterodiol and enterolactone. J Chromatogr B Analyt Technol Biomed Life Sci 777:289–309

Wang L, Chen J, Thompson LU (2005) The inhibitory effect of flaxseed on the growth and metastasis of estrogen receptor negative human breast cancer xenograftsis attributed to both its lignan and oil components. Int J Cancer 116:793–798

Ward WE, Chen J, Thompson LU (2001) Exposure to flaxseed or its purified lignan during suckling only or continuously does not alter reproductive indices in male and female offspring. J Toxicol Environ Health A 64:567–577

Ward WE, Jiang FO, Thompson LU (2000) Exposure to flaxseed or purified lignan during lactation influences rat mammary gland structures. Nutr Cancer 37:187–192

Welshons WV, Murphy CS, Koch R et al (1987) Stimulation of breast cancer cells in vitro by the environmental estrogen enterolactone and the phytoestrogen equol. Breast Cancer Res Treat 10:169–175

Wen W, Lu J, Zhang K et al (2008) Grape seed extract inhibits angiogenesis via suppression of the vascular endothelial growth factor receptor signaling pathway. Cancer Prev Res (Phila Pa) 1:554–561

Woo JH, Li D, Wilsbach K et al (2007) Coix seed extract, a commonly used treatment for cancer in China, inhibits NFkappaB and protein kinase C signaling. Cancer Biol Ther 6:2005–2011

World Cancer Research Fund/American Institute for Cancer Research (2007) Food, nutrition, physical activity, and the prevention of cancer: a global perspective. AICR, Washington, DC

Yager JD, Davidson NE (2006) Estrogen carcinogenesis in breast cancer. N Engl J Med 354: 270–282

Yi T, Cho SG, Yi Z et al (2008) Thymoquinone inhibits tumor angiogenesis and tumor growth through suppressing AKT and extracellular signal-regulated kinase signaling pathways. Mol Cancer Ther 7:1789–1796

Yokota T, Matsuzaki Y, Koyama M et al (2007) Sesamin, a lignan of sesame, down-regulates cyclin D1 protein expression in human tumor cells. Cancer Sci 98:1447–1453

Yoon SO, Park SJ, Yun CH et al (2003) Roles of matrix metalloproteinases in tumor metastasis and angiogenesis. J Biochem Mol Biol 36:128–137

Yu B, Khan G, Foxworth A et al (2006) Maternal dietary exposure to fiber during pregnancy and mammary tumorigenesis among rat offspring. Int J Cancer 119:2279–2286

Chapter 9
Nuts as Part of a Whole Diet Approach to Cancer Prevention

Paul A. Davis

Abstract This review presents a case for tree nuts as an important food in terms of their effects on cancer and their role in a whole food approach to cancer prevention. The review will assess the limited number of currently published experimental and epidemiological reports examining the relationship(s) between tree nuts and cancer. In addition because of limited experimental literature on tree nuts, the review will also use as a stopgap, the reported effects of constituents known to be present in nuts and their anti-cancer activity as a means to make the case for nuts in cancer prevention. The strength of the conclusions that can be drawn are limited, particularly given the increasing recognition that difficulties arise in using single ingredients to assess food based cancer and other health effects. However, in summary, this review assembles significant evidence that is consistent with but not conclusive proof of nuts' efficacy in cancer prevention.

Keywords Nuts · Chemoprevention · Whole diet approach

Contents

P.A. Davis (✉)
Department of Nutrition, College of Agricultural and Environmental Sciences, University of California, Davis, Davis, CA 95616, USA
e-mail: padavis@ucdavis.edu

M. Mutanen, A.-M. Pajari (eds.), *Vegetables, Whole Grains, and Their Derivatives in Cancer Prevention*, Diet and Cancer 2, DOI 10.1007/978-90-481-9800-9_9,
© Springer Science+Business Media B.V. 2011

9.1 Introduction

Almonds, walnuts and other tree nuts represent a unique type of foodstuff whose consumption results in a higher fat intake that is more commonly associated with meat rich Western diet while providing nutrients that are associated with a plant derived diet. This unique combination in nuts has proven to be a significant detriment when fat is the sole or major metric for assessing a food's healthiness. This is particularly evident as studies demonstrate that high fat diets such as the Mediterranean diet, primarily derived from plant based foods, actually provide protective effects for several chronic diseases.

This article has as its goal to review the evidence, experimental or epidemiological that has been generated to address the question of the effect of nuts on cancer. However a literature search using the terms nuts and cancer turns up relatively few such studies. The Food, Nutrition, Physical Activity, and the Prevention of Cancer: a Global Perspective issued in 2007 reviewed the literature linking nuts and seeds to cancer and concluded that the evidence was too limited in amount, consistency, or quality to draw any conclusions regarding the effects of nut and seed consumption on cancer (World Cancer Research Fund 2007). By way of response, this article will adopt a two-fold approach to expand the potential basis for associating nut consumption with positive effects on cancer. One branch will consist of highlighting the limited number of reports that have directly addressed the effects of nuts. The other approach will be to highlight selected studies that have used specific or related constituents present or likely present in nuts on cancer. These will be combined using a whole diet approach in cancer prevention to discuss the evidence available to affect risk of cancer and other Western-type diseases by replacing foods with unfavorable composition with foods with more favorable composition such as tree nuts. The overall goal of the review is to present evidence, both direct and indirect that adding nuts to a diet to replace or displace other foodstuffs has or will have positive effects on cancer.

9.2 Nuts in Cancer Prevention

9.2.1 Main Composition of Tree Nuts

Tree nuts are nutrient-dense foods that are widely consumed, albeit at differing levels, and have been present in human diets since pre-agricultural times (Sabate et al. 2006). Their elevated nutrient density is a result of their high lipid levels, composed of monounsaturated (MUFA) and polyunsaturated fatty acids (PUFA) with low saturated fat (Ros and Mataix 2006; Venkatachalam and Sathe 2006). Nuts, most particularly walnuts, are especially a rich source of ALA (6.81 g/75 g walnuts). Tree nuts also contain an appreciable amount, 10–25% of calories, of plant protein (Brufau et al. 2006).

Nuts are a good source of dietary fiber, as a standard serving of tree nuts will provide 5–10% of daily fiber requirements (Coates and Howe 2007). Tree nuts are also source vitamins including folic acid, niacin, vitamins B6 and E, and minerals such as calcium, magnesium, copper, zinc, and phosphorus (Brufau et al. 2006). They are a rich source of vitamin E derivates with almonds and hazelnuts having the highest concentrations of α-tocopherol, while Brazil nuts, pecans, pistachios, and walnuts contain high levels of vitamin E in the forms of β- and γ-tocopherols. Phytosterols are found in all tree nuts, especially pistachios, pine nuts, almonds, and cashews with β-sitosterol as the most abundant. Of the polyphenolic compounds in nuts, 80% are phenolic acids, with walnuts and pecans having the highest levels that compare favorably with a wide variety of fruits (Wu et al. 2004; Chen and Blumberg 2008). Hazelnuts and pecans have the highest total flavonoid content with over 500 mg/100 g and they along with pistachios and almonds contain multiple proanthocyanidins at levels similar to those in dark chocolate, berries, red wine and grape juice. The high content of unsaturated fatty acids, protein with a low lysine to arginine ratio, dietary fiber, and a range of vitamins, minerals and other bioactive compounds make tree nuts likely to beneficial in cancer as well as other diet affected diseases.

9.2.2 Evidence Behind Nuts and Cancer

There are a few published epidemiologic studies that have considered nut intake and risk of cancer (Pickle et al. 1984; Kune et al. 1987; Singh and Fraser 1998; Jain et al. 1999; Petridou et al. 2002). The results have ranged from no association (Pickle et al. 1984) to a beneficial one in women only (Kune et al. 1987). An overriding reason for this inconsistency is that any relationship is likely vitiated as a result of flawed nut and seed intake assessment methodology. Unfortunately, very few studies have specifically assessed the intake of nuts and seeds alone, let alone specific nuts. Most studies have assessed their intake after incorporating them as part of larger and heterogeneous groups.

The European Prospective Investigation into Cancer and Nutrition (EPIC) examined the association of colorectal cancer risk with nuts and seeds intakes as determined from dietary questionnaire (Jenab et al. 2004). The resulting data set had a 2−1 ratio of women to men with a total of 855 (327 men, 528 women) colon and 474 (215 men, 259 women) rectal cancer cases. No whole group association between higher intake of nuts and seeds and risk of colorectal, colon, and rectal cancers were found. However, in women, there was a significant inverse association with colon cancer at the highest intake of nuts and seeds versus the non-consumer. The overall conclusion was that the results are consistent with an effect of nuts but the exact extent they were attributable to nuts and seeds themselves, or nuts and seeds acting as a healthier diet pattern marker remained unclear.

There is only one study that examined the relationship between nut consumption and cancer, specifically prostate cancer in humans. The study by Spaccarotella et al. had as its primary goal to evaluate the effects of consuming 75 g/d of walnuts on metabolic factors related to prostate cancer along with cardiovascular disease in men at risk for these diseases (Spaccarotella et al. 2008). They reported that while the subjects' tocopherol ratio was significantly improved with walnut consumption, the primary markers of prostate health (prostate specific antigen, PSA and urinary symptoms) were not changed significantly by the 8-week dietary intervention. Moreover there was a nonsignificant increase in the ratio of free PSA: total PSA, the use of which in combination with total PSA has been suggested to improve specificity of diagnosis and decrease false-positives (Catalona et al. 1997). The authors described that the results were disappointing. PSA levels are, however, known to be depressed by abdominal obesity and high serum triglyceride levels (Kim et al. 2008) both of which appear to be present in the population studied by Spaccarotella et al. (2008).

As regard to animal studies, there is only one publication on the effect of almond feeding on chemical induced colon carcinogenesis in rats (Davis and Iwahashi 2001). In this study the effect of almond was investigated in a colon cancer model using male F344 rats that were given subcutaneous injections of azoxymethane (15 mg/kg body weight) twice 1 week apart. The rats were randomized between the cellulose or wheat bran controls or whole almonds, defatted almond meal or almond oil groups. The almond diets were design to give 53% of energy from fat from whole almonds, partially defatted almond meal (~35% fat) or almond oil substituted into AIN-76A diet. After 26 weeks of ad lib feeding, animals were injected with bromodeoxyuridine 1 h prior to determine gastrointestinal (GI) labeling index and then sacrificed. The groups fed with whole almond had the number of colonic aberrant crypt foci (ACF) and labeling index significantly lower than wheat bran and cellulose diet groups (−30 and −40%, respectively). This study on almonds and GI cancer was then followed up using the ApcMin mouse, a genetic GI tumor animal cancer model (Yamada and Mori 2007) but failed to replicate a positive effect in terms of polyp numbers (Davis et al. 2003). However, GI tissue gene analysis showed that p27 kip1, a cyclin-dependent kinase inhibitor, was induced by almond feeding in these animals. A p27 kip1 is a tumor suppressor and it is induced by compounds that have been shown to be chemopreventive (Eto 2006 et al. 2007; Aggarwal BB, Banerjee S et al. 2007). Crucially, p27 kip1 signaling has been reported to act via signals of the Wnt/β-catenin pathway (Hulit et al. 2006) that likely explains the absence of a positive almond effect on polyp numbers as the Wnt/β-catenin pathway is specifically disturbed in the ApcMin mouse.

Very recently, both Hardman et al. and Davis et al. have examined the role of walnut consumption in breast cancer and prostate cancer animal models, respectively (Davis et al. 2009; Ion et al. 2009). Their preliminary reports, as abstracts, indicated that in both types of cancer, the inclusion of whole walnuts into experimental diets had beneficial effects.

9.2.3 Evidence for Cancer Related Benefits in the Main Components of Nut

9.2.3.1 α-Linolenic Acid and Possible Benifits of Lipids in Tree Nuts

In addition to epidemiological evidence suggesting a positive linkage of nuts to reduced cancer, there have been epidemiology-based reports that suggest the opposite. These arose in relationship to the potential negative effects of α-linolenic acid

(ALA) on prostate cancer. This is because nuts, most particularly walnuts are a rich source of ALA (6.81 g/75 g walnuts). These studies examined the relationship between prostate cancer incidence or prevalence and intake or blood levels of ALA and reported that ALA increased risk of prostate cancer (Brouwer et al. 2004). However, more recent reports suggest that there is no association between ALA intake and risk of prostate cancer (Koralek et al. 2006; Simon et al. 2007). In another study of 161 men with prostate cancer, 30 days treatment with flaxseed suggested a significant protective effect on tumour proliferation rate (Demark-Wahnefried et al. 2008).

$n-3$ fatty acids have been shown to inhibit the promotion and progression stage of prostate carcinogenesis in animal models and cell culture studies. Larsson et al. (2004) has published a review on potential mechanisms. The mechanisms that mediate ALA as compared to the effects of other $n-3$ fatty acids on carcinogenesis are incompletely understood since humans can convert ALA into eicosapentaenoic acid and to some extent to docosahexaenoic acid. Most studies have been done with eicosapentaenoic and docosahexaenoic acids. Mechanisms proposed include (1) altered arachidonic acid levels that change eicosanoid biosynthesis, which results in altered inflammation and immune responses to cancer cells along with altered cell proliferation, and apoptosis; (2) alterations in signal transduction e.g. insulin sensitivity and membrane fluidity and transcription factor activity, perhaps via increased or decreased production of free radicals and reactive oxygen species, leading to changes in gene expression accompanied by changes in metabolism, cell growth, and differentiation; and (3) altered steroid metabolism, which leads to reduced estrogen-stimulated cell growth.

With respect to nut consumption and lipid signaling changes, Garg and coworkers have reported that in a human feeding trial, consumption of macadamia nuts reduced plasma LTB4 by 22% (Garg et al. 2007). This is of note as LTB4 levels have been shown to be elevated in cancers such as prostate cancer (Larre et al. 2008) and down-regulation of LTB4 levels has been shown to inhibit the development of intestinal polyps in ApcMin mice (Shen et al. 2007). LTB4 has been shown to stimulate proliferation of human colon carcinoma cells in vitro (Qiao et al. 1995; Bortuzzo et al. 1996). Blocking its receptor inhibits cancer cell growth (Kuramoto et al. 20008) and many cancer chemopreventive agents induce the metabolism of LTB4 (Primiano et al. 1999). This suggests that macadamia nuts may have an effect on colon and prostate cancer.

Another potential link between nut consumption and cancer is via fatty acid effects on oncogenes such as HER2, an oncogene whose overexpression is linked to human cancer, especially breast cancer pathogenesis (Moasser 2007). Menendez and coworkers have published several articles documenting the ability of ALA and oleic acid as well as olive oil polyphenols to modulate HER2 (Menendez and Lupu 2006; Menendez et al. 2006, 2009) via their ability to induce transcriptional repression of Her-2/neu. The effect of oleate was shown to act by affecting PEA3 protein at the promoter level (Menendez et al. 2006).

The high level of omega-3-PUFAs in nuts is important in terms of cancer as these fatty acids have been shown up-regulate the genes involved in insulin sensitivity (PPARγ), glucose transport (GLUT-2/GLUT-4), and insulin receptor signaling (IRS-1/IRS-2). Moreover, omega-3-PUFAs increase adiponectin, an anti-inflammatory and insulin-sensitizing adipokine, and induces AMPK phosphorylation, a fuel-sensing enzyme and a gatekeeper of energy balance (Gonzalez-Periz et al. 2009). These data suggest that including nuts in diets likely has beneficial effects for cancer by reducing insulin levels (Mavropoulos et al. 2006). HER receptor family crosstalks with the IGF signaling system as substantial apoptosis was only seen after complete blockade of both IGF and HER signaling pathways (Haluska et al. 2008). This crosstalk may explain the disappointing clinical activity in ovarian cancer upon targeting only the HER family of receptors (Haluska et al. 2008). High circulating IGF-I concentrations are associated with a moderately increased risk for prostate cancer and the insulin-like growth factor-I (IGF-I) pathway components have been shown to be dysregulated (Cox et al. 2009). Critically, the IGF pathway is responsive to and modifiable by diet as demonstrated by its association with many dietary and lifestyle factors (Roddam et al. 2008). The recent report by Davis et al. with respect to beneficial effects of walnuts on prostate cancer reported that plasma IGF-1 levels were significantly reduced in walnut consumption group that exhibited reduced tumor growth rate and size (Davis et al. 2009).

9.2.3.2 Phytochemicals

The content of tocochromanols such as a tocopherol is high in different nuts walnuts being particularly rich in γ-tocopherol. Several in vitro studies have demonstrated that γ-tocopherol can inhibit prostate cancer cell growth (Yu et al. 2008). Recently, Takahashi and coworkers using the TRAP rat model of prostate cancer, similar to the TRAMP mouse model, reported that while α-tocopherol was ineffective, γ-tocopherol significantly suppressed the sequential progression from high-grade prostatic intraepithelial neoplasia to adenocarcinoma in a dose-dependent manner (Takahashi et al. 2009). However, results from EPIC study results showed no association between plasma tocopherol levels and prostate cancer risk (Key et al. 2007). Wright and coworkers have reported that while supplemental vitamin E did not protect against, increased consumption of γ-tocopherol from foods was associated reduced prostate cancer risk (Wright et al. 2007). Disappointing results of the SELECT study suggest that tocopherol metabolism and cancer is more complex than initially appreciated and may, as noted, depend on not only the levels but the kinds of tocopherols.

9.2.3.3 Phytosterols

Nuts are high in phytosterols, a group a group of >200 naturally occurring plant sterols that have been shown to lower serum cholesterol and inhibit dietary cholesterol absorption (Piironen et al. 2000; Nashed et al. 2005). Multiple nut types have appreciable amounts of phytosterols ranging from 95 mg/100 g) in Brazil nuts to 280 mg/100 g in pistachios. These levels are comparable to chocolate and flaxseed. Several studies suggest phytosterols, especially beta-sitosterol, are protective from colon, prostate, and breast cancer. Animal studies have investigated the effect of dietary phytosterols on human breast cancer cells xenografted in mice (Awad, Downie et al. 2000). In animals fed phytosterols, human breast cancer tumor xenografts size was 33% smaller with 20% fewer metastases to lymph nodes and lungs after 8 weeks. In in vitro studies, both HT-29 human colon cancer cells (Awad et al. 1996) as well as human prostate cancer cells, LNCaP showed that tumor growth was inhibited by beta-sitosterol (von Holtz et al. 1998). The exact mechanism by which phytosterols offer cancer protection is not known. Potential mechanisms that have been suggested range from phytosterols being incorporated in the cell membrane, altering membrane fluidity and the activity of membrane-bound enzymes, phytosterols directly altering tumor growth signals transduction or phytosterols affecting the level of fecal sterols by altering conversion of cholesterol and primary bile acids to coprostanol and secondary bile acids by bacterial action in the large intestine.

9.2.3.4 Phenolic Compounds

Nuts especially walnuts contain a variety of phenolic compounds which includes ellagic acid. Ellagic acid has been shown to effectively induce apoptosis and inhibit angiogenesis in culture (Narayanan et al. 1999; Labrecque et al. 2005) as well as inducing down-regulation of IGF-II and increasing p21waf1/Cip1 in colon cancer cells (Narayanan and Re 2001). The linkage of phenolics to anticancer activity suggests that nuts might be effective against cancer. Ellagitannins and their hydrolysis product, ellagic acid, have been shown to inhibit prostate cancer cell growth through cell-cycle arrest and stimulation of apoptosis (Castonguay et al. 1997; Albrecht et al. 2004; Lansky et al. 2005). In addition, they inhibit NF-κB controlled inflammatory pathways along with other inflammatory pathways as well as inhibiting angiogenesis. Feeding ECGC, another phenolic compound found in nuts produced less tumor growth in an ovarian cancer xenograft animal (Spinella et al. 2006) and accentuates the positive effects of a cox-2 inhibitor in prostate cancer (Adhami et al. 2007). The effectiveness of these compounds and their common mechanisms in multiple cancers suggests that nuts which contain these compounds may also be useful for cancer such as breast cancer.

9.2.3.5 Others

Nuts are rich in phytates and inositol hexaphosphate (IP6), a polyphosphorylated carbohydrate that is present in high amounts in nuts, ranging from 2.63 mg/g in macadamia nuts to 6.70 mg/g in walnuts and 9.23 mg/g in almonds (Venkatachalam and Sathe 2006). Shamsuddin and coworkers first reported the cancer preventive ability of IP6 in carcinogen-induced colon cancer models (Vucenik and Shamsuddin 2006) and IP6 has shown significant activity in prostate, colon, pancreas, liver, and breast cancer models (Jenab and Thompson 2002; Somasundar et al. 2005; Tian 2006; Vucenik et al. 1998) and IP6. Roy and colleagues have reported in vitro and in vivo studies that demonstrate antitumor, antiproliferative, and apoptotic effects of IP6 (Roy et al. 2009). Of note the major molecular targets affected by IP6 were identified as p21 and p27 (Cip and Kip family) proteins, which were also identified as being elevated by almonds in the almond fed ApcMin mice study (Davis et al. 2003). Roy et al.'s study combined with other previous studies with IP6 (rephrase) lead Roy et al. to suggest clinical investigation of IP6 in patients with prostate cancer (Roy et al. 2009). It would appear likely that using nuts high in IP6 in cancer models would show effects on cancer.

PPARα, β/δ, γ, LXRα, β, RXRα, β, γ, PXR and FXR receptors are important nutrient sensors and regulators of gene expression to achieve metabolic homeostasis. Vanden Heuvel and coworkers have shown that extracts from walnut, pistachio and peanut were able to decrease inflammatory markers in cell culture (Vanden Heuvel et al. 2006). Walnut extract activated all PPARs tested while having little or no effect on LXRβ. In the case of pistachios, whole oil as well as the lipid extract predominantly activated PPARα but with minimal effects on the other PPARs, RXR or LXR. Comparing the effects of a variety of nuts with similar analysis done on activation by fatty acids showed that nuts showed a complex pattern that suggests that neither component alone drives the system's response (Davis et al. 2008). Of note, Tontonoz and Spiegelmann (2008) consider PPARγ as a tumor suppressor gene. They base this on the fact that PPARγ+/− mice had a markedly increase frequency of colon tumors upon treatment with azoxymethane (Girnun et al. 2002). Moreover, when the PPARγ+/− mice were crossed with the tumor-prone mice bearing a mutation in the *Apc* gene, results showed that the tumor suppressor function of PPARγ was dependent on the *Apc* gene.

9.3 Whole Diet Approach in Cancer Prevention

9.3.1 Common Mechanisms Related to Western-Type Diseases

Inflammation and oxidative stress represent a common mechanism that underlies the pathogenesis of atherosclerosis, diabetes, and cancer. The orchestration of inflammatory processes has become better defined, and in situations of prolonged or unrelenting inflammation, has been shown to provide critical ingredients for disease development and progression. For example, obesity and cancer have been linked. Obesity, particularly visceral obesity, is closely linked to the development of the metabolic syndrome, type 2 diabetes mellitus, and atherosclerotic cardiovascular disease, all characterized by chronic inflammatory states (O'Keefe et al. 2008). The processes underlying these i.e. production of cell growth promoting cytokines, induction of epithelial and macrophage cyclooxygenase-2 (COX-2), and generation of mutagenic reactive oxygen species (ROS) and reactive nitrogen species (RNS) are interrelated and makes it likely that the effects of inflammation are due to their concerted action to promote carcinogenesis. Foods affecting these pathways are likely to have effects on multiple diseases. Thus results found in CVD related studies of nuts may be applicable to cancer as well.

As an example, the Ros group has published several studies using whole diets containing walnuts showing an improvement in CVD risk markers in patients and, specifically, improved endothelial function due to walnut intake (Ros et al. 2004; Cortes et al. 2006). Endothelin is a well known mediator of inflammation and oxidative stress and our recent animal study demonstrated that walnut feeding reduced aortic endothelin messenger levels in a hamster model of atherosclerosis (Davis et al. 2006). The effect of walnuts on endothelin and this signaling molecule's effect on inflammation and oxidative stress makes it likely that walnut consumption alters (inhibit) those disease processes where inflammation and oxidative stress represent a common mechanism.

9.3.2 Do Nuts Belong in a Healthy Diet?

As noted earlier, a major if not majority constituent in all cases, of nuts are fats. There is a determination in the US Government's food regulatory framework that high fat (>30% of calories from fat) content foods cannot be considered as providing any health benefits i.e. to be healthy. Currently, 21 C.F.R. § 101.73(e) states that diets high in total fat are associated with an increased cancer risk, although the FDA intends to reevaluate the scientific evidence on dietary lipids and cancer risk to determine if the totality of the scientific evidence continues to meet their own standards of significant scientific agreement. The issue of unhealthiness of fats is of considerable import to nuts as they are and are viewed as high fat foods. The repeated efforts to demonstrate a relationship between fat intake and breast cancer starkly illustrate the difficulties that arise in trying to link fat intake to cancer causation as well as the persistence of this particular paradigm. In a very recent summary of the various studies to date regarding breast cancer and fat, Michels et al. concluded that the percentage of energy from fat during midlife and later life is not an important risk factor (Michels et al. 2007). They suggested that energy balance has a major impact on breast cancer risk and that this was mainly mediated through childhood growth rates and weight gain in adult life. Other studies have suggested that a high carbohydrate diet, the obverse diet of a high fat diet, may raise cancer risk, specifically prostrate cancer (Leitzmann 2005). A significant amount of the scientific arguments made to support that elevated fat intake and cancer are related are the result of the conflation of two very different questions i.e. the link between fat intake and obesity and the link between obesity and cancer. For the latter, data clearly demonstrates that obesity is linked to elevated cancer. In fact, Food, Nutrition, Physical Activity, and the Prevention of Cancer: a Global Perspective has now judged the evidence as convincing with respect to excess body fat raising the risk for cancer of the colon, kidney, pancreas, adenocarcinoma of the esophagus and endometrium as well as post-menopausal breast cancer (World Cancer Res Fund 2007). However the former, i.e. the linkage between fat intake and obesity is by no means proven. It is widely recognized that obesity results from excess energy input relative to energy output. But research using weight loss (Astrup et al. 2004; McAuley et al. 2006; Westman et al. 2007) to assess the effect of calories from carbohydrates, protein and fats have been equivocal. Moreover, studies assessing the association in the general population between carbohydrate, protein and lipid intakes and BMI and waist circumference, indicators of overweight and obesity have been inconclusive (Roberts et al. 2002; Liu et al. 2003; Howarth et al. 2005; Halkjaer et al. 2006). Even a very recent large population study was unable to show any link between fat intake and obesity after fully statistically adjusting their models (Ahluwalia et al. 2009). Moreover, total fat consists of different fatty acid families, e.g., SFAs, MUFAs, and $n-3$ and $n-6$ PUFAs. While studies suggest that different fatty acids have different effects on carcinogenesis, these associations remain difficult to firmly establish in human epidemiological studies (Tsubura et al. 2009).

9.3.3 Nuts Versus Its Components in Cancer Prevention

Finally, while this review has sought to link consumption of nuts and reduced cancer risk, one of the approaches adopted, i.e. citing studies in other foods, which have tested components that are the same or similar to those found in nuts raises an issue that remains at the heart of unraveling the diet-cancer links. That is the degree to which the findings represent the action of multiple components acting in concert to produce the effects noted. The reductionist approach to diet-cancer interactions i.e. the central assumption that specific components are responsible for the effects noted and can be identified is likely incomplete. This limitation has been repeatedly demonstrated as substances when delivered as supplements or pills produce results that differ markedly in their disease-related effects compared to when these same components are consumed as food. Several recent large studies clearly highlight this. The Women's Health Initiative tracked multivitamin use in more than 161,000 postmenopausal women and after a median follow-up of 8.0 and 7.9 years in the clinical trial and observational study cohorts, respectively, showed no evidence that multivitamins reduced the risk of common cancers, CVD, or total mortality in postmenopausal women (Neuhouser et al. 2009). The well-documented beneficial effects of Mediterranean-style diets on endothelial dysfunction and markers of vascular inflammation (Trichopoulou et al. 2003) are in contrast to the absence of documented beneficial effects for individual components (Esposito et al. 2004; Genkinger et al. 2004). With respect to cancer, despite Mutanen et al.'s report showing that berries high in ellagic acid were effective against gastrointestinal cancer in an animal study, they found that pure ellagic acid had no effect on the number or size of adenomas in the distal or total small intestine in Apc- mutated Min/+ mice (Mutanen et al. 2008). Not only that but ellagic acid increased adenoma size in the duodenum when compared with the control diet ($p < 0.05$). In addition, 2 relatively recent studies have reported that tocopherol used as a supplement either provided no benefit or actually increased overall mortality risk or coronary heart failure, respectively (Miller et al. 2005; Bjelakovic et al. 2007). The observed health benefits of diets rich in fruits, vegetables, and whole grains are not reproduced by specific compounds. Other studies have consistently shown that single components are unable to provide the benefits ascribed to them when consumed as part of food e.g. calcium and vitamin D had no influence on women's risk of breast cancer (Kavanaugh, Trumbo et al. 2009; Neuhouser, Wassertheil-Smoller et al. 2009). Temple et al. have reported in their review of more than 200 cohort and case-control studies of fruit and vegetable intake and cancer, that they found support for a teamwork concept of fruit and vegetable intake i.e. that an intake of wide variety was required for optimal protection and that it was unlikely there were specific compounds responsible (Temple and Gladwin 2003). Most recently, the hugely expensive SELECT trial on selenium and vitamin E on prostate cancer in patients was halted in September 2008 when its independent data and safety monitoring committee determined that no benefit from either study agent was convincingly demonstrated ($p < 0.0001$) (Lippman et al. 2009). Remarkably α-tocopherol alone was selected as the vitamin E supplement despite evidence that α-tocopherol alone was unlikely to be effective. This arises as α-tocopherol and γ-tocopherol levels have been shown interact with respect to prostate cancer risk (Helzlsouer et al. 2000; Huang et al. 2003). Moreover, a study from the mid-1980s had shown that increasing α-tocopherol intake results in declines in γ-tocopherol levels (Handelman et al. 1985). These data suggest that the α-tocopherol supplement based trial could actually increase prostate cancer risk by driving γ-tocopherol levels down. And this is what in fact appears to have occurred, as an increased prostate cancer risk in men supplemented with α-tocopherol was found (Lippman et al. 2009). Bjelakovic et al. have recently reported that based on a meta-analysis of 20 randomized trials assessing antioxidants supplementation in over 200,000 participants, they could find no evidence that the studied antioxidant supplements prevented gastrointestinal cancers but rather seemed to increase overall mortality (Bjelakovic et al. 2008). Finally, in a very recent review, de Kok et al. again noted that multiple studies have demonstrated that purified phytochemicals did not necessarily exert the same beneficial health effect as when the compound source was a food or even a complete specific diet (de Kok et al. 2008). De Kok et al. concluded that combinations of dietary chemopreventive agents result in significant activities at concentrations where any single agent was inactive, that some food items or diets show cancer preventive effects which cannot be explained based on individual bioactive ingredients and, that, despite the molecular mechanism(s) behind the observed combinatorial effects being ill defined, synergistic effects should be further explored (de Kok et al. 2008; Demark-Wahnefried et al. 2008).

9.4 Conclusions

This review suggests, by using both the limited number of studies available and extrapolating from the effects of constituents of nuts, that tree nuts have likely to have significant anticancer effects. Overall, as recognized by the Food, Nutrition, Physical Activity, and the Prevention of Cancer: a Global Perspective, studies have show some intriguing potential positive relationships between nuts and cancer but data limitations prevent the identification of nut-specific effects. The potential of a positive association between nuts and cancer then leads to the urgent need for more studies but only if stringent approaches to better identify and quantify the intake of specific nuts and seeds are implemented. Therefore nuts should be included in a healthy diet; moreover they should be included in a whole food approach to cancer prevention. This latter note is recognition that there is the need to test the effects of whole nuts as well as whole diets, given the difficulties that arise when focusing on single ingredients (Jacobs et al. 2009). In conclusion, this chapter has hopefully provided renewed impetus to explore tree nuts, this age-old foodstuff, and their place in promoting health via positive effects on cancer derived from the unique package of nutrients they bring to the table. Also it identifies the need for conclusive demonstrations of the actual effects of nut consumption on cancer as well as other diseases via further studies

References

Adhami VM, Malik A et al (2007) Combined inhibitory effects of green tea polyphenols and selective cyclooxygenase-2 inhibitors on the growth of human prostate cancer cells both in vitro and in vivo. Clin Cancer Res 13:1611–1619

Aggarwal BB, Banerjee S et al (2007) Curcumin induces the degradation of cyclin E expression through ubiquitin-dependent pathway and up-regulates cyclin-dependent kinase inhibitors p21 and p27 in multiple human tumor cell lines. Biochem Pharmacol 73:1024–1032

Ahluwalia N, Ferrieres J et al (2009) Association of macronutrient intake patterns with being overweight in a population-based random sample of men in France. Diabetes Metab 35: 129–136

Albrecht M, Jiang W et al (2004) Pomegranate extracts potently suppress proliferation, xenograft growth, and invasion of human prostate cancer cells. J Med Food 7:274–283

Astrup A, Meinert Larsen T et al (2004) Atkins and other low-carbohydrate diets: hoax or an effective tool for weight loss? Lancet 364:897–899

Awad AB, Chen YC et al (1996) beta-Sitosterol inhibits HT-29 human colon cancer cell growth and alters membrane lipids. Anticancer Res 16:2797–2804

Awad AB, Downie A et al (2000) Dietary phytosterol inhibits the growth and metastasis of MDA-MB-231 human breast cancer cells grown in SCID mice. Anticancer Res 20:821–824

Bjelakovic G, Nikolova D et al (2007) Mortality in randomized trials of antioxidant supplements for primary and secondary prevention: systematic review and meta-analysis. JAMA 297: 842–857

Bjelakovic G, Nikolova D et al (2008) Systematic review: primary and secondary prevention of gastrointestinal cancers with antioxidant supplements. Aliment Pharmacol Ther 28:689–703

Bortuzzo C, Hanif R et al (1996) The effect of leukotrienes B and selected HETEs on the proliferation of colon cancer cells. Biochim Biophys Acta 1300:240–246

Brouwer IA, Katan MB, et al (2004) Dietary alpha-linolenic acid is associated with reduced risk of fatal coronary heart disease, but increased prostate cancer risk: a meta-analysis. J Nutr 134: 919–922

Brufau G, Boatella J et al (2006) Nuts: source of energy and macronutrients. Br J Nutr 96(Suppl 2):S24–28

Castonguay A, Gali HU et al (1997) Antitumorigenic and antipromoting activities of ellagic acid, ellagitannins and oligomeric anthocyanin and procyanidin. Int J Oncol 10:367–373

Catalona WJ, Smith DS et al (1997) Prostate cancer detection in men with serum PSA concentrations of 2.6–4.0 ng/mL and benign prostate examination. Enhancement of specificity with free PSA measurements. JAMA 277:1452–1455

Chen CY, Blumberg JB (2008) Phytochemical composition of nuts. Asia Pac J Clin Nutr 17(Suppl 1):329–332

Coates AM, Howe PR (2007) Edible nuts and metabolic health. Curr Opin Lipidol 18:25–30

Cortes B, Nunez I et al (2006) Acute effects of high-fat meals enriched with walnuts or olive oil on postprandial endothelial function. J Am Coll Cardiol 48:1666–1671

Cox ME, Gleave ME et al (2009) Insulin receptor expression by human prostate cancers. Prostate 69:33–40

Davis P, Iwahashi C et al (2003) Whole almonds activate gastrointestinal (GI) tract antiproliferative signaling in APC(min) (multiple intestinal neoplasia) mice. FASEB J 17:A1153

Davis P, Valacchi G et al (2006) Walnuts reduce aortic ET-1 mRNA levels in hamsters fed a high-fat, atherogenic diet. J Nutr 136:428–432

Davis PA, Gohil K et al (2009) Walnut feeding effects on prostate tumor size and growth in TRAMP mice. 20th Annual AICR research conference on food, nutrition, physical activity and cancer, AICR, Washington, DC

Davis PA, Iwahashi CK (2001) Whole almonds and almond fractions reduce aberrant crypt foci in a rat model of colon carcinogenesis. Cancer Lett 165:27–33

Davis PA, Jenab M et al (2008) Tree nut and peanut consumption in relation to chronic and metabolic diseases including allergy. J Nutr 138:1757S–1762S

de Kok TM, van Breda SG et al (2008) Mechanisms of combined action of different chemopreventive dietary compounds: a review. Eur J Nutr 47(Suppl 2):51–59

Demark-Wahnefried W, Polascik TJ et al (2008) Flaxseed supplementation (not dietary fat restriction) reduces prostate cancer proliferation rates in men presurgery. Cancer Epidemiol Biomarkers Prev 17:3577–3587

Esposito K, Marfella R et al (2004) Effect of a mediterranean-style diet on endothelial dysfunction and markers of vascular inflammation in the metabolic syndrome: a randomized trial. JAMA 292:1440–1446

Eto I (2006) Nutritional and chemopreventive anti-cancer agents up-regulate expression of p27Kip1, a cyclin-dependent kinase inhibitor, in mouse JB6 epidermal and human MCF7, MDA-MB-321 and AU565 breast cancer cells . Cancer Cell Int 6:20

Garg ML, Blake RJ et al (2007) Macadamia nut consumption modulates favourably risk factors for coronary artery disease in hypercholesterolemic subjects. Lipids 42:583–587

Genkinger JM, Platz EA et al (2004) Fruit, vegetable, and antioxidant intake and all-cause, cancer, and cardiovascular disease mortality in a community-dwelling population in Washington County, Maryland. Am J Epidemiol 160:1223–1233

Girnun GD, Smith WM et al (2002) APC-dependent suppression of colon carcinogenesis by PPARgamma. Proc Natl Acad Sci USA 99:13771–13776

Gonzalez-Periz A, Horrillo R et al (2009) Obesity-induced insulin resistance and hepatic steatosis are alleviated by {omega}-3 fatty acids: a role for resolvins and protectins. FASEB J 23: 1946–1957

Halkjaer J, Tjonneland A et al (2006) Intake of macronutrients as predictors of 5-y changes in waist circumference. Am J Clin Nutr 84:789–797

Haluska P, Carboni JM et al (2008) HER receptor signaling confers resistance to the insulin-like growth factor-I receptor inhibitor, BMS-536924. Mol Cancer Ther 7: 2589–2598

Handelman GJ, Machlin LJ et al (1985) Oral alpha-tocopherol supplements decrease plasma gamma-tocopherol levels in humans. J Nutr 115:807–813

Helzlsouer KJ, Huang HY, et al (2000) Association between alpha-tocopherol, gamma-tocopherol, selenium, and subsequent prostate cancer. J Natl Cancer Inst 92:2018–2023

Howarth NC, Huang TT et al (2005) Dietary fiber and fat are associated with excess weight in young and middle-aged US adults. J Am Diet Assoc 105:1365–1372

Huang HY, Alberg AJ et al (2003) Prospective study of antioxidant micronutrients in the blood and the risk of developing prostate cancer. Am J Epidemiol 157:335–344

Hulit J, Lee RJ et al (2006) p27Kip1 repression of ErbB2-induced mammary tumor growth in transgenic mice involves Skp2 and Wnt/beta-catenin signaling. Cancer Res 66: 8529–8541

Ion G, Akinsete JA et al (2009) Walnut consumption decreases mammary gland tumor incidence, multiplicity and growth in the C(3)1Tag transgenic mouse. 2009 AACR Annual Meeting, AACR, Denver, LB–247

Jacobs DR Jr, Gross MD, Tapsell LC (2009) Food synergy: an operational concept for understanding nutrition. Am J Clin Nutr 89(5):1543S–1548S

Jain MG, Hislop GT et al (1999) Plant foods, antioxidants, and prostate cancer risk: findings from case-control studies in Canada. Nutr Cancer 34:173–184

Jenab M, Ferrari P et al (2004) Association of nut and seed intake with colorectal cancer risk in the European Prospective Investigation into Cancer and Nutrition. Cancer Epidemiol Biomarkers Prev 13:1595–1603

Jenab M, Thompson LU (2002) Purified and endogenous phytic acid in wheat bran affects early biomarkers of colon cancer risk. IARC Sci Publ 156:387–389

Kavanaugh CJ, Trumbo PR et al (2009) Qualified health claims for calcium and colorectal, breast, and prostate cancers: The U.S. Food and Drug Administration's evidence-based review. Nutr Cancer 61:157–164

Key TJ, Appleby PN et al (2007) Plasma carotenoids, retinol, and tocopherols and the risk of prostate cancer in the European Prospective Investigation into Cancer and Nutrition study. Am J Clin Nutr 86:672–681

Kim YJ, Cho YJ et al (2008) The association between metabolic syndrome and prostate-specific antigen levels. Int J Urol 15:905–909

Koralek DO, Peters U et al (2006) A prospective study of dietary alpha-linolenic acid and the risk of prostate cancer (United States). Cancer Causes Control 17:783–791

Kune S, Kune GA et al (1987) Case-control study of dietary etiological factors: the Melbourne Colorectal Cancer Study. Nutr Cancer 9:21–42

Kuramoto M, Sakata Y et al (2008) Preparation of leukotriene B(4) inhibitory active 2- and 3-(2-aminothiazol-4-yl)benzo[*b*]furan derivatives and their growth inhibitory activity on human pancreatic cancer cells. Org Biomol Chem 6:2772–2781

Labrecque L, Lamy S et al (2005) Combined inhibition of PDGF and VEGF receptors by ellagic acid, a dietary-derived phenolic compound. Carcinogenesis 26:821–826

Lansky EP, Jiang W et al (2005) Possible synergistic prostate cancer suppression by anatomically discrete pomegranate fractions. Invest New Drugs 23:11–20

Larre S, Tran N et al (2008) PGE2 and LTB4 tissue levels in benign and cancerous prostates. Prostaglandins Other Lipid Mediat 87:14–19

Larsson SC, Kumlin M et al (2004) Dietary long-chain *n*–3 fatty acids for the prevention of cancer: a review of potential mechanisms. Am J Clin Nutr 79:935–945

Leitzmann MF (2005) Is there a link between macronutrient intake and prostate cancer? Nat Clin Pract Oncol 2:184–185

Lippman SM, Klein EA et al (2009) Effect of selenium and vitamin E on risk of prostate cancer and other cancers: the Selenium and Vitamin E Cancer Prevention Trial (SELECT). JAMA 301:39–51

Liu S, Willett WC et al (2003) Relation between changes in intakes of dietary fiber and grain products and changes in weight and development of obesity among middle-aged women. Am J Clin Nutr 78:920–927

Mavropoulos JC, Isaacs WB et al (2006) Is there a role for a low-carbohydrate ketogenic diet in the management of prostate cancer? Urology 68:15–18

McAuley KA, Smith KJ et al (2006) Long-term effects of popular dietary approaches on weight loss and features of insulin resistance. Int J Obes (Lond) 30:342–349

Menendez JA, Lupu R (2006) Mediterranean dietary traditions for the molecular treatment of human cancer: anti-oncogenic actions of the main olive oil's monounsaturated fatty acid oleic acid (18:1*n*–9). Curr Pharm Biotechnol 7:495–502

Menendez JA, Papadimitropoulo A et al (2006) A genomic explanation connecting Mediterranean diet, olive oil and cancer: oleic acid, the main monounsaturated fatty acid of olive oil, induces formation of inhibitory PEA3 transcription factor-PEA3 DNA binding site complexes at the Her-2/neu (erbB-2) oncogene promoter in breast, ovarian and stomach cancer cells. Eur J Cancer 42:2425–2432

Menendez JA, Vazquez-Martin A et al (2009) Extra-virgin olive oil polyphenols inhibit HER2 (erbB-2)-induced malignant transformation in human breast epithelial cells: relationship between the chemical structures of extra-virgin olive oil secoiridoids and lignans and their inhibitory activities on the tyrosine kinase activity of HER2. Int J Oncol 34: 43–51

Menendez JA, Vazquez-Martin A et al (2006) HER2 (erbB-2)-targeted effects of the omega-3 polyunsaturated fatty acid, alpha-linolenic acid (ALA; 18:3n–3), in breast cancer cells: the fat features of the Mediterranean diet as an anti-HER2 cocktail. Clin Transl Oncol 8:812–820

Michels KB, MohllajeAP et al (2007) Diet and breast cancer: a review of the prospective observational studies. Cancer 109: 2712–2749

Miller ER, Pastor-Barrius R et al (2005) Meta-analysis: high-dosage vitamin E supplementation may increase all-cause mortality. Ann Intern Med 142:37–46

Moasser MM (2007) The oncogene HER2: its signaling and transforming functions and its role in human cancer pathogenesis. Oncogene 26:6469–6487

Mutanen M, Pajari AM et al (2008) Berries as chemopreventive dietary constituents – a mechanistic approach with the ApcMin/+ mouse. Asia Pac J Clin Nutr 17(Suppl 1):123–125

Narayanan BA, Geoffroy O et al (1999) p53/p21(WAF1/CIP1) expression and its possible role in G1 arrest and apoptosis in ellagic acid treated cancer cells. Cancer Lett 136:215–221

Narayanan BA, Re GG (2001) IGF-II down regulation associated cell cycle arrest in colon cancer cells exposed to phenolic antioxidant ellagic acid. Anticancer Res 21:359–364

Nashed B, Yeganeh B et al (2005) Antiatherogenic effects of dietary plant sterols are associated with inhibition of proinflammatory cytokine production in apo E-KO mice. J Nutr 135: 2438–2444

Neuhouser ML, Wassertheil-Smoller S et al (2009) Multivitamin use and risk of cancer and cardiovascular disease in the Women's Health Initiative cohorts. Arch Intern Med 169:294–304

O'Keefe JH, Gheewala NM, O'Keefe JO (2008) Dietary strategies for improving post-prandial glucose, lipids, inflammation, and cardiovascular health. J Am Coll Cardiol 51(3):249–255

Petridou E, Kedikoglou S et al (2002) Diet in relation to endometrial cancer risk: a case-control study in Greece. Nutr Cancer 44:16–22

Pickle LW, Greene MH et al (1984) Colorectal cancer in rural Nebraska. Cancer Res 44:363–369

Piironen V, Lindsay DG et al (2000) Plant sterols: Biosynthesis, biological function and their importance to human nutrition. J Sci Food Agric 80:939–966

Primiano T, Kensler TW et al (1999) Induction of leukotriene B4 metabolism by cancer chemopreventive agents. Adv Exp Med Biol 469:599–605

Qiao L, Kozoni V et al (1995) Selected eicosanoids increase the proliferation rate of human colon carcinoma cell lines and mouse colonocytes in vivo. Biochim Biophys Acta 1258:215–223

Roberts SB, McCrory MA et al (2002) The influence of dietary composition on energy intake and body weight. J Am Coll Nutr 21:140S–145S

Roddam AW, Allen NE et al (2008) Insulin-like growth factors, their binding proteins, and prostate cancer risk: analysis of individual patient data from 12 prospective studies. Ann Intern Med 149:461–471

Ros E, Mataix J (2006) Fatty acid composition of nuts – implications for cardiovascular health. Br J Nutr 96(Suppl 2):S29–35

Ros E, Nunez I et al (2004) A walnut diet improves endothelial function in hypercholesterolemic subjects: a randomized crossover trial. Circulation 109:1609–1614

Roy S, Gu M et al (2009) p21/Cip1 and p27/Kip1 Are essential molecular targets of inositol hexaphosphate for its antitumor efficacy against prostate cancer. Cancer Res 69:1166–1173

Sabate J, Ros E et al (2006) Nuts: nutrition and health outcomes. Preface. Br J Nutr 96(Suppl 2):S1–2

Shen G, Khor TO et al (2007) Chemoprevention of familial adenomatous polyposis by natural dietary compounds sulforaphane and dibenzoylmethane alone and in combination in ApcMin/+ mouse. Cancer Res 67:9937–9944

Simon JA, Tanzman JS et al (2007) Lack of effect of walnuts on serum levels of prostate specific antigen: a brief report. J Am Coll Nutr 26:317–320

Singh PN, Fraser GE (1998) Dietary risk factors for colon cancer in a low-risk population. Am J Epidemiol 148:761–774

Somasundar P, Riggs, DR et al (2005) Inositol hexaphosphate (IP6): a novel treatment for pancreatic cancer. J Surg Res 126:199–203

Spaccarotella KJ, Kris-Etherton PM et al (2008) The effect of walnut intake on factors related to prostate and vascular health in older men. Nutr J 7:13.

Spinella F, Rosano L et al (2006) Green tea polyphenol epigallocatechin-3-gallate inhibits the endothelin axis and downstream signaling pathways in ovarian carcinoma. Mol Cancer Ther 5:1483–1492

Takahashi S, Takeshita K et al (2009) Suppression of prostate cancer in a transgenic rat model via gamma-tocopherol activation of caspase signaling. Prostate 69:644–651

Temple NJ, Gladwin KK (2003) Fruit, vegetables, and the prevention of cancer: research challenges. Nutrition 19:467–470

Tian WX (2006) Inhibition of fatty acid synthase by polyphenols. Curr Med Chem 13: 967–977

Tontonoz P, Spiegelman BM (2008) Fat and beyond: the diverse biology of PPARgamma. Annu Rev Biochem 77:289–312

Trichopoulou A, Costacou T et al (2003) Adherence to a Mediterranean diet and survival in a Greek population. N Engl J Med 348:2599–2608

Tsubura A, Yuri T et al (2009) Role of fatty acids in malignancy and visual impairment: epidemiological evidence and experimental studies. Histol Histopathol 24:223–234

Vanden Heuvel JP, Thompson JT et al (2006) Differential activation of nuclear receptors by per-fluorinated fatty acid analogs and natural fatty acids: a comparison of human, mouse, and rat peroxisome proliferator-activated receptor-alpha, -beta, and -gamma, liver X receptor-beta, and retinoid X receptor-alpha. Toxicol Sci 92:476–489

Venkatachalam M, Sathe SK (2006) Chemical composition of selected edible nut seeds. J Agric Food Chem 54:4705–4714

von Holtz RL, Fink CS et al (1998) Beta-Sitosterol activates the sphingomyelin cycle and induces apoptosis in LNCaP human prostate cancer cells. Nutr Cancer 32:8–12

Vucenik I, Shamsuddin AM (2006) Protection against cancer by dietary IP6 and inositol. Nutr Cancer 55:109–125

Vucenik I, Zhang ZS et al (1998) IP6 in treatment of liver cancer. II. Intra-tumoral injection of IP6 regresses pre-existing human liver cancer xenotransplanted in nude mice. Anticancer Res 18:4091–4096

Westman EC, Feinman RD et al (2007) Low-carbohydrate nutrition and metabolism. Am J Clin Nutr 86:276–284

World Cancer Research Fund/American Institute for Cancer Research (2007) Food, nutrition, physical activity, and the prevention of cancer: a global perspective. AICR, Washington, DC

Wright ME, Weinstein SJ et al (2007) Supplemental and dietary vitamin E intakes and risk of prostate cancer in a large prospective study. Cancer Epidemiol Biomarkers Prev 16:1128–1135

Wu X, Beecher GR et al (2004) Lipophilic and hydrophilic antioxidant capacities of common foods in the United States. J Agric Food Chem 52:4026–4037

Yamada Y, Mori H (2007) Multistep carcinogenesis of the colon in Apc(Min/+) mouse. Cancer Sci 98:6–10

Yu W, Park SK et al (2008) RRR-gamma-tocopherol induces human breast cancer cells to undergo apoptosis via death receptor 5 (DR5)-mediated apoptotic signaling. Cancer Lett 259:165–176

Chapter 10
Whole Grains and Their Constituents in the Prevention of Colon Cancer

Anne-Maria Pajari

Abstract Cereal grains are important stable food worldwide. When used as whole-grain products, they provide a good source, not only of energy and protein, but minerals, vitamins, phytochemicals and dietary fibre. Since 1970s, evidence has been accumulating to suggest that high consumption of whole grains protects against cardiovascular diseases and certain types of cancers, particularly colon cancer. This chapter gives first a brief overview of the epidemiological evidence regarding whole grains and colon cancer and then reviews the substantial number of experimental studies which have investigated the effects of different whole grains and their constituents on colon carcinogenesis in animal models. Lastly, the underlying mechanisms whereby whole grains mediate their effects on colon cancer development will be discussed.

Keywords Cereal grain · Colon cancer · Butyrate · Bile acids · Phytoestrogens

Contents

A. Pajari (✉)
Division of Nutrition, Department of Food and Environmental Sciences, University of Helsinki, Helsinki 00014, Finland
e-mail: anne-maria.pajari@helsinki.fi

M. Mutanen, A.-M. Pajari (eds.), *Vegetables, Whole Grains, and Their Derivatives in Cancer Prevention*, Diet and Cancer 2, DOI 10.1007/978-90-481-9800-9_10,
© Springer Science+Business Media B.V. 2011

10.1 Introduction

Since the era of agriculture began approximately 10, 000 years ago, cereal grains have become the foundation of human diets around the world. In many societies, cereals are staple food and provide a major source of dietary energy and protein. The main cereal grains grown today are wheat, oats, rye, barley, maize (corn), rice, millets and sorghum, of which wheat and rice are the two most important grains used as human food worldwide. By definition, grains are one-seeded fruits of cultivated cereal grasses. The grain is composed of the starchy endosperm, the nutrient-rich germ, and the outer layers of the grain, often called as bran. Bran is not an exact term but refers merely to a by-product comprising the outer coverings of a grain, derived from refining process of common cereals (Fulcher and Duke 2002).

Whole grains are rich in many nutrients (Table 10.1). In general, the composition of all cereals is similar so that they contain carbohydrates in the range of 55–71%, proteins 6–15% and lipids 1–7%. Particularly the bran part of whole grains is a very good source of dietary fibre, originally defined as intrinsic plant cell wall polysaccharides consisting of cellulose, hemicellulose, and lignin (Trowell 1976). Whole grains also provide vitamin E, folate and other vitamin Bs, minerals and trace elements such as zinc, magnesium and selenium, as well as a number of phytochemicals such as phytates, tannins, enzyme inhibitors, phytosterols, lignans (diphenolics), phenolic acids and polyphenolics.

As dietary fibre, vitamins, minerals and phytochemicals are concentrated in the bran and germ, removing these parts during refining of grains results in substantially reduced nutritional values of refined grain products in comparison to whole-grain products. The inventions in milling technology in the 19th century led to the situation where consumption of whole grains was largely replaced by refined grains in industrialised countries. This change among other changes in dietary practices and in lifestyle related to urbanisation has been associated with the increased rates of cardiovascular diseases and certain types of cancers worldwide.

10.2 Epidemiological Evidence on Whole Grains and Colon Cancer

World Cancer Research Found (WCRF) and American Institute for Cancer Research (AICR) published their latest comprehensive review on the epidemiological evidence on food, nutrition and cancer in 2007. Somewhat surprisingly, the report

Table 10.1 Composition of some whole-grain flours (g/100 g raw)

	Wheat	Rice	Maize	Oats	Rye	Barley
Energy (kcal)	309	321	335	355	277	313
Protein	10.6	6.1	8.5	14.5	8.8	8.3
Lipids, total	2.2	0.7	1.6	7.3	1.9	2.0
Saturated fatty acids	0.2	<0.1	0.2	0.7	0.2	0.3
Monounsaturated	0.3	0.1	0.4	1.6	0.2	0.2
Polyunsaturated	0.9	0.1	0.7	1.6	0.6	0.7
Sterols (mg)	74.4	72.3	89.5	40.9	95.4	62.1
Carbohydrate	70.6	78.8	77.6	67.0	69.3	72.0
Starch	60.0	70.0	69.6	55.7	53.0	63.5
Sugars	0.7	1.4	0.6	1.3	2.4	0.9
Dietary fibre	9.9	7.4	7.4	10.0	13.9	7.6
Insoluble	8.9	6.3	NA	4.6	11.4	6.6
Soluble	1.0	1.1	NA	1.1	2.2	1.0
Minerals (mg)						
Sodium	2.0	6.0	3.0	2.0	5.0	4.0
Potassium	390	260	162	410	500	360
Magnesium	127	110	40	134	114	89
Calcium	26	11	5.0	43	30	23
Phosphorus	350	250	84	430	356	300
Iron	5.2	3.6	1.1	6.3	4.9	4.5
Zinc	3.6	1.6	0.7	4.5	3.3	2.8
Iodine (μg)	5.0	5.0	NA	20	5.0	5.0
Selenium (μg)	9.5	23.0	7.8	8.6	2.8	8.6
Vitamins (mg)						
Vitamin C	0.0	0.0	0.0	0.0	0.0	0.0
Vitamin A (μg)	0.4	0.0	10.7	0.0	0.5	0.0
Vitamin D (μg)	0.0	0.0	0.0	0.0	0.0	0.0
Vitamin E	1.0	0.6	0.2	0.9	1.0	0.3
Vitamin K (μg)	2.6	0.8	0.3	2.1	5.9	2.2
Folate (μg)	50	20	48	46	72	19
Niacin	5.0	4.3	1.0	0.8	0.2	5.5
Riboflavin	0.15	0.03	0.05	0.09	0.16	0.12
Thiamin	0.35	0.05	0.14	0.33	0.31	0.40
B12 (μg)	0.0	0.0	0.0	0.0	0.0	0.0
Pyridoxine	0.11	0.61	0.26	0.13	0.17	0.10
Carotenoids (μg)	224.1	0.0	1515	177.0	219.7	162.4

NA, not available

Source: Composition data from Fineli, the Finnish Food Composition Database. Helsinki: National Institute for Health and Welfare. Available from: http://www.fineli.fi

summarises the evidence regarding cereal grains and cancer to be too limited in amount, consistency, or quality to draw any conclusions (WCRF/AICR 2007). One reason for this may be the limitations in assessing actual dietary intake of whole grains in epidemiological studies. The definition of whole-grain products varies in food frequency questionnaires, typically including cereal brans and any dark breads and crackers. The accuracy of quantitation in questionnaires also differs and sometimes only a preference of using whole-grain instead of refined flour products has been asked.

Nevertheless, epidemiological research on whole grain consumption in relation to cancer risk has been carried out. Two well-known meta-analyses by Jacobs et al. (1995 and 1998) studied the association between whole grain intake and cancers at several sites. The first analysis included one prospective and 14 case-control studies of colorectal, gastric and endometrial cancers, and the second analysis included 40 case-control studies and 20 tumour types. The strongest evidence was found for the role of whole-grain products in reducing the risk for gastrointestinal cancers, including colorectal and gastric cancers. Recently, Schatzkin et al. (2007, 2008) reported results of a large prospective cohort study which showed that intakes of whole-grain products and fibre from grains are associated with lower risk of colorectal and small intestinal cancers. In a smaller cohort of Swedish women, high consumption of whole grains was associated with lower risk of colon but not rectal cancer (Larsson et al. 2005). Interestingly, consumption of hard whole-grain rye bread and intake of cereal fibre were inversely associated with colon cancer risk in this study. Women in the top quintile of cereal fibre intake had a 27% reduction in colon cancer risk compared to those in the bottom quintile, indicating that fibre partly explained the protective effect of whole grains (Larsson et al. 2005). Similarly, Slattery et al. (2004) found that rectal cancer was inversely associated with intakes of whole-grain products and dietary fibre, particularly insoluble fibre.

Whole-grain foods are a good source of especially insoluble dietary fibre and contribute significantly to total fibre intake. A substantial number of epidemiological studies have been conducted to study the relation of dietary fibre intake to cancer risk. The WCRF/AICR report (2007) summarises results from altogether sixteen cohort and 91 case-control studies carried out on fibre-rich foods and colorectal cancer. The expert panel regards the evidence consistent to suggest that dietary fibre probably protects against colorectal cancer (WCRF/AICR 2007). Strong evidence supporting the role of fibre in preventing colon cancer comes from the results of the European Prospective Investigation into Cancer and Nutrition (EPIC) study which consisted of 22 subcohorts in ten European countries with a large range of intakes of dietary fibre (Bingham et al. 2003). In EPIC, total dietary fibre intake was associated with lower colorectal cancer risk. After correcting fibre intake from the dietary questionnaire with intake from the 24-h recall, the reduction in risk was 40% for the highest intake group when compared to the lowest. The EPIC results have been challenged by the results from the Pooling Project of Prospective Studies of Diet and Cancer which found no significant association between dietary fibre intake and colon cancer after adjusting for other risk factors (Park et al. 2005). One plausible reason for the discrepancy between the study results may be differences in study populations and their dietary practices including the heterogeneous nature of dietary fibre consumed. Most cohorts in the Pooling Project come from the USA, whereas EPIC cohorts are strictly European. In EPIC study, fibre from cereals showed strongest inverse relation to colorectal cancer, while in US populations fibre from vegetables, fruits and beans contributes more than cereal fibre to the total fibre intake (Schatzkin et al. 2007).

10.3 Effects of Whole-grain Cereals and Their Constituents on Colon Carcinogenesis in Experimental Animals

10.3.1 Wheat and Its Constituents

Wheat and particularly wheat bran has been extensively studied in experimental animal models of colon cancer (Table 10.2). The early studies have focused on the role of wheat bran as a concentrated source of dietary fibre, mostly insoluble, and presumed that the anticarcinogenic effects of wheat bran are due to its dietary fibre content. In these studies, diets with rather high levels of wheat bran (15–20% w/w) in combination of high or low fat content and of different fat types have been fed to carcinogen-treated rats during and after carcinogen administration (Table 10.2). In most cases wheat bran feeding has resulted in a reduction of the incidence of colon tumours and, somewhat less frequently, also a reduction in the multiplicity of colon tumours regardless of the type or quantity of fat in the diet (for example Wilson et al. 1977; Reddy et al. 1981). Results seem to be partly dependent on the carcinogen used (Watanabe et al. 1979) and wheat bran tends to be more protective when given after carcinogen treatment (Barnes et al. 1983). One study actually reports a strong enhancing effect on tumorigenesis of wheat bran when given during carcinogen administration, i.e. at the initiation stage (Jacobs 1983). More recently, lower levels of wheat bran have been shown to reduce the number of preneoplastic aberrant crypt foci (ACF) as well as tumour incidence and multiplicity in azoxymethane (AOM)-treated rats (Alabaster et al. 1993, 1995, Table 10.2).

In 1990s the development of genetically modified mouse models brought new tools for cancer research, including the Multiple intestinal neoplasia (Min) mouse and the Apc[delta716] mouse which develop spontaneous intestinal tumours owing to a germ line mutation in the Adenomatous polyposis coli (Apc) tumour suppressor gene. Compared to carcinogen-treated rats, these mice provide a closer resemblance to human colon cancer pathobiology (Preston et al. 2008) even though majority of tumours develop in the distal small intestine. Wheat bran has been tested in three studies using Apc-mutated mice (Table 10.2). Hioki et al. (1997) found that 20% wheat bran in a high-fat diet reduced the number of polyps by 36% in the small intestine and by 64% in the colon but had no effect on polyp size in Apc[delta716] mice. In another study, feeding high-fat diets containing 5 or 10% of dietary fibre from wheat bran to Min mice resulted in a reduction in the number of tumours in the small intestine but not in the colon (Yu et al. 2001). We have studied the effects of a moderate level of wheat bran (10% w/w providing dietary fibre approximately 5% of weight) on intestinal tumorigenesis in Min mice and found a non-significant reduction in adenoma numbers in the small intestine when compared to the high-fat non-fibre control (Mutanen et al. 2000). When taking into consideration results obtained by using both carcinogen-treated rats and Apc-mutated mice, wheat bran consistently inhibits colon carcinogenesis (Table 10.2).

Table 10.2 Effects of whole-grains and their constituents on colon carcinogenesis in experimental animals

Type of cereal/Reference	Model	Experimental diet	Effect in comparison to control treatment
Wheat bran Wilson et al. (1977)	DMH-treated male rats	Semipurified high corn oil or high beef fat diets supplemented with 20% of wheat bran compared to the non-fibre control diet	Rats fed wheat bran had lower incidence of colon tumours regardless of the type of dietary fat
Wheat bran Watanabe et al. (1979)	Female rats treated with MNU or AOM	Semipurified diets with 15% (w/w) wheat bran, pectin or alfalfa compared to the non-supplemented control diet	Lower incidence of AOM-induced colon tumours but no effect on MNU-induced tumours by wheat bran feeding
Wheat bran Reddy and Mori (1981)	DMAB-treated male rats	Semipurified diets with 5% Alphacel or 5% Alphacel plus 15% wheat bran	Lower incidence and multiplicity of colon and small intestinal tumours in rats fed wheat bran
Wheat bran Reddy et al. (1981)	AOM-treated male rats	Semipurified diets containing 5% fat and 15% wheat bran or citrus fibre	Lower incidence and multiplicity of colon and small intestinal tumours in rats fed wheat bran
Wheat bran Barnes et al. (1983)	DMH-treated male rats	High-fat diets containing 20% (w/w) of wheat, rice, maize or soybean bran compared to the non-fibre control	Rats fed wheat bran at post-initiation stage had lower incidence of colon tumours.
Wheat bran Jacobs (1983)	DMH-treated male rats	A diet supplemented with 20% wheat bran compared to the non-fibre control	Wheat bran given during carcinogen administration resulted in increased numbers of benign and malignant tumours, whereas wheat bran given after carcinogen exposure resulted in reduction in benign tumour numbers.
Wheat bran Sinkeldam et al. (1990)	MNNG-treated male rats	3 × 3 factorial design with differing levels of wheat bran (fibre) and lard (fat)	Complex interactions with wheat bran and lard; a reduction in tumour numbers by wheat bran only in high fat context
Wheat bran Alabaster et al. (1993)	AOM-treated rats	A high-fat, low Ca diet with low (1%), medium (4%) or high (8%) fibre levels from wheat bran	Increasing the dietary fibre concentration of wheat bran from 1 to 8% reduced the number of colon tumours/group.

Table 10.2 (continued)

Type of cereal/Reference	Model	Experimental diet	Effect in comparison to control treatment
Wheat bran, oat bran McIntry et al. (1993)	DMH-treated male rats	Diets containing 10% w/w dietary fibre from wheat bran, oat bran or guar gum compared to the non-fibre control	No effect of wheat bran in comparison to the control; a reduction in the number of tumours per rat when compared to oat bran or guar gum.
Wheat bran Alabaster et al. (1995)	AOM-treated male rats	A high-fat (20% w/w) low wheat bran fibre (1%) diet compared to a high-fat, high wheat bran fibre (8%) diet	Rats fed high wheat bran diet developed less ACF/rat and had lower colon tumour incidence.
Wheat bran Young et al. (1996)	DMH-treated rats	A basic diet low in fibre/resistant starch supplemented with potato starch or with potato starch and wheat bran fibre (10%)	Addition of wheat bran prevented the potato starch-induced increases in tumour incidence, multiplicity and size.
Wheat bran, oat bran Zoran et al. (1997)	AOM-treated rats	Diets providing 6% of dietary fibre from either wheat bran (12% w/w) or oat bran (30% w/w) compared to each other	Rats fed wheat bran had lower incidence of colon tumours when compared to the oat bran fed rats (27% vs. 52%).
Microfibril wheat bran Takahashi et al. (1999)	AOM-treated female mice	A modified AIN76 diet supplemented with 20% (w/w) of microfibril wheat bran, wheat bran or cellulose	Mice fed microfibril wheat bran had lower number of tumours per mouse and lower incidence of carcinomas in situ compared to the cellulose group.
Wheat bran Hioki et al. (1997)	Apc-mutated male and female mice	A high-fat (20% w/w) low-fibre diet (2.5% wheat bran) compared to a low-fat (5%) high-fibre diet (20% wheat bran)	Mice fed low-fat, high wheat bran diet had 36% fewer polyps in the small intestine and 64% fewer polyps in the colon than control mice.
Wheat bran Yu et al. (2001)	Apc Min male and female mice	ModifiedAIN93G-diets with high-fat content (20%) and 5–10% of fibre from wheat bran, cellulose or guar gum	Mice fed wheat bran fibre at 5 or 10% had lower number of small intestinal tumours compared to controls fed high-fat low-fibre diet.

Table 10.2 (continued)

Type of cereal/Reference	Model	Experimental diet	Effect in comparison to control treatment
Wheat bran fractions Reddy et al. (2000)	AOM-treated male rats	AIN-76-based, high-fat diet with 10% of wheat bran compared to diets with dephytinized or defatted wheat bran or the latters fortified with 2% bran oil or 0.4% phytate	Removal of both phytate and bran oil was required for attenuating the anticarcinogenic effect of wheat bran. It was recovered by supplementing with the bran oil or with phytate and bran oil together but not with phytate alone.
Different wheat constituents Drankhan et al. (2003)	Apc Min mice	Two low-fat whole-wheat (45–50%) and two wheat bran diets compared to low-fat moderate fibre (6% cellulose) control diet	Wheat diets with high phenolic contents resulted in lower number of tumours and smaller tumour burden than the control diet or the wheat diets with low phenolic contents.
Wheat aleurone flour McIntosh et al. (2001)	AOM-treated male rats	A semipurified AIN93G-based high-fat diet supplemented with wheat aleurone flour at 16 and 33% w/w	Rats fed wheat aleurone flour at 33% had a tendency ($p = 0.06$) to have fewer colon adenomas than the controls.
Wheat bran oil and its fractions Sang et al. (2006)	Apc Min male mice	AIN93-G diet supplemented with 2% of wheat bran oil, 2% of wheat bran phytochemicals or 2% of wheat bran nonpolar lipids.	Wheat bran oil resulted in lower tumour number and inhibited formation of large tumours in the small intestine. Phytochemicals and nonpolar lipids were less effective.
Phytate in wheat bran Jenab and Thompson (1998)	AOM-treated male rats	AIN93G-diet supplemented with 25% of wheat bran, 25% dephytinized wheat bran (DWB), 25% DWB plus 1% phytic acid or 1% phytic acid.	Wheat bran with or without phytic acid had no effect on the number or size of colon ACF. Supplementation of diet with pure phytic acid reduced both number and size of colonic ACF.
Oat bran Jacobs and Lupton (1986)	DMH-treated male rats	A fibre-free basal diet supplemented with 20% (w/w) oat bran, or 10% of pectin, cellulose or guar gum.	Oat bran supplementation resulted in a 4-fold increase in the incidence and also increased the number of adenocarcinomas in the proximal colon in comparison to the control group.

Table 10.2 (continued)

Type of cereal/Reference	Model	Experimental diet	Effect in comparison to control treatment
Rye bran Davies et al. (2000)	AOM-treated male rats	A high-fat, low Ca diet supplemented with 30% (w/w) rye bran. Control diet was adjusted for fibre.	The rye supplemented group had decreased numbers of large ACF and colon tumours compared to the control group.
Rye bran Van Kranen et al. (2003)	Apc Min male and female mice	A high-fat, low Ca diet supplemented with 30% (w/w) rye bran. Control diet was adjusted for fibre.	Female mice fed rye bran diet had increased numbers of small intestinal tumours.
Wheat, oat and rye bran Mutanen et al. (2000)	Apc Min male mice	A high-fat, non-fibre AIN93G diet supplemented with 10% (w/w) of wheat, oat, or rye bran or inulin.	No effects in comparison to the non-fibre high-fat control. Mice fed rye bran had the lowest tumour number and differed from the inulin-fed mice which had the highest tumour number.
Rye bran and rye bran fractions Oikarinen et al. (2003)	Apc Min mice	A high-fat, non-fibre AIN93G diet supplemented with 10% of rye bran or rye bran fractions concentrated either with insoluble or soluble fibre.	Mice fed rye bran or the fraction containing insoluble fibre did not differ from the controls. Mice fed the soluble fraction had significantly more and larger tumours than the controls.
Barley brans McIntosh et al. (1993) and McIntosh et al. (1996)	DMH-treated male rats	AIN76A-based high-fat (20%) diet supplemented with 5% dietary fibre from two different barley brans and spent barley grain.	No effect on tumour incidence and multiplicity in comparison to a cellulose containing diet.
Rice bran Verschoyle et al. (2007)	Apc Min mice	AIN93G diet supplemented with 10 or 30% of rice bran or 30% of low-fibre rice bran	30% rice bran resulted in a reduction in the number of adenomas in the small intestine and in the colon.
Rice germ Kawabata et al. (1999)	AOM-treated rats	A basal diet supplemented with 2.5% (w/w) of rice germ or GABA-enriched defatted rice germ	Rice germ reduced the incidence of colon adenocarcinomas during the initiation phase and both rice germs decreased the frequency of colon adenocarcinomas during post-initiation.

Table 10.2 (continued)

Type of cereal/Reference	Model	Experimental diet	Effect in comparison to control treatment
Fermented brown rice Katyama et al. (2002)	AOM-treated rats	Fermented brown rice at 2.5 and 5% in a diet during the initiation and post-initiation phases	Rats fed 5% of fermented brown rice had lower incidence and multiplicity of colon adenocarcinomas compared to the controls.
Kurosu from rice Shimoji et al. (2003, 2004)	AOM-treated male rats	Kurosu, a vinegar from unpolished rice, at levels of 0.05 and 0.1% in drinking water	Both levels of Kurosu administration reduced the incidence and multiplicity of colon adenocarcinomas.
Rice and maize bran Barnes et al. (1983)	DMH-treated male rats	High-fat diets containing 20% (w/w) of wheat, rice, maize or soybean bran compared to the non-fibre control	Rats fed maize bran had increased numbers of colon tumours including adenocarcinomas. Rice bran fed rats did not differ from the controls.
Maize bran Reddy et al. (1983)	DMAB-treated male rats	Semipurified diet supplemented with 15% (w/w) of maize bran	The incidence and the multiplicity of colon tumours was increased in rats fed maize bran.
Maize bran Madar et al. (1993)	DMH-treated male rats	A low-fat fibre-free control diet supplemented with 18 or 25% of maize	Maize fibre at 25% of diet decreased the tumour incidence and tumour yield.

Apart from the dietary fibre component, other constituents in wheat and wheat bran have been considered as being responsible for the cancer preventive effects of wheat (Table 10.2). McIntosh et al. (2001) tested the effects of wheat aleurone flour, a good source of fibre, proteins, minerals, vitamins and phenolic compounds, on colon carcinogenesis in AOM-treated rats. Aleurone flour at 33% (w/w), providing 5 g/100 g of dietary fibre, had a tendency to reduce colon adenoma burden, which was similar in magnitude to the effect seen with 16% of wheat bran providing the same level of dietary fibre. In another study, Min mice fed wheat varieties with high orthophenolic content had lower number of tumours and smaller tumour burden than Min mice fed the AIN93 control diet (Drankhan et al. 2003). Wheats with low phenolic content had no effect, suggesting that phenolic compounds may be partly responsible for the anti-carcinogenic effects of wheat. Reddy et al. (2000) studied the anti-carcinogenic effects of the phytate and oil components of wheat bran by feeding AOM-treated rats with dephytinized or defatted wheat bran, or the dephytinized and defatted fractions fortified with either phytates or oil or both. Interestingly, removal of both phytates and bran oil was required for attenuating the anti-carcinogenic effect of wheat bran, which was recovered by supplementing with the bran oil or with phytate and bran oil together but not with phytate alone (Reddy et al. 2000). In line with these results, supplementation of AIN93 diet with 2% (w/w) of wheat bran oil resulted in an inhibition of intestinal tumorigenesis by 36% in the Min mouse (Sang et al. 2006), which gives further support for cancer preventive properties of wheat bran oil. The role of phytate in wheat bran was also studied by Jenab and Thompson (1998) who found that dephytinized wheat bran alone or fortified with pure phytic acid had only a marginal effect on ACF formation in AOM-treated rats even though pure phytic acid administered alone was able to reduce the number and size of colon ACF (Jenab and Thompson 1998). Many studies have evaluated the effect of pure phytic acid on colon carcinogenesis in carcinogen-treated rats (see Vucenik and Shamsuddin 2003). A usual finding has been that phytic acid reduces the incidence and size of colon tumours when administered in drinking water at 1–2% (Ullah and Shamsuddin 1990) but has no effect or a marginal effect when administered at the same level in diet (Hirose et al. 1991).

10.3.2 Oats, Rye, and Barley and Their Constituents

In comparison to other cereal grains, oats contain less dietary fibre and considerable part of oat fibre is classified as soluble fibre (Table 10.1). The effects of oat bran on colon carcinogenesis have been studied less frequently than those of wheat bran, presumably because an early study showed that 20% (w/w) oat bran enhances carcinogen-induced colon tumorigenesis by resulting in a 4-fold increase in the incidence and also an increase in the number of proximal colon adenocarcinomas when compared to the non-fibre control (Jacobs and Lupton 1987, Table 10.2). In the study of McIntry et al. (1993), rats fed diet containing 10% of dietary fibre from oat bran did not differ from the non-fibre controls but had a tendency for increased number of tumours and differed significantly from the wheat bran fed rats with lowest tumour

number among the dietary groups studied. Similar effects of oat bran on colon carcinogenesis in rats and Min mice have been reported by others (Zoran et al. 1997;
Mutanen et al. 2000). In conclusion, oat bran as well as other soluble fibres such as
pectin and guar gum have increased rather than decreased the number and incidence
of colonic tumours in animal models (Jacobs and Lupton 1986; McIntry et al. 1993;
Zoran et al. 1997; Mutanen et al. 2000).

Whole-grain rye products are traditionally consumed in large quantities in
Northern and Eastern Europe. Rye is the best source of dietary fibre among cereals and rye fibre is mostly insoluble (Table 10.1). Rye also contains lignans, a type
of phytoestrogens postulated to have anticarcinogenic properties. The effect of rye
bran on intestinal tumorigenesis was studied in Min mice by feeding a high-fat diet
with 10% of rye bran (Mutanen et al. 2000; Table 10.2). The number of intestinal
tumours and the incidence of colon tumours in rye fed mice showed a tendency
to be lower than in mice fed control diet (26 vs. 35 tumours/mouse; 33% vs. 71%
mice with colon polyps) but the differences did not reach statistical significance.
However, in later studies 10% of rye bran had no effect on tumour number in Min
mice and a soluble extract from rye bran, mainly containing pentosans and fruc-
tans, actually enhanced tumorigenesis (Oikarinen et al. 2003). Another study tested
the effect of rye lignans on colon carcinogenesis in AOM-treated rats (Davies et al.
1999). Rats fed a high-fat diet supplemented with 30% of rye bran had significantly
less tumours per animal than rats fed the control diet, which was suggested to stem
from rye lignans as the diets were adjusted for their fibre and phytate content. A
rye diet with the same composition was also fed to Min mice, starting the exposure
to the rye diet while the pups were still in utero, but no effect on tumour development was observed in male mice and an enhancement of small intestinal tumours in
female mice (van Kranen et al. 2003). The plant lignans matairesinol and secoiso-
larisirecinol, also present in rye, were given as pure compounds at 0.02% (w/w) in
diet to Min mice but neither of them were able to inhibit intestinal tumourigenesis
in this animal model (Pajari et al. 2006). Taken together, rye bran has shown some
anti-cancer activity in carcinogen-treated rats but less in the Min mouse.

The effect of barley on colon carcinogenesis has seldom been studied and no
definitive conclusions are therefore possible (Table 10.2). McIntosh et al. (1993
and 1996) studied the effects of 5% of dietary fibre from spent barley grains
or two barley brans with different content of soluble and insoluble fibre in 1,2-
dimethylhydratzine (DMH)-treated rats. They found no difference in the incidence
or multiplicity of tumours in barley-fed rats when compared to cellulose-fed rats.
The different barley components resulted in mixed results in comparison to each
other. Kanauchi et al. (2008) reported that germinated barley was protective against
formation of colonic ACF in AOM-treated rats.

10.3.3 Rice, Maize (corn) and Their Constituents

A number of studies have tested the anti-carcinogenic effects of rice and its constituents (Table 10.2). In an early study, DMH-treated rats fed 20% of rice bran in
a high-fat diet did not differ from the control rats fed non-fibre diet (Barnes et al.

1983). A higher level of rice bran (30%), however, was effective in reducing the number of adenomas in the small intestine and colon of Min mice by altogether 51% (Verschoyle et al. 2007). In the same study low-fibre rice bran at 30% in the diet was not able to affect adenoma development, indicating that the fibre content of the bran was mainly responsible for the anti-tumorigenic effects. Interestingly, fermented brown rice at 5% during post-initiation phase suppressed the incidence (44% vs. 18%) and multiplicity of adenocarcinomas in the colon of AOM-treated rats (Katayama et al. 2002). Similarly, defatted rice-germ and γ-aminobutyric acid – enriched rice germ at 2.5% reduced the incidence of tumours and number of adenocarcinomas in the large intestine of AOM-treated rats (Kawabata et al. 1999). Kurosu, vinegar produced from unpolished rice, was shown to inhibit ACF formation (Shimoji et al. 2003) and to decrease both the incidence and number of adenocarcinomas in the colon of carcinogen-treated rats (Shimoji et al. 2004). Kurosu contains dihydroferulic acid and dihydrosinapic acids, which are derivatives of ferulic acid, a phenolic compound suggested possessing anti-carcinogenic activity. Rice bran and germ as well as other grains are good sources of ferulic acid. The effect of pure ferulic acid on colon carcinogenesis has been reported twice; ferulic acid was shown to inhibit the formation of colonic aberrant crypts (Wargovich et al. 2000) and reduce the incidence of tumours in AOM-treated rats (Kawabata et al. 2000) but only during the initiation phase, suggesting a moderate protective effect of ferulic acid against colon carcinogenesis.

Only few studies have investigated the effect of maize (corn) on colonic tumour development (Table 10.2). Two early studies reported a clear promotive effect of maize bran on colon cancer so that 15 or 20% (w/w) of maize bran resulted in an increase in the tumour incidence and/or tumour numbers in the colon of DMAB or DMH-treated rats (Reddy et al. 1983; Barnes et al. 1983). In contrast to these two studies, Madar et al. (1993) reported a decrease in the tumour incidence and tumour yield in the colon of rats fed 25% maize fibre. There is no clear explanation for the mixed results which leaves the effect of maize on colon carcinogenesis controversial.

10.4 Mechanisms of Action of Whole Grains and Their Constituents in Colon Cancer

Many of the mechanisms mediating the protective effects of whole grains are related to dietary fibre and will be discussed more thoroughly in Sections 10.4.1 and 10.4.2. In addition to the fibre content, whole grains contain a number of other substances that may have cancer preventive effects, including vitamins, trace minerals, and phenolic compounds such as phytic acids and phytoestrogens. Of these compounds, vitamin E, selenium, phenolic acids, and phytate have been proposed to function as antioxidants, protecting cells from oxidative damage (Slavin et al. 1999). Phenolic compounds may also induce the detoxification systems, specifically the phase II conjugation reactions. The mechanisms related to phytoestrogens will be dealt with in Section 10.4.3.

10.4.1 Production of Butyrate

One of the much favoured mechanisms whereby whole grains are thought to prevent colon carcinogenesis is through the fermentation products of the dietary fibre in whole grains, such as butyrate, propionate, and acetate. Of these short-chain fatty acids (SCFA), butyrate has been suggested to play an important role in colon cancer prevention. Butyrate is the principal energy source of colonic epithelial cells (Roediger 1982) and it also takes part in the regulation of cell proliferation, differentiation, and apoptosis. The effects of butyrate on these cellular processes have often been opposite in normal colonocytes relative to neoplastic colonic cells. In normal colonocytes butyrate has been shown to increase cell proliferation (Sakata 1987; Lupton and Kurtz 1993), whereas in colon cancer cell lines butyrate has promoted expression of differentiation markers (Whitehead et al. 1986) and induced apoptosis (Hague et al. 1995).

Studies in experimental animals have given controversial results of the protective effect of butyrate *in vivo*. McIntry et al. (1991) demonstrated that rats fed wheat bran maintained relatively high butyrate concentrations in the luminal contents along the entire length of their large intestine, particularly in the distal colon. In a further study they showed that wheat bran reduced colonic tumour development and that tumour mass was negatively correlated with faecal butyrate concentration in carcinogen-treated rats (McIntry et al. 1993). They concluded that the protective effect of wheat bran is due to its ability to maintain butyrate production in the distal colon where the majority of tumours occur. In contrast, Zoran et al. (1997) compared the effects of oat bran and wheat bran in a rat colon cancer model and found no relationship between tumour formation and high butyrate concentrations in the distal colon. Rats fed oat bran had significantly higher butyrate concentrations in both the proximal and distal colon but also significantly more tumours than wheat bran-fed rats.

Butyrate as such has also been administered to carcinogen-treated rats with mixed results. Sodium butyrate dissolved in drinking water at 1–2% enhanced significantly colonic tumour formation in DMH-treated rats (Freeman 1986), whereas butyrate as tributyrin at 5% or as slow-release sodium butyrate pellets at 1.5% in a high-fat diet had no effect on AOM-induced colon carcinogenesis despite of causing a 10-fold increase in faecal butyric acid (Deschner et al. 1990; Caderni et al. 2001). No change in the level of apoptosis or p21 protein in the tumours was seen by feeding sodium butyrate pellets either (Caderni et al. 2001). Two more recent studies give some indirect support for the anti-carcinogenic effects of butyrate. Kameue et al. (2004) observed that feeding sodium gluconate increased cecal concentrations of butyrate and decreased the incidence and number of colon tumours induced by AOM- and deoxycholic acid. In another study, administration of butyrate producing bacteria *Butyrivibrio fibrisolvens* resulted in an increase in the rate of butyrate production and reduced the number of colonic ACF in DMH-treated rats (Ohkawara et al. 2005).

Despite of the lack of protective effect of butyrate against colon tumorigenesis in most of the animal experiments, butyrate is still under intense investigation. This is because butyrate has been identified as belonging to histone deacetylase inhibitors, a group of compounds considered as promising candidates for cancer prevention and treatment (Myzak and Dashwood 2006). Butyrate treatment of colon cancer cells *in vitro* results in the inhibition of histone deacetylases, leading to higher acetylation of histones with a more open chromatin conformation, which allows transcription factor access to DNA. By this mechanism butyrate has been shown to result changes in the expression of genes regulating cell differentiation, cell cycle arrest and apoptosis, such as induction of the cell cycle inhibitor p21$^{waf1/kip1}$ (Archer et al. 1998; Wilson et al. 2006), downregulation of cyclin D1 and upregulation of cyclin D3 (Siavoshian et al. 2000), and induction of the death receptor 5/TRAIL-R2 accompanied by the activation of caspases (Nakata et al. 2004). Butyrate also potentially modulates immune function of the gut (Fusunyan et al. 1999) and may affect metastatic capacity of colon cancer cells (Li et al. 2004).

The majority of sporadic colorectal cancers as well as the familial adenomatosis polyposis syndrome are initiated by mutations in the APC gene, which leads to the constitutive activation of the Wnt/β-catenin pathway (Kinzler andVogelstein 1996). As an anti-carcinogenic agent, butyrate would be expected to downregulate the hyperactive β-catenin signalling in colon cancer cells. However, the opposite seems to be true. Butyrate was shown to greatly induce the transcriptional activity of β-catenin in ten different colorectal cancer cell lines (Bordonaro et al. 2008). Paradoxically, hyper-activation of β-catenin was associated with suppression of clonal growth and enhanced apoptosis. Induction of apoptosis does not necessarily result in inhibition of tumorigenesis *in vivo*. In the study by Augenlicht et al. (1999), elimination of the SCFA metabolism by a *Scad* mutation in Apc-mutated mice led to a major reduction in apoptosis in the colonic mucosa but had no effect on the incidence or number of intestinal tumours. There was also a high variability in the response to butyrate among the colon cancer cell subtypes tested (Bordonaro et al. 2008), implicating that in some colon cancer cell subtypes butyrate might even promote colon carcinogenesis. This view is supported by observations from *in vivo* studies. Feeding inulin, a highly fermentable dietary fructo-oligosaccharide, resulted in an increased concentration of faecal butyrate (Gråsten et al. 2002) but also promoted the development and growth of intestinal tumours in the Min mouse, which was accompanied by increased levels of β-catenin in the tumour tissue (Pajari et al. 2003). In conclusion, the relationship between butyrate and colon carcinogenesis is very complex and may vary depending on the concentration and timing of administration of butyrate during the carcinogenic process. With regard to whole grains, other bioactive constituents and/or dietary fibre components present may affect the production of butyrate from whole-grain fibres and its effects on tumorigenesis.

10.4.2 Modulation of Bile Acid Metabolism

Over 95% of primary bile acids, predominantly cholic and chenodeoxycholic acids is reabsorbed in the terminal ileum and returned to the liver through the portal vein (Nagengast et al. 1995). The remaining 2–5% continues into the colon where they are converted by anaerobic bacteria to secondary bile acids, such as deoxy-cholic acid and lithocholic acid. The bacterial enzyme thought to be responsible for the conversion is 7α-dehydroxylase (Reddy et al. 1996). The secondary bile acids are postulated to have detrimental effects on the colonic epithelium and thus promote colon cancer. Animal studies have demonstrated that bile acids are capable of inducing hyperproliferation of colonic epithelial cells (Lapre' and Van der Meer 1992) and promoting colon tumourigenesis (Reddy et al. 1977; McSherry et al. 1989). An early human study by Reddy and Wynder (1973) also described a positive association between the incidence of colon cancer and faecal bile acid excretion.

High-fat Western diets are thought to promote tumourigenesis by increasing bile acid excretion, and thereby luminal concentrations of secondary bile acids in the colon (Nagengast et al. 1995). Dietary fibre from whole grains may prevent colon tumourigenesis by increasing stool bulk, which binds and dilutes bile acids, and reduces transit time of the faeces. This results in a shorter exposure of colonic epithelium to bile acids as well as to other potentially toxic compounds. Bacterial fermentation of fibre produces SCFAs that decrease luminal pH and thereby inhibit the conversion of primary to secondary bile acids (Ridlon et al. 2006).

The experimental evidence concerning the bile acid hypothesis has not been entirely supportive. Though a diet high in corn oil resulted in elevated levels of secondary bile acids in faeces of carcinogen-treated rats (Reddy et al. 1996), diets high in saturated fats, such as butter and beef tallow, did not increase the concentration of faecal bile acids (Chang et al. 1994; Morotomi et al. 1997). In another study, dietary fat as maize oil had no effect on faecal bile acids but 8% of dietary fibre from oat, rye or barley brans were all effective in lowering faecal bile acid concentrations, which was mainly caused by greater faecal mass on the bran diets (Gallaher et al. 1992). The effects of cereal brans on bile acids and other putative faecal risk markers of colon cancer have also been studied in a number of human interventions. In the study by Reddy et al. (1989) healthy subjects consumed a 10 g supplement of wheat bran, oat bran or cellulose for 5 weeks. Compared to their respective control diet periods, those in the wheat bran and cellulose groups had a significantly lower concentration of secondary and total bile acids in the faeces. Similarly, supplementation of 13.5 g/d of wheat bran fibre for 9 months resulted in a significant reduction in faecal concentrations of total and deoxycholic acids in colon cancer patients (Alberts et al. 1996). A 4-week intervention on either a high-fibre wheat or high-fibre rye diet had no effect on faecal bile acids even though both diets decreased faecal pH and increased faecal output in healthy, overweight men (McIntosh et al. 2003). By contrast, Gråsten et al. (2000) observed in healthy volunteers that consuming whole-meal rye bread as a minimum of 20% of the daily energy intake led to increased faecal output, shortened the mean transit time and decreased the concentrations of total and secondary bile acids. Based on the human interventions, whole-grain wheat and rye products seem to be able to decrease the concentration of faecal bile acids, owing to the bulking effect of whole grains.

Bile acids are known to affect several cellular pathways involved in colon carcinogenesis. They have been shown to induce the activity of the transcription factor AP-1 in a dose-dependent manner which was associated with increased expression of the c-Jun and c-Fos (Hirano et al. 1996; Glinghammar et al. 1999). In colon cancer cells, deoxycholic acid results in activation of epidermal growth factor receptor and its downstream signalling to Raf-1 and extracellular signal-regulated kinase (Im and Martinez 2004), activation of beta-catenin signalling accompanied by increased expression of uPA, uPAR and cyclin D (Pai et al. 2004), and elevated COX-2 expression leading to 10-fold increase in the production of prostaglandin E2 (Zhang et al. 1998). Bile acids have also been demonstrated to induce protein kinase C (PKC) activity in human and rat colon tissues (Pongracz et al. 1995; Pence et al. 1995) and colon cancer cell lines (Huang et al. 1992), and to enhance bacterial production of luminal diacylglycerol, a physiological activator of PKC (Morotomi et al. 1990). Interestingly, feeding 10% of wheat, rye or oat bran in a high-fat diet resulted in different effects on the mucosal PKC activity and isoenzyme profiles in rat colon (Pajari et al. 2000), indicating that PKC enzymes may be involved in mediating the effects of whole grains on colon carcinogenesis.

10.4.3 Phytoestrogens

Whole grains, especially rye and wheat, contain plant lignans, which are converted by gut bacteria to the mammalian lignans enterolactone and enterodiol (Adlercreutz and Mazur 1997). Lignans belong to phytoestrogens, a group of compounds that can bind weakly to the oestrogen receptor. Therefore they may have either a mild oestrogen-like action or they may antagonise oestrogen action. Phytoestrogens may have relevance in colon cancer prevention because age-related hypermethylation of the oestrogen receptor gene is thought to be one of the molecular pathways leading to colon cancer (Issa et al. 1994). In colon cancer cells, hypermethylation results in inactivation of the oestrogen receptor gene, which is accompanied by deregulated growth (Issa et al. 1994). Circulating oestrogens have been shown to modulate the expression of oestrogen receptor in several tissues (Tata et al. 1993), suggesting that blood levels of oestrogens or phytoestrogens might be able to attenuate the inactivating effect of hypermethylation on the oestrogen receptor gene. This hypothesis is supported by some epidemiological studies which have shown that postmenopausal oestrogen replacement is associated with a reduced risk of colon cancer (Giovannucci and Platz 1999).

Lignans also have oestrogen receptor-independent effects in colon cancer cell lines. Enterolactone and enterodiol have been shown to inhibit proliferation (Sung et al 1998) and enterolactone to induce apoptosis in colon cancer cells (Danbara et al. 2005). In animal models, the effects of whole-grain lignans on colon carcinogenesis have been modest as only one study showed protection of rye lignans against colon tumour development (Davies et al. 1999, Table 10.2). Results from two case-control studies have been more encouraging; one reported a significant reduction in colorectal adenoma risk in the subjects with high plasma concentrations of enterodiol (Kuijsten et al. 2006) and the other one reported that dietary intake of lignans is inversely associated with colorectal cancer risk (Cotterchio et al. 2006).

10.5 Controlled Clinical Trials

Over the past two decades, several clinical trials have been conducted using the recurrence of colon or rectal adenomas as an end point in order to test the protective effect of wheat bran or a fibre-rich diet on colon cancer. Adenomas are regarded as good surrogates as most colon carcinomas arise from adenomatous polyps. The results of two early clinical trials have suggested that wheat bran supplement may offer some protection against colorectal cancer. In an early study by DeCosse et al. (1989), familial adenomatous polyposis patients that received a daily supplementation of 22.5 g wheat bran together with 4 g ascorbic acid and 400 mg α-tocopherol had, in comparison to the low-fibre control group, consistently but non-significantly lower numbers of rectal polyps assessed at several visits during the 4-year trial. Australian Polyp Prevention Project reported no effect of a daily supplement of 25 g wheat-bran for 48 months on the recurrence of colon adenomas but observed a significant reduction in the risk of large adenomas by a combination of wheat bran and low-fat diet (MacLennan et al. 1995). However, a large clinical trial in the USA found no evidence of a protective effect of any kind on colon adenoma recurrence by a daily supplement of 13.5 g wheat bran for 3 years (Alberts et al. 2000). A more recent, small trial in Japan reported that a supplement of 25 g wheat-bran biscuits providing 17.5 g dietary fibre daily for 4 years had no significant effect on colon adenoma recurrence (Ishikawa et al. 2005). Interestingly, supplementation with isphagula husk, also known as psyllium, was shown to significantly increase the risk of adenoma recurrence in the colon with odds ratio 1.67 (95% CI 1.01−2.76, $p = 0.028$), which is in line with the animal data indicating that highly fermentable fibres may in some occasions promote colon carcinogenesis (Bonithon-Kopp et al. 2000).

Two trials have studied the effect of a low-fat, high-fibre diet on colon adenoma recurrence. In Toronto Polyp Prevention trial, the recurrence of colon adenomas in patients following a diet providing on average 25% of energy from fat and 35 g dietary fibre per day did not differ from the recurrence in the control group on a diet providing 33% of energy from fat and 16 g dietary fibre per day (McKeown-Eyssen et al. 1994). Unexpectedly, men in the low-fat high-fibre group had an increase (relative risk 1.6) and women a decrease (relative risk 0.7) in polyp recurrence, suggesting possible gender-specific effects. Because of a small study size this result may be a chance observation. Polyp Prevention Trial in the USA consisted of nearly 2,000 subjects who were randomised either to a control group to follow their usual diet or to the intervention group to follow a diet low in fat (20% of energy from fat), high in fibre (18 g/1,000 kcal) and high in fruits and vegetables (3.5 servings/1,000 kcal) (Schatzkin et al. 2000). The unambiguous result from this large trial was that a diet low in fat and high in fibre, fruits and vegetables failed to reduce the recurrence of colon adenomas.

Overall, the results from these clinical trials show that wheat bran supplements or high-fibre diets do not protect against the recurrence of new adenomas in the colon. However, it would be a gross oversimplification to conclude that wheat bran or dietary fibre is useless in colon cancer prevention. Colon carcinogenesis is a multistep process which may take several decades to evolve from a preneoplastic epithelium to adenoma, to carcinoma and finally to metastatic disease. Clinical trials have usually lasted for 3–4 years, which might be too short time to see real effects. Lanza et al. (2007) did an attempt to address this question by carrying out an additional 4-year follow-up with a subset of participants of the Polyp Prevention Trial. The result, however, remained the same as after the first 4 years, i.e. no change in polyp recurrence by the diet. Still, even 8 years of intervention might not be long enough, particularly so if it only covers one stage of carcinogenesis. Another problem in the trial was that the intervention group increased their fat intake and decreased their fibre intake with time even though they still differed from the control group (Lanza et al. 2007). Compliance is a general problem in trials; for example Alberts et al. (2000) observed that by the third year of the study, only 74% of the subjects in the high-fibre group consumed over 75% of their daily wheat bran supplement. It could also be that the dietary goals or the level of supplements in trials have been insufficient.

10.6 Conclusions

Early studies presumed that the cancer-preventive effects of whole grains are due to their high dietary fibre content. Most of these studies typically tested the effect of diets containing high levels of wheat and other brans on colon tumorigenesis in rats during and after carcinogen administration. The most consistent though not always statistically significant result from these studies was that wheat bran, mainly containing insoluble cellulose-type fibre, protected against colon tumorigenesis, particularly when given at post-initiation stage. Oat bran, containing substantial amounts of soluble fibre, had no protective effect and in some cases promoted colon carcinogenesis. In subsequent studies with Apc-mutated mice, wheat and oat bran have basically given similar results as in carcinogen-treated rats earlier. Rye and rice brans have also been studied using Apc-muteted mice. Rye has offered a modest protection against colon tumorigenesis in some studies and no effect in others, whereas rice has resulted in a clear inhibition in tumour development when given at relatively high levels in the diet. Only few studies have evaluated the effects of barley and maize on colon tumorigenesis and the results have been mixed.

In addition to dietary fibre, whole grains contain phytochemicals such as phytates, ferulic acid, lignans, and phytosterols, which may explain at least partly the cancer-preventive effects of whole grains seen in animal models. However, when these phytochemicals have been studied as extracts or pure compounds, none of them have exceeded the effects seen with the original whole-grain product. In many cases, the anti-tumorigenic activity has been lost as a result from the fractionation process.

There are several mechanisms which may explain the anti-carcinogenic effects of whole grains. Dietary fibre in whole grains contributes to faecal bulking and thus reduces transit time, which dilutes potential toxic substances in the faeces, such as secondary bile acids, and shortens the exposure time of these substances with the colonic mucosa. Though being rather simple in nature this mechanism may be an important mediator of the protective effects of whole grains. Butyrate, the fermentation product of dietary fibre, has been recognised as a histone deasetylase inhibitor which affects many cell signalling pathways regulating cell maturation, cell cycle arrest, and apoptosis. The effect of bytyrate on colon cancer cells with upregulated β-catenin signalling has been complex, suggesting that butyrate may in some cases have cancer-promotive effects on cells.

Based on the promising results in animal models, the effect of wheat bran supplementation on the recurrence of adenomatous colon polyps has been tested in several clinical trials. The results from these trials have, however, been disappointing as wheat bran supplements have been unable to prevent the recurrence of new adenomas to a significant extent. It is worth remembering that these trials cover a limited period of carcinogenic process, may have problems with the compliance and have used a single dose of wheat bran.

References

Adlercreutz H, Mazur W (1997) Phyto-oestrogens and Western diseases. Ann Med 29:95–120

Alabaster O, Tang ZC, Frost A et al (1993) Potential synergism between wheat bran and psyllium: enhanced inhibition of colon cancer. Cancer Lett 75:53–58

Alabaster O, Tang ZC, Frost A et al (1995) Effect of β-carotene and wheat bran fiber on colonic aberrant crypt and tumor formation in rats exposed to azoxymethane and high dietary fat. Carcinogenesis 16:127–132

Alberts DS, Martínez ME, Roe DJ et al (2000) Lack of effect of a high-fiber cereal supplement on the recurrence of colorectal adenomas. N Engl J Med 342:1156–1162

Alberts DS, Ritenbaugh C, Story JA et al (1996) Randomized, double-blinded, placebo-controlled study of effect of wheat bran fiber and calcium on fecal bile acids in patients with resected adenomatous colon polyps. J Natl Cancer Inst 88:81–92

Archer SY, Meng S, Shei A et al (1998) p21[WAF1] is required for butyrate-mediated growth inhibition of human colon cancer cells. Proc Natl Acad Sci USA 95:6791–6796

Augenlicht LH, Anthony GM, Church TL et al (1999) Short-chain fatty acid metabolism, apoptosis, and Apc-initiated tumorigenesis in the mouse gastrointestinal mucosa. Cancer Res 59:6005–6009

Barnes DS, Clapp NK, Scott DA et al (1983) Effects of wheat, rice, corn, and soybean bran on 1,2-dimethylhydrazine-induced large bowel tumorigenesis in F344 rats. Nutr Cancer 5:1–9

Bingham SA, Day NE, Luben R et al (2003) Dietary fibre in food and protection against colorectal cancer in the European Prospective Investigation Into Cancer and Nutrition (EPIC): an observational study. Lancet 361:1496–1501

Bonithon-Kopp C, Kronborg O, Giacosa A et al (2000) Calcium and fibre supplementation in prevention of colorectal adenoma recurrence: a randomised intervention trial. Lancet 356:1300–1306

Bordonaro M, Lazarova DL, Sartorelli AC (2008) Butyrate and Wnt signaling: a possible solution to the puzzle of dietary fiber and colon cancer risk? Cell Cycle 7:1178–1183

Caderni G, Luceri C, De Filippo C et al (2001) Slow-release pellets of sodium butyrate do not modify azoxymethane (AOM)-induced intestinal carcinogenesis in F344 rats. Carcinogenesis 22:525–527

Chang W-C, Lupton JR, Frølich W et al (1994) A very low intake of fat is required to decrease fecal bile acid concentrations in rats. J Nutr 124:181–187

Cotterchio M, Boucher BA, Manno M et al (2006) Dietary phytoestrogen intake is associated with reduced colorectal cancer risk. J Nutr 136:3046–3053

Danbara N, Yuri T, Tsujita-Kyutoku M et al (2005) Enterolactone induces apoptosis and inhibits growth of Colo 201 human colon cancer cells both in vitro and in vivo. Anticancer Res 25:2269–2276

Davies MJ, Bowey EA, Adlercreutz H (1999) Effects of soy or rye supplementation of high-fat diets on colon tumour development in azoxymethane-treated rats. Carcinogenesis 20:927–931

DeCosse JJ, Miller HH, Lesser ML (1989) Effect of wheat fiber and vitamins C and E on rectal polyps in patients with familial adenomatous polyposis. J Natl Cancer Inst 81:1290–1297

Deschner EE, Ruperto JF, Lupton JR et al (1990) Dietary butyrate (tributyrin) does not enhance AOM-induced colon tumorigenesis. Cancer Lett 52:79–82

Drankhan K, Carter J, Madl R et al (2003) Antitumor activity of wheats with high ortophenolic content. Nutr Cancer 47:188–194

Freeman HJ (1986) Effects of differing concentrations of sodium butyrate on 1,2-dimethylhydrazine-induced rat intestinal neoplasia. Gastroenterology 91:596–602

Fulcher RG, Duke RTK (2002) Whole-grain structure and organization: implications for nutritionists and processors. In: Marquart L, Slavin JL, Fulcher RG (eds) Whole-grain foods in health and disease. American Association of Cereal Chemists, St Paul, MN 10: 9–45

Fusunyan RD, Quinn JJ, Fujimoto M et al (1999) Butyrate switches the pattern of chemokine secretion by intestinal epithelial cells through histone acetylation. Mol Med 5:631–640

Gallaher DD, Locket PL, Gallaher CM (1992) Bile acid metabolism in rats fed two levels of corn oil and brans of oat, rye and barley and sugar beet fiber. J Nutr 122:473–481

Giovannucci E, Platz EA (1999) Colorectal cancer: the problems. In: Schmiegel W, Schölmerich J (eds) Colorectal cancer: molecular mechanisms, premalignant state and its prevention (Falk symposium 109). Kluwer Academic, Dortrecht

Glinghammar B, Holmberg K, Rafter J (1999) Effects of colonic lumenal components on AP-1-dependent gene transcription in cultured human colon carcinoma cells. Carcinogenesis 20: 969–976

Gråsten SM, Juntunen KS, Poutanen KS et al (2000) Rye bread improves bowel function and decreases the concentrations of some compounds that are putative colon cancer risk markers in middle-aged women and men. J Nutr 130:2215–2221

Gråsten SM, Pajari AM, Liukkonen KH et al (2002) Fibers with different solubility charasterictics alter similarly the metabolic activity of intestinal microbiota in rats fed cereal brans and inulin. Nutr Res 22:1435–1444

Hague PR, Elder DJE, Hicks DJ et al (1995) Apoptosis in colorectal tumor cells: induction by the short chain fatty acids butyrate, propionate, and acetate, and the bile salt deoxycholate. Int J Cancer 60:400–406

Hioki K, Shivapurkar N, Oshima H et al (1997) Suppression of intestinal polyp development by low-fat and high-fiber diet in Apc$^{\Delta716}$ knockout mice. Carcinogenesis 18:1863–1865

Hirano F, Tanaka H, Makino Y et al (1996) Induction of the transcription factor AP-1 in cultured human colon adenocarcinoma cells following exposure to bile acids. Carcinogenesis 17: 427–433

Hirose M, Ozaki K, Takaba K et al (1991) Modifying effects of the naturally occurring antioxidants gamma-oryzanol, phytic acid, tannic acid and n-tritriacontane-16, 18-dione in a rat wide-spectrum organ carcinogenesis model. Carcinogenesis 12:1917–1921

Huang XP, Fan XT, Desjeux JF et al (1992) Bile acids, non-phorbol-ester-type tumor promoters, stimulate the phosphorylation of protein kinase C substrates in human platelets and colon cell line HT29. Int J Cancer 52:444–450

Im E, Martinez JD (2004) Ursodeoxycholic acid (UDCA) can inhibit deoxycholic acid (DCA)-induced apoptosis via modulation of EGFR/Raf-1/ERK signaling in human colon cancer cells. J Nutr 134:483–436

Ishikawa H, Akedo I, Otani T et al (2005) Randomized trial of dietary fiber and Lactobacillus casei administration for prevention of colorectal tumors. Int J Cancer 116:762–767

Issa J-P, Ottaviano YL, Celano P (1994) Methylation of the oestrogen receptor CpG island links ageing and neoplasia in human colon. Nat Genet 7:536–540

Jacobs LR (1983) Enhancement of rat colon carcinogenesis by wheat bran consumption during the stage of 1,2-dimethylhydrazine administration. Cancer Res 43:4057–4061

Jacobs DR Jr, Marquart L, Slavin J et al (1998) Whole grain intake and cancer: an expanded review and meta-analysis. Nutr Cancer 30:85–96

Jacobs DR Jr, Slavin J, Marquart L (1995) Whole grain intake and cancer: a review of the literature. Nutr Cancer 24:221–229

Jacobs LR, Lupton JR (1986) Relationship of between colonic luminal pH, cell proliferation and colon carcinogenesis in 1,2-dimethylhydratzine treated rats fed high fibre diets. Cancer Res 46:1727–1734

Jenab M, Thompson L (1998) The influence of phytic acid in wheat bran on early biomarkers of colon carcinogenesis. Carcinogenesis 19:1087–1092

Kameue C, Tsukahara T, Yamada K et al (2004) Dietary sodium gluconate protects rats from large bowel cancer by stimulating butyrate production. J Nutr 134:940–944

Kanauchi O, Mitsuyama K, Andoh A et al (2008) Modulation of intestinal environment by prebiotic germinated barley foodstuff prevents chemo-induced colonic carcinogenesis in rats. Oncol Rep 20:793–801

Katayama M, Yoshimi N, Sakata K et al (2002) Preventive effect of fermented brown rice and rice bran against colon carcinogenesis in male F344 rats. Oncol Rep 9:817–822

Kawabata K, Tanaka T, Murakami T et al (1999) Dietary prevention of azoxymethane-induced colon carcinogenesis with rice-germ in F344 rats. Carcinogenesis 20:2109–2115

Kawabata K, Yamamoto T, Hara A et al (2000) Modifying effects of ferulic acid on azoxymethan-induced colon carcinogenesis. Cancer Lett 157:15–21

Kinzler KW, Vogelstein B (1996) Lessons from hereditary colon cancer. Cell 87:159–170

Kuijsten A, Arts IC, Hollman PC et al (2006) Plasma enterolignans are associated with lower colorectal adenoma risk. Cancer Epidemiol Biomarkers Prev 15:1132–1136

Lanza E, Yu B, Murphy G et al (2007) The polyp prevention trial continued follow-up study: no effect of a low-fat, high-fiber, high-fruit, and -vegetable diet on adenoma recurrence 8 years after randomization. Cancer Epidemiol Biomarkers Prev 16:1745–1752

Lapre JA, Van der Meer R (1992) Diet-induced increase of colonic bile acids stimulates lytic activity of fecal water and proliferation of colonic cells. Carcinogenesis 13:41–44

Larsson SC, Giovannucci E, Bergkvist L et al (2005) Whole grain consumption and risk of colorectal cancer: a population-based cohort of 60,000 women. Br J Cancer 92:1803–1807

Li X, Mikkelsen IM, Mortensen B et al (2004) Butyrate reduces liver metastasis of rat colon carcinoma cells in vivo and resistance to oxidative stress in vitro. Clin Exp Metastasis 21:331–338

Lupton JR, Kurtz PP (1993) Relationship of colonic luminal short-chain fatty acids and pH to in vivo cell proliferation. J Nutr 123:1522–1530

MacLennan R, Macrae F, Bain C et al (1995) Randomized trial of intake of fat, fiber, and beta carotene to prevent colorectal adenomas. J Natl Cancer Inst 87:1760–1766

Madar Z, Timar B, Nyska A et al (1993) Effects of high-fiber diets on pathological changes in DMH-induced rat colon cancer. Nutr Cancer 20:87–96

McIntosh GH, Jorgensen L, Royle P (1993) The potential of an insoluble dietary fiber-rich source from barley to protect from DMH-induced intestinal tumors in rats. Nutr Cancer 19:213–221

McIntosh GH, Leu RKL, Royle PJ et al (1996) A compartive study of the influence of differing barley brans on DMH-induced intestinal tumours in male Sprague-Dawley rats. J Gastroenterol Hepatol 11:113–119

McIntosh GH, Noakes M, Royle PJ et al (2003) Whole-grain rye and wheat foods and markers of bowel health in overweight middle-aged men. Am J Clin Nutr 77:967–974

McIntosh GH, Royle PJ, Pointing G (2001) Wheat aleurone flour increases cecal beta-glucuronidase activity and butyrate concentration and reduces colon adenoma burden in azoxymethane-treated rats. J Nutr 131:127–131

McIntry A, Gibson PR, Yong GP (1993) Butyrate production from dietary fibre and protection against large bowel cancer in a rat model. Gut 34:386–391

McIntry A, Young GP, Taranto T (1991) Different fibers have different regional effects on luminal contents of rat colon. Gastroenterology 101:1274–1281

McKeown-Eyssen GE, Bright-See E, Bruce WR et al (1994) A randomized trial of a low fat high fibre diet in the recurrence of colorectal polyps. J Clin Epidemiol 47:525–536

McSherry CK, Cohen BI, Bokkenheuser VD et al (1989) Effects of calcium and bile acid feeding on colon tumors in the rat. Cancer Res 49:6039–6043

Morotomi M, Guillem JG, LoGorfo P et al (1990) Production of diacylglyserol, an activator of protein kinase C, by human intestinal microflora. Cancer Res 50:3595–3599

Morotomi M, Sakaitani Y, Satou M et al (1997) Effects of a high-fat diet on azoxymethane-induced aberrant crypt foci and fecal biochemistry and microbial activity in rats. Nutr Cancer 27:84–91

Mutanen M, Pajari AM, Oikarinen SI (2000) Beef induces and rye bran prevents the formation of intestinal polyps in Apc(Min) mice: relation to beta-catenin and PKC isozymes. Carcinogenesis 21:1167–1173

Myzak MC, Dashwood RH (2006) Histone deacetylases as targets for dietary cancer preventive agents: lessons learned with butyrate, diallyl disulfide, and sulforaphane. Curr Drug Targets 7:443–452

Nagengast FM, Gruppen MJAL, van Munster IP (1995) Role of bile acids in colorectal carcinogenesis. Eur J Cancer 31A:1067–1070

Nakata S, Yoshida T, Horinaka M et al (2004) Histone deacetylase inhibitors upregulate death receptor 5/TRAIL-R2 and sensitize apoptosis induced by TRAIL/APO2-L in human malignant tumor cells. Oncogene 23:6261–6271

Ohkawara S, Furuya H, Nagashima K et al (2005) Oral administration of butyrivibrio fibrisolvens, a butyrate-producing bacterium, decreases the formation of aberrant crypt foci in the colon and rectum of mice. J Nutr 135:2878–2883

Oikarinen S, Heinonen S, Karppinen S (2003) Plasma enterolactone or intestinal Bifidobacterium levels do not explain adenoma formation in multiple intestinal neoplasia (Min) mice fed with two different types of rye-bran fractions. Br J Nutr 90:119–125

Pai R, Tarnawski AS, Tran T (2004) Deoxycholic acid activates beta-catenin signaling pathway and increases colon cell cancer growth and invasiveness. Mol Biol Cell 15:2156–2163

Pajari AM, Oikarinen S, Gråsten S et al (2000) Diets enriched with cereal brans or inulin modulate protein kinase C activity and isozyme expression in rat colonic mucosa. Br J Nutr 84: 635–643

Pajari AM, Rajakangas J, Päivärinta E et al (2003) Promotion of intestinal tumor formation by inulin is associated with an accumulation of cytosolic beta-catenin in Min mice. Int J Cancer 106:653–660

Pajari AM, Smeds AI, Oikarinen S et al (2006) The plant lignans matairesinol and secoisolariciresinol administered to Min mice do not protect against intestinal tumor formation. Cancer Lett 233:309–314

Park Y, Hunter DJ, Spiegelman D et al (2005) Dietary fiber intake and risk of colorectal cancer: a pooled analysis of prospective cohort studies. JAMA 294:2849–2857

Pence BC, Dunn DM, Zhao C et al (1995) Chemopreventive effects of calcium but not aspirin supplementation in cholic acid-promoted colon carcinogenesis: correlation with intermediate endpoints. Carcinogenesis 16:757–765

Pongracz J, Clark P, Neoptolemos JP et al (1995) Expression of protein kinase C isoenzymes in colorectal cancer tissue and their differential activation by different bile acids. Int J Cancer 61:35–39

Preston SL, Leedham SJ, Oukrif D et al (2008) The development of duodenal microadenomas in FAP patients: the human correlate of the Min mouse. J Pathol 214:294–301

Reddy B, Engle A, Katsifis S et al (1989) Biochemical epidemiology of colon cancer: effect of types of dietary fiber on fecal mutagens, acid, and neutral sterols in healthy subjects. Cancer Res 49:4629–4635

Reddy BS, Hirose Y, Cohen LA et al (2000) Preventive potential of wheat bran fractions against experimental colon carcinogenesis: implications for human colon cancer prevention. Cancer Res 60:4792–4797

Reddy BS, Maeura Y, Wayman M (1983) Effect of dietary corn bran and autohydrolyzed lignin on 3,2'-dimethyl-4-aminobiphenyl-induced intestinal carcinogenesis in male F344 rats. J Natl Cancer Inst 71:419–423

Reddy BS, Mori H (1981) Effect of dietary wheat bran and dehydrated citrus fiber on 3,2'-dimethyl-4-aminobiphenyl-induced intestinal carcinogenesis in F344 rats. Carcinogenesis 2:21–25

Reddy BS, Mori H, Nicolais M (1981) Effect of dietary wheat bran and dehydrated citrus fiber on azoxymethane-induced intestinal carcinogenesis in Fischer 344 rats. J Natl Cancer Inst 66: 553–557

Reddy BS, Simi B, Patel N et al (1996) Effect of amount and types of dietary fat on intestinal bacterial 7α-dehydroxylase and phosphatidylinositol-specific phospholipase C and colonic mucosal diacylglycerol kinase and PKC activities during different stages of colon tumor promotion. Cancer Res 56:2314–2320

Reddy BS, Watanabe K, Weisburger JH et al (1977) Promoting effect of bile acids in colon carcinogenesis in germ free and conventional F344 rats. Cancer Res 37:3238–3242

Reddy BS, Wynder EL (1973) Large bowel carcinogenesis: fecal constituents of populations with diverse incidence rates of colon cancer. J Natl Cancer Inst 50:1437–1442

Ridlon JM, Kang DJ, Hylemon PB (2006) Bile salt biotransformations by human intestinal bacteria. J Lipid Res 47:241–259

Roediger WW (1982) Utilization of nutrients by isolated epithelial cells of the rat colon. Gastroenterology 83:424–429

Sakata T (1987) Stimulatory effect of short chain fatty acids on epithelial cell proliferation in rat intestine: a possible explanation for trophic effects of fermentable fibre, gut microbes, and luminal trophic factors. Br J Nutr 58:95–103

Sang S, Ju J, Lambert JD (2006) Wheat bran oil and its fractions inhibit human colon cancer cell growth and intestinal tumorigenesis in Apcmin/+ mice. J Agric Food Chem 54:9792–9797

Schatzkin A, Lanza E, Corle D et al (2000) Lack of effect of a low-fat, high-fiber diet on the recurrence of colorectal adenomas. N Engl J Med 342:1149–1155

Schatzkin A, Mouw T, Park Y et al (2007) Dietary fiber and whole-grain consumption in relation to colorectal cancer in the NIH-AARP Diet and Health Study. Am J Clin Nutr 85: 1353–1360

Schatzkin A, Park Y, Leitzman MF et al (2008) Prospective study of dietary fiber, whole grain foods, and small intestinal cancer. Gastroenterology 135:1163–1167

Shimoji Y, Kohno H, Nanda K et al (2004) Extract of Kurosu, a vinegar from unpolished rice, inhibits azoxymethane-induced colon carcinogenesis in male F344 rats. Nutr Cancer 49: 170–173

Shimoji Y, Sugie S, Kohno H et al (2003) Extract of vinegars Kurosu from unpolished rice inhibits the development of colon aberrant crypt foci induced by azoxymethane. J Exp Clin Cancer Res 22:591–597

Siavoshian S, Segain JP, Kornprobst M et al (2000) Butyrate and trichostatin A effects on the proliferation/differentiation of human intestinal epithelial cells: induction of cyclin D3 and p21 expression. Gut 46:507–514

Sinkeldam EJ, Kuper CF, Bosland MC et al (1990) Interactive effects of dietary wheat bran and lard on N-methyl-N'-nitro-N-nitrosoguanidine-induced colon carcinogenesis in rats. Cancer Res 50:1092–1096

Slattery ML, Curtin KP, Edwards SL et al (2004) Plant foods, fiber, and rectal cancer. Am J Clin Nutr 79:274–281

Slavin J, Martini MC, Jackobs DR Jr et al (1999) Plausible mechanisms for the protectiveness of whole grains. Am J Clin Nutr 70:459S–463S

Sung MK, Lautens M, Thompson LU (1998) Mammalian lignans inhibit the growth of estrogen-independent human colon tumor cells. Anticancer Res 18:1405–1408

Takahashi T, Satou M, Watanabe N et al (1999) Inhibitory effect of microfibril wheat bran on azoxymethane-induced colon carcinogenesis in CF1 mice. Cancer Lett 141:139–146

Tata JR, Baker BS, Machuca I et al (1993) Autoinduction of nuclear receptor genes and its significance. J Steroid Biochem Mol Biol 46:105–119

Trowell H (1976) Definition of dietary fiber and hypotheses that it is a protective factor in certain diseases. Am J Clin Nutr 29:417–427

Ullah A, Shamsuddin AM (1990) Dose-dependent inhibition of large intestinal cancer by inositol hexaphospate in F344 rats. Carcinogenesis 11:2219–2222

van Kranen HJ, Mortensen A, Sørensen IK et al (2003) Lignan precursors from flaxseed or rye bran do not protect against the development of intestinal neoplasia in ApcMin mice. Nutr Cancer 45:203–210

Verschoyle RD, Greaves P, Cai H et al (2007) Evaluation of the cancer chemopreventive efficacy of rice bran in genetic mouse models of breast, prostate and intestinal carcinogenesis. Br J Cancer 96:248–254

Vucenik I, Shamsuddin AM (2003) Cancer inhibition by inositol hexaphosphate (IP6) and inositol: from laboratory to clinic. J Nutr 133:3778S–3784S

Wargovich MJ, Jimenez A, McKee K et al (2000) Efficacy of potential chemopreventive agents on rat colon aberrant crypt formation and progression. Carcinogenesis 21:1149–1155

Watanabe K, Reddy BS, Weisburger JH et al (1979) Effect of dietary alfalfa, pectin, and wheat bran on azoxymethane-or methylnitrosourea-induced colon carcinogenesis in F344 rats. J Natl Cancer Inst 63:141–145

Whitehead RH, Young GP, Bhathal PS (1986) Effects of short chain fatty acids on a new human colon carcinoma cell line (LIM1215). Gut 27:1457–1463

Wilson AJ, Byun DS, Popova N et al (2006) Histone deacetylase 3 (HDAC3) and other class I HDACs regulate colon cell maturation and p21 expression and are deregulated in human colon cancer. J Biol Chem 281:13548–13558

Wilson RB, Hutcheson DP, Wideman L (1977) Dimethylhydrazine-induced colon tumors in rats fed diets containing beef fat or corn oil with and without wheat bran. Am J Clin Nutr 30: 176–181

World Cancer Research Fund/American Institute for Cancer Research (2007) Food, nutrition, physical activity, and the prevention of cancer: a global perspective. AICR, Washington DC

Young GP, McIntry A, Albert V et al (1996) Wheat bran suppresses potato starch -potentiated colorectal tumorigenesis at the aberrant crypt stage in a rat model. Gastroenterology 110: 508–514

Yu CF, Whitley L, Carryl O et al (2001) Differential dietary effects on colonic and small bowel neoplasia in C57BL/6 J Apc Min/+ mice. Dig Dis Sci 46:1367–1380

Zhang F, Subbaramaiah K, Altorki N et al (1998) Dihydroxy bile acids activate the transcription of cyclooxygenase-2. J Biol Chem 273:2424–2428

Zoran DL, Turner ND, Taddeo SS et al (1997) Wheat bran diet reduces tumor incidence in a rat model of colon cancer independent of effects on distal luminal butyrate concentrations. J Nutr 127:2217–2225

Index

CPSIA information can be obtained
at www.ICGtesting.com
Printed in the USA
LVOW01*1710310317
529199LV00012B/172/P